Indications in Vascular and Endovascular Surgery

Indications in Vascular and Endovascular Surgery

Edited by

R. M. GREENHALGH MA MD MChir FRCS

Professor of Surgery
Head of Department of Vascular Surgery
Imperial College School of Medicine
Charing Cross Hospital
London

W. B. SAUNDERS COMPANY LTD
London · Philadelphia · Toronto · Sydney · Tokyo

W. B. Saunders Company Ltd 24–28 Oval Road
London NW1 7DX

The Curtis Center
Independence Square West
Philadelphia, PA 19106-3399, USA

Harcourt Brace & Company
55 Horner Avenue
Toronto, Ontario M8Z 4X6, Canada

Harcourt Brace & Company, Australia
30-52 Smidmore Street
Marrickville, NSW 2204, Australia

Harcourt Brace & Company, Japan
Ichibancho Central Building, 22-1 Ichibancho
Chiyoda-ku, Tokyo, 102, Japan

A catalogue record for this book is available from the British Library.

ISBN 0-7020-2445-7

Editorial and Production Services by Jane Duncan
10 Barley Mow Passage, London W4 4PH

Typeset by Phoenix Photosetting, Chatham, Kent
Printed in Great Britain at the University Press, Cambridge

Contents

DISTAL RECONSTRUCTION QUESTIONS AND INDICATIONS

VENOUS QUESTIONS AND INDICATIONS

Contributors

O. ABDUL-KHOUDOUD, MD
Surgical Resident
The Union Memorial Hospital
3333 North Calvert Street
Suite 570
Baltimore
MD 21218, USA

B. AL-SOUFI, MD
Department of Surgery
The Union Memorial Hospital
3333 North Calvert Street
Suite 570
Baltimore
MD 21218, USA

J. ANDERSON, MBBS FACS FRACS
Consultant, Vascular Surgeon
Vascular Surgery Department
Royal Perth Hospital
Wellington Street Campus
PO Box X2213
Perth
Western Australia 6001
Australia

M. ANTONINI, MD
Istituto di Anestesiologia e Rianimazion
Dell'Universita di Roma 'La Sapienza'
Policlinico Umberto 1
0061 Rome, Italy

M.P. ARMON, FRCS
Specialist Registrar
E16 University Hospital
Queen's Medical Centre
Nottingham NG7 2UH, UK

J.D. BEARD, ChM FRCS MB BS BSc
Consultant
Sheffield Vascular Institute
Northern General Hospital
Herries Road
Sheffield S5 7AU, UK

J.-P. BECQUEMIN, MD
Department of Vascular Surgery
Henri Mondor Hospital
University Paris XII
Creteil 94000, France

M. BELKIN, MD
Department of Surgery
Harvard Medical School
Brigham and Women's Hospital
75 Francis Street
Boston MA 02115, USA

P.R.F. BELL, MD FRCS
Professor of Surgery
University of Leicester
Robert Kilpatrick Building
Leicester Royal Infirmary
Leicester LE2 7LX, UK

D. BERGQVIST, MD PhD
Professor of Vascular Surgery
Department of Surgery
Academic Hospital
S-751 85 Uppsala
Sweden

D. BERRAHAL, MD
Department of Vascular Surgery
Henri Mondor Hospital
University Paris XII
Creteil 94000, France

G.M. BIASI, MD FACS
Professor of Vascular Surgery
Chief, Division of Vascular Surgery
Bassini Teaching Hospital
Via M. Gorki 50
20092 Cinisello Balsamo
Milan, Italy

J.R. BOYLE, FRCS
Specialist Registrar
Clinical Sciences Building
Leicester Royal Infirmary
Leicester LE2 7LX, UK

A.W. BRADBURY, MB BSc MD FRCSE
Consultant Vascular Surgeon
Department of Surgery
The Royal Infirmary of Edinburgh
Edinburgh EH3 9YW
Scotland

J. BRENNAN, MS FRCS
Consultant Vascular Surgeon
Vascular Surgery Unit
Royal Liverpool Hospital
Prescot Street
Liverpool L7 8XP, UK

A.S. BROWN, FRCS Ed
Vascular Research Fellow
Northern Vascular Centre
Freeman Hospital
Newcastle upon Tyne
NE7 7DN, UK

K.G. BURNAND, MS FRCS
Professor of Vascular Surgery
Department of Surgery
St Thomas' Hospital UMDS
Lambeth Palace Road
London SE1 7EH, UK

S.M. BYRD, RVT
Irvine Laboratory for Cardiovascular
    Investigation and Research
Department of Vascular Surgery
Division of Anaesthetics, Surgery and
    Intensive Care
Imperial College School of Medicine
St Mary's Hospital
London W2 1NY, UK

W.B. CAMPBELL, MS FRCP FRCS
Consultant Surgeon
Exeter Vascular Service
Department of Surgery
Royal Devon and Exeter Hospital
Exeter EX2 5DW, UK

R.T.A. CHALMERS, MD FRCSEd
Senior Registrar
Regional Vascular Unit
St Mary's Hospital
Praed Street
London W2 1NY, UK

D. CLAIR, MD
Department of Surgery
Uniformed Services University of the
    Health Sciences
Malcolm Grow Medical Center
1050 West Perimeter Road
Andrews Air Force Base
MD 20031, USA

F.J. CRIADO, MD FACS
Chief, Division of Vascular Surgery
Director Endovascular Program
The Union Memorial Hospital
3333 North Calvert Street
Suite 570, Baltimore
MD 21218, USA

J.N. CRINNION, FRCS
Irvine Laboratory for Cardiovascular
    Investigation and Research
Department of Vascular Surgery
Division of Anaesthetics, Surgery and
    Intensive Care
Imperial College School of Medicine
St Mary's Hospital
London W2 1NY, UK

J. CRON, MD
Department of Vascular Surgery
Henri Mondor Hospital
University Paris XII
Creteil 94000, France

A.H. DAVIES, MA DM FRCS
Senior Lecturer/Honorary Consultant
Department of Vascular Surgery
Imperial College School of Medicine
Charing Cross Hospital
Fulham Palace Road
London W6 8RF, UK

J. DEAL, MD MRCP DCH
Consultant Paediatric Nephrologist
Department of Medical Paediatrics
St Mary's Hospital
Praed Street, London W2 1NY, UK

A. DHADWAL, MB ChB
Senior House Officer
Regional Vascular Unit
St Mary's Hospital
Praed Street
London W2 1NY

S. DHANJIL, RVT AVT MSD DMU
Irvine Laboratory for Cardiovascular
    Investigation and Research
Department of Vascular Surgery
Division of Anaesthetics, Surgery and
    Intensive Care
Imperial College School of Medicine
St Mary's Hospital
London W2 1NY, UK

M.C. DONALDSON, MD
Department of Surgery
Harvard Medical School
Brigham and Women's Hospital
75 Francis Street, Boston
MA 02115, USA

P. FIORANI, MD
Professor of Surgery
Cattedra de Chirurgia Vascolare
Dell'Universita di Roma 'La Sapienza'
Policlinico Umberto 1
0061 Rome, Italy

G. FISHWICK, FRCS FRCR
Consultant Interventional Radiologist
Clinical Sciences Building
Leicester Royal Infirmary
Leicester LE2 7LX, UK

P.A. GAINES, MRCP FRCR
Consultant Vascular Radiologist
The Sheffield Vascular Institute
Northern General Hospital
Herries Road
Sheffield S5 7AU, UK

W.V. GARRETT, MD
Department of Surgery
Baylor University Medical Center
Dallas, TX, USA

A.E.B. GIDDINGS, MD FRCS
Consultant Surgeon
King's College, Guy's and St Thomas'
    Hospitals London
Honorary Consultant Surgeon
Royal Surrey County Hospital
Egerton Road
Guildford
Surrey, UK

K. GRABITZ, MD
Professor of Vascular Surgery
Department of Vascular Surgery and
    Kidney Transplantation
Heinrich-Heine University
Moorenstrasse 5
D-40225 Düsseldorf
Germany

R.M. GREENHALGH, MA MD MChir FRCS
Professor of Surgery
Head of Department of Vascular Surgery
Imperial College School of Medicine
Charing Cross Hospital
Fulham Palace Road
London W6 8RF, UK

M. GRIFFIN, DCR DMU
Irvine Laboratory for Cardiovascular
    Investigation and Research
Department of Vascular Surgery
Division of Anaesthetics, Surgery and
    Intensive Care
Imperial College School of Medicine
St Mary's Hospital
London W2 1NY, UK

E.J. GUSSENHOVEN, MD PhD
Department of Experimental
    Echocardiography
University Hospital Rotterdam
Dr Molewaterplein 40
3015 GD Rotterdam
The Netherlands

A.W. HALLIDAY, MS FRCS
Consultant Vascular Surgeon
Epsom General Hospital
Dorking Road
Epsom, Surrey, UK

G. HAMILTON, FRCS
Consultant Vascular Surgeon
Royal Free Hospital School of Medicine
Pond Street
London NW3 2QG, UK

P.L. HARRIS, MD FRCS
Consultant Vascular Surgeon
Vascular Surgery Unit
Royal Liverpool Hospital
Prescot Street
Liverpool L7 8XP, UK

D. HARTLEY, FAIR
Radiographer
Vascular Surgery Department
Royal Perth Hospital
Wellington Street Campus
PO Box X2213
Perth
Western Australia 6001, Australia

S. HATLINGHUS, MD
Consultant Radiologist
Department of Radiology
University Hospital of Trondheim
N-7006 Trondheim
Norway

E.S. HAUG, MD
Registrar
Department of Surgery
University Hospital of Trondheim
N-7006 Trondheim
Norway

P. HEILBERGER, MD
Department of Surgery
Nuremberg Southern Hospital
Breslauer Strasse 201
D 90471 Nuremberg
Germany

D. HEWIN, FRCS
Specialist Registrar
Exeter Vascular Service
Department of Surgery
Royal Devon and Exeter Hospital
Exeter EX2 5DW, UK

B.R. HOPKINSON, ChM FRCS
Professor and Head of Division
   of Vascular Surgery
E16 University Hospital
Queen's Medical Centre
Nottingham NG7 2UH, UK

A.T. IRVINE
Consultant Radiologist
St Thomas's Hospital
Lambeth Palace Road
London SE1 7EH, UK

S. KARACAGIL, MD PhD
Associate Professor of Surgery
Department of Surgery
Academic Hospital
S-751 85 Uppsala
Sweden

H. KOBEITER, MD
Department of Radiology
Henri Mondor Hospital
University Paris XII
Creteil 94000
France

A. KROESE, MD
Department of Vascular Surgery
Aker Hospital
0514 Oslo
Norway

M. LAWRENCE-BROWN, FRCS FRCSE FRACS
Vascular Surgeon
Vascular Surgery Department
Royal Perth Hospital
Wellington Street Campus
PO Box X2213, Perth
Western Australia 6001, Australia

E.C. LIPSITZ, MD
Fellow in Vascular Surgery
Montefiore Medical Center
Albert Einstein College of Medicine
111 East 210th Street
Bronx, NY 10467-2490, USA

A.-M. LÖFBERG, MD
Consultant
Department of Diagnostic Radiology
Academic Hospital
S-751 85 Uppsala
Sweden

B. LUTHER, MD
Associate Professor of Vascular Surgery
Department of Vascular Surgery and
   Kidney Transplantation
Heinrich-Heine University
Moorenstrasse 5
D 40225 Düsseldorf
Germany

J.A. MANNICK, MD
Department of Surgery
Harvard Medical School
Brigham and Women's Hospital
75 Francis Street
Boston, MA 02115, USA

F.J. MEYER, MA FRCS
Lecturer in Surgery
Department of Surgery
St Thomas's Hospital
Lambeth Palace Road
London SE1 7EH, UK

P.M. MINGAZZINI, MD
Division of Vascular Surgery
Bassini Teaching Hospital
Via M. Gorki 50
20092 Cinisello Balsamo
Milan, Italy

B.T. MÜLLER, MD
Vascular Surgeon
Department of Vascular Surgery and
   Kidney Transplantation
Heinrich-Heine University
Moorenstrasse 5
D 40225 Düsseldorf, Germany

H.O. MYHRE, MD PhD
Professor and Chairman
Department of Surgery
University Hospital of Trondheim
N-7006 Trondheim, Norway

A.N. NICOLAIDES, MS FRCS
Professor of Vascular Surgery
Director
Irvine Laboratory for Cardiovascular
   Investigation and Research
Department of Vascular Surgery
Division of Anaesthetics, Surgery and
   Intensive Care
Imperial College School of Medicine
St Mary's Hospital
London W2 1NY, UK

B.L. NOEL, BSN RN
Department of Surgery
Baylor University Medical Center
Dallas, TX, USA

L. NORGREN, MD
Professor of Vascular Surgery
Department of Surgery
University Hospital
S221 85 Lund, Sweden

D.M. NOTT, BSc MD FRCS
Consultant Surgeon
Department of Surgery
Chelsea and Westminster Hospital
London SW10 9NH, UK

T. OHKI, MD
Assistant Professor of Surgery
Director Vascular Surgery Research
   Laboratory
Montefiore Medical Center
Albert Einstein College of Medicine
111 East 210th Street
Bronx, NY 10467-2490 USA

J.C. PARODI, MD
Director
Instituto Cardiovascular de Buenos Aires
Blanco Encalada 1543/47
1428 Capital Federal
Buenos Aires, Argentina

G.J. PEARL, MD
Department of Surgery
Baylor University Medical Center
Dallas, TX, USA

N. QUINEY, BSc FRCA
Consultant Anaesthetist
Royal Surrey County Hospital
Egerton Road, Guildford
Surrey, UK

H.A. RACHED, MD
Cattedra de Chirurgia Vascolare
Dell'Universita di Roma 'La Sapienza'
Policlinico Umberto 1
0061 Rome, Italy

D. RAITHEL, MD
Professor of Vascular Surgery
Nuremberg Southern Hospital
Breslauer Strasse 201
D 90471 Nuremberg, Germany

J.R. ROCHESTER, MD FRCS (Gen) BM
Senior Registrar
University Department of Surgery
University of Otago
PO Box 913
Dunedin
New Zealand

J.D.G. ROSE, FRCP FRCR
Consultant Vascular Radiologist
Northern Vascular Centre
Freeman Hospital
Newcastle upon Tyne,
NE7 7DN, UK

C.V. RUCKLEY, MB ChM FRCSE FRCPE
Professor of Vascular Surgery
Vascular Surgery Unit
Royal Infirmary of Edinburgh
Edinburgh EH3 9YW
Scotland

W. SANDMANN, MD
Professor and Chairman
Department of Surgery
Director, Department of Vascular Surgery
    and Kidney Transplantation
Heinrich-Heine University
Moorenstrasse 5
D 40225 Düsseldorf
Germany

G. SANDBAEK, MD
Department of Vascular Surgery
Aker Hospital
0514 Oslo
Norway

E. SBARIGIA, MD
Cattedra de Chirurgia Vascolare
Dell'Universita di Roma 'La Sapienza'
Policlinico Umberto 1
0061 Rome, Italy

P. SBRAGA, MD
Cattedra de Chirurgia Vascolare
Dell'Universita di Roma 'La Sapienza'
Policlinico Umberto 1
0061 Rome, Italy

C. SCHUNN, MD
Department of Surgery
Nuremberg Southern Hospital
Breslauer Strasse 201
D 90471 Nuremberg
Germany

T.V. SHCROEDER, MD DMSc
Professor of Surgery
Department of Vascular Surgery
Rigshospitalet 3111
University of Copenhagen
9 Blegdamsvej
DK 2100, Copenhagen
Denmark

K. SIEUNARINE, FRACS FRCSE
Consultant Vascular Surgeon
Department of Surgery
Harvard Medical School
Brigham and Women's Hospital
75 Francis Street
Boston, MA 02115, USA

B.L. SMITH III, MD
Department of Surgery
Baylor University Medical Center
Dallas, TX, USA

J. SMITH, FRCS
Research Fellow and Honorary Registrar
Department of Surgery
Imperial College School of Medicine
Charing Cross Hospital
Fulham Palace Road
London W6 8RF, UK

M.S. SOBEH, FRCS
Consultant Vascular and Transplant
    Surgeon
Royal London Hospital
Whitechapel
London, UK

F. SPEZIALE, MD
Cattedra de Chirurgia Vascolare
Dell'Universita di Roma 'La Sapienza'
Policlinico Umberto 1
0061 Rome, Italy

L.E. STAXRUD, MD
Department of Vascular Surgery
Aker Hospital
0514 Oslo
Norway

T. STRØMHOLM, MD
Registrar
Department of Surgery
University Hospital of Trondheim
N-7006 Trondheim
Norway

W.P. STUART, MB ChB FRCSE
Research Fellow
Vascular Surgery Unit
Royal Infirmary of Edinburgh
Edinburgh EH3 9YW
Scotland

C.M. TALKINGTON, MD
Department of Surgery
Baylor University Medical Center
Dallas, TX, USA

O. TEIXEIRA, MD
Department of Vascular Surgery
Henri Mondor Hospital
University Paris XII
Creteil 94000
France

S.M. THOMAS, MRCP FRCR
Endovascular Fellow
The Sheffield Vascular Institute
Northern General Hospital
Herries Road
Sheffield S5 7AU, UK

J.E. THOMPSON, MD
3075 Stanford Avenue
Dallas
Texas 75225, USA

M.M. THOMPSON, MD, FRCS
University of Leicester
Robert Kirkpatrick Building
Leicester Royal Infirmary
Leicester LE2 7LX, UK

M. TWENA, MD
Chief Surgical Resident
The Union Memorial Hospital
3333 North Calvert Street
Suite 570, Baltimore
MD 21218, USA

A. VAN DER LUGT, MD PhD
Department of Radiology
University Hospital Rotterdam
Dr Molewaterplein 40
3015 GD Rotterdam
The Netherlands

W. VAN LANKEREN, MD
Department of Experimental
   Echocardiography
University Hospital Rotterdam
Dr Molewaterplein 40
3015 GD Rotterdam
The Netherlands

M.R.H.M. VAN SAMBEEK, MD
Department of Vascular Surgery
University Hospital Rotterdam
Dr Molewaterplein 40
3015 GD Rotterdam
The Netherlands

G. VAN SCHIE, MD
Vascular Surgery Department
Royal Perth Hospital
Wellington Street Campus
PO Box X2213
Perth
Western Australia 6001, Australia

H. VAN URK, MD PhD
Department of Vascular Surgery
University Hospital Rotterdam
Dr Molewaterplein 40
3015 GD Rotterdam
The Netherlands

F.J. VEITH, MD
Professor of Surgery
Chief of Vascular Surgical Services
Montefiore Medical Center
Albert Einstein College of Medicine
111 East 210th Street
Bronx, NY 10467-2490, USA

C.D. VIZZA, MD
Cattedra di Cardiologia
Dell'Universita di Roma 'La Sapienza'
Policlinico Umberto 1
0061 Rome, Italy

J. WESCHE, MD PhD
Senior Registrar
Department of Surgery
University Hospital of Trondheim
N-7006 Trondheim, Norway

A.D. WHITTEMORE, MD
Department of Surgery
Harvard Medical School;
Brigham and Women's Hospital
75 Francis Street
Boston, MA 02115, USA

J.H.N. WOLFE, MS FRCS
Consultant Vascular Surgeon
Regional Vascular Unit
St Mary's Hospital
Praed Street
London W2 1NY, UK

M.G. WYATT, MSc MD FRCS
Consultant Vascular Surgeon
Northern Vascular Centre
Freeman Hospital
Newcastle upon Tyne
NE7 7DN, UK

S.W. YUSUF, DM FRCS
Clinical Endovascular Fellow
Department of Surgery
Division of Vascular Surgery
E Floor West Block
University Hospital Nottingham
Nottingham NG7 2UH, UK

A. ZACCARIA, MD
Cattedra de Chirurgia Vascolare
Dell'Universita di Roma 'La Sapienza'
Policlinico Umberto 1
0061 Rome, Italy

Preface

It is ten years since our successful book *Indications in Vascular Surgery* was published with reprints. It was an extremely popular title. Since that time, it has become clear that there are endovascular and endoscopic opportunities as alternative approaches to vascular surgery and therefore the title of this publication includes endovascular techniques. Frequently a choice has to be made between the two.

Thus the authors have been asked to take a topic and to consider the place of the vascular or endovascular approach. Each author was asked to concentrate on indications of use of a procedure, not the results of their life's work. A common format for each chapter was suggested including:the author's choice of procedure; the alternatives available; evidence for the author's choice where relevant; what trials support the author's view; what future trials would be helpful.

You will be able to judge whether the authors have performed according to this format. I asked Professor Peter Bell, Professor Brian Hopkinson and Professor Vaughan Ruckley to join me in making comments at the end of each chapter, as to whether it was felt that these aims had been achieved. Some subjects were much easier than others. This was in no sense intended to cause conflict between author and commentator. Nevertheless, it is important to clarify what is known and what is accepted and what we need to learn in the future. The aim was to determine where randomized controlled clinical trials have or have not been performed and whether they should or should not be in the future. This approach of commentary after the chapters is rather new and I hope it makes for good reading. Only time will tell whether I dare try it again. I am extremely grateful to the authors and to Peter Bell, Brian Hopkinson and Vaughan Ruckley for helping in this controversial way. Sometimes authors have wished to answer 'unjustified' commentary and I regret that this was hardly possible because of time.

I would like to record my thanks to Sean Duggan for more than 10 years of collaborating as my publisher and editorial director. This could be the last book we will do together in partnership. I have always greatly appreciated Sean and I recognize his gentle, courteous and artistic skills. It hurts very much losing the opportunity of working with Sean Duggan in the future on this series of books. Sue Hamblin has been the person who has made it possible to bring the chapters together and for me to edit these books in a very painless way. She is at a critical stage with her family at the moment and my fingers are crossed that in the future she will be able to return and help once again, but for the moment, we wish Sean and Sue a happy time away from the hurly burly of the deadlines of these chapters and this annual book.

R.M. Greenhalgh

INVESTIGATION INDICATIONS

Indications for Non-invasive Vascular Investigations

James N. Crinnion, Surinder Dhanjil, Sheila M. Byrd, Maura Griffin and Andrew N. Nicolaides

INTRODUCTION

Non-invasive vascular investigations have now become essential for the management of patients with vascular disorders. They consist of imaging techniques, physiological measurements or a combination of the two. They provide information about the presence or absence of vascular disease, its anatomical extent and functional severity. Such information answers questions posed by the clinician so that appropriate clinical decisions can be made on patient management without any need for invasive and expensive investigations such as angiography.

Because of the expertise and quality control required in the performance of these non-invasive tests, they are now performed in specialized 'non-invasive' vascular laboratories by trained vascular technologists. In contrast to a 'technician' who performs a test and supplies the results to the doctor for interpretation, a vascular technologist is defined as the specialist who when confronted with the questions posed by the clinician performs a series of observations and measurements which he/she interprets and provides the answers.

In the past there have been many questions as to the value of some non-invasive tests, their appropriateness and cost effectiveness. In the current climate of rapidly evolving technology there is a corresponding and parallel change in vascular investigative techniques. Many tests become obsolete as new and more accurate ones become available. Also, new tests are initially used in research and do not enter the clinical arena until it has been clearly shown that they influence decisions on the management of patients in a way that is at least as accurate, quicker and/or less expensive than existing investigations.

This chapter discusses what are considered to be the current indications for performing the most commonly used non-invasive vascular investigations. The indications for non-invasive investigation of lower limb arterial disease, cerebrovascular disease and venous disease will be described. In each disease category the information provided and the accuracy of the relevant non-invasive tests will be discussed. The clinical indications for each test and how the test result may influence patient management is considered.

LOWER LIMB ARTERIAL DISEASE

Ankle brachial pressure index (ABPI)

The measurement of ankle and brachial systolic pressures using continuous wave Doppler ultrasound is an established procedure that can be performed by doctors or nurses in outpatient departments or in the ward. It provides an indirect but accurate measure of distal limb perfusion. In normal individuals at rest the ABPI has a mean value of 1.11 (0.9–1.2).[1] In arterial occlusive disease blood flow is diverted through collateral channels which have a high resistance. As a result there is an abnormal pressure gradient across the collateral bed which reduces distal perfusion and the measured ABPI. Measurement of ABPI before and after a standard 1-min treadmill exercise test with Doppler velocity tracings is a specialist investigation performed in the vascular laboratory. In normal individuals there is an increase or no change in the ankle systolic pressure following such exercise, but in patients with occlusive disease there is a further fall in the ABPI, the magnitude and duration of which is proportional to the severity of disease.[2,3] Doppler velocity tracings provide information about the site of arterial stenosis/occlusion and whether it is suprainguinal, infrainguinal or both. A treadmill exercise test can provide the following further objective information; (1) the maximum walking time at a constant work load, (2) the site, time of onset and severity of pain, and (3) the walking pattern as symptoms occur.

Indications for exercise testing

The resting ABPI is usually sufficient to establish the diagnosis of occlusive disease and its severity. It may also be adequate to assess disease progression and the effect of angioplasty or surgery. In several clinical scenarios additional exercise testing provides important clinical information.

Absolute indications for post-exercise ankle pressures

1. Pain on walking suggestive of intermittent claudication in the presence of pedal pulses
In a patient with ischaemic claudication there will always be a fall in the ABPI following exercise indicating the presence of a haemodynamically significant stenosis. The absence of a decrease or an increase in ankle pressure following a standard treadmill test excludes the presence of haemodynamically significant occlusive disease and will spare the patient from further vascular investigations.

2. Intermittent claudication in the presence of arterial occlusive disease (absent pulses) and the presence of additional pathology (sciatica, arthritis)
If the patient stops because of pain without a fall in the ankle pressure it is highly likely that the pain is caused by pathology other than the arterial disease. Treating the arterial lesion in such patients will not relieve symptoms.

Relative indications

1. To have a baseline for follow-up of patients with occlusive vascular disease particularly those managed medically

2. To have documentation of the patient's walking ability/distance
Often it is difficult to appreciate the degree of disability from direct questioning and a treadmill test provides objective data.

3. To document the effect of intervention upon walking distance
Many patients with intermittent claudication have multisegment disease and correction of occlusive disease in one segment may not greatly increase the resting ABPI. However, the response of the ankle systolic pressure and its recovery following a standard treadmill exercise can be used to objectively evaluate the results of arterial surgery or angioplasty.

Duplex scanning

The combination of Doppler ultrasound with B mode ultrasonic imaging is currently the principle method for the investigation of vascular disease. The recent addition of colour flow imaging to duplex ultrasonography has greatly increased the speed of examination, and the aorta to calf vessels may be examined by an experienced technologist in 30 minutes.[4]

Arterial occlusions are detected by an absence of flow on colour and pulsed Doppler imaging. Stenoses are graded by measuring peak systolic velocity ratio in which the velocity within a stenosis is compared with that just proximal to the stenotic segment.[4] The sonographer is able to use this information to construct an anatomical and haemodynamic map of the lower limb arterial supply.

Accuracy

Iliac disease
Although the depth of this segment makes it difficult to insonate it can be imaged successfully by an experienced technologist in over 90% of patients.[5,6] There is a good correlation between duplex ultrasonography and arteriography in detecting significant lesions in this region, and the sensitivity and specificity of duplex ultrasound in identifying haemodynamically significant stenoses are 80 and 95% respectively, and for the detection of occlusions 94 and 99%.[7] However, both arteriography and duplex scanning may miss up to 25% of significant lesions when compared with intra-arterial pressure measurements which are considered by many to be the 'gold standard' for the detection of haemodynamically significant lesions.[8]

Femoropopliteal segment
These vessels can be imaged in virtually all patients including the profunda femoris artery. The sensitivity and specificity for the detection of a significant stenosis (>50%) in this region are 82 and 96% respectively, and for detecting occlusions 90 and 97% respectively.[7]

Infrapopliteal arteries
Tibial vessels may be imaged successfully by duplex ultrasound in around 90% of patients and may accurately identify both stenoses and occlusions.[9,10] Arterial wall calcification may, however, cause technical problems in imaging these vessels especially in diabetics.

Indications

1. Selection of patients with intermittent claudication for percutaneous transluminal angioplasty

Angioplasty is often considered as the treatment of choice for patients with claudication who have significant handicap. However, only a proportion of these patients will have lesions suitable for balloon dilatation. Duplex scanning may identify those patients who are likely to benefit from angioplasty (severe stenosis or occlusion less than 10 cm long) and exclude those with long occlusions or multilevel disease in whom angioplasty is not a practical therapeutic option. Angiography is required in only about 20% of patients in whom visualization of the whole arterial tree is not feasible with duplex scanning. Although arterial surgery has been performed safely on the basis of duplex scanning alone, preoperative angiography is generally considered mandatory.[11]

2. Graft surveillance

It is widely accepted that patients with infrainguinal bypass grafts should have routine duplex scanning to identify intragraft stenoses and/or proximal (inflow) or distal (outflow) progression of the atherosclerotic disease which may precipitate graft failure. Prompt balloon dilatation or surgical intervention can prevent graft occlusion and limb loss.

EXTRACRANIAL CEREBROVASCULAR DISEASE

Carotid duplex

Recent large clinical trials from North America and Europe have proved that carotid endarterectomy can reduce the risk of stroke in both symptomatic[12,13] and asymptomatic[14] patients with high-grade stenosis of the internal carotid artery. In these studies the degree of stenosis was assessed by carotid angiography. Although angiography provides accurate measurements it may be associated with a combined stroke and death rate of 1–2%,[14,15] and therefore an accurate non-invasive test which can be used to select patients for surgery is highly desirable.

Modern colour duplex imaging grades internal carotid artery disease on the basis of both velocity criteria and the measurement of plaque thickness and residual lumen using high resolution B mode ultrasound.[16] Using duplex velocity criteria alone the overall accuracy of detecting a 70–99% internal carotid is around 90% (sensitivity 91%, specificity 87%).[17] Similar results can be obtained with transverse section measurements of residual lumen using B mode ultrasound[18,19] and a combination of both modalities offers the best method to ensure accuracy.[16] It is important to appreciate that a few false negative and false positive results occur with carotid duplex and it is particularly difficult to distinguish between a 99% stenosis and total occlusion.[16] Poor duplex examinations due to calcification and coiling of vessels, borderline cases (55–75% stenosis), and possible occlusions should be considered for angiography.[16]

Vertebral sonography

Duplex scanning of the vertebral arteries has received less attention than the carotid vessels because surgical intervention is not popular and because of technical problems in their imaging. Nevertheless ischaemic events in the vertebral territory occur frequently and the vertebrobasilar supply is pivotal in providing collateral flow in the presence of carotid occlusive disease. The patency of the vertebral supply is usually assessed routinely as part of the colour duplex survey of patients suspected of having extracranial cerebrovascular disease. Satisfactory images of the vertebral artery during its course in the neck can usually be obtained by conventional colour Doppler imaging and the intracranial course of the vertebral vessels may be imaged by transcranial Doppler examination.[20]

Transcranial Doppler sonography[21,22]

Transcranial Doppler examination is capable of providing anatomical and physiological data about the cerebral vessels. This new technique was first described in 1982 and was initially performed with non-imaging transducers. Its accuracy was dependent on the user's knowledge of the anatomy and the ability to imagine the Circle of Willis while obtaining Doppler samples from designated vessels. Individual vessels were identified by assessment of sample volume depth, probe angulation, flow direction and the spatial relationships of the vessels to each other. The ultrasound signal from the insonated vessel is displayed as a spectral waveform from which blood flow measurements such as mean flow velocity and pulsatility index may be derived.[23] The recent introduction of colour flow imaging to transcranial Doppler has allowed direct visualization of the spatial relationships and anatomical location of the intracranial vessels. It is likely that transcranial colour flow imaging will replace non-imaging transducers in the future.

Transcranial Doppler may be used to continually assess changes in cerebral blood flow during functional stimulation of the intracranial circulation, and provides a real time method of monitoring cerebral blood flow during carotid endarterectomy. It is of particular value in evaluating the haemodynamic effects of extracranial occlusive disease upon intracranial blood flow (e.g. internal carotid artery occlusion, subclavian steal syndrome). In some centres a 50% reduction in middle cerebral artery velocity is an indication to use a shunt during carotid endarterectomy.

Cerebral reactivity using transcranial Doppler[24]

Cerebrovascular reactivity refers to the responses of the cerebral arterial tree and total cerebral blood flow to specific vasoactive agents. The major physiological modulator of cerebrovascular resistance is CO_2 with hypercapnia promoting an increase in cerebral blood flow via arteriolar dilatation. Changes in the cerebral blood flow in response to CO_2 inhalation can be detected as changes in the mean flow velocity in the intracerebral vessels using transcranial Doppler. In normal individuals there is an approximate 80% change in mean flow velocity between extremes of hypocapnia and hypercapnia. Absent or diminished (<10%) cerebral reactivity to CO_2 inhalation is an indication of increased risk of stroke.[25] An assessment of CO_2 reactivity is indicated in the presence of unilateral internal carotid occlusion or bilateral stenoses > 80% in diameter.

Indications

Neurological symptoms

1. Carotid disease

A recent hemispheric transient ischaemic attack (distinct focal neurological dysfunction), monocular blindness (amaurosis fugax) persisting less than 24 hours, or a non-disabling stroke with persistence of symptoms and signs are absolute indications for a carotid duplex scan. The subsequent risk of major stroke and death in these groups of patients who also have a 70–99% stenosis of the ipsilateral internal carotid artery can be significantly reduced by carotid endarterectomy.[12,13] In many centres patients with significant internal carotid artery stenoses (detected by duplex scanning) proceed directly to carotid endarterectomy without confirmatory angiography, provided intracerebral pathology (haemorrhage, tumour, large aneurysm) has been excluded by computerized tomography or magnetic resonance imaging, and lesions of the great vessels are considered unlikely in the presence of good carotid pulses and absence of bruits at the base of the neck. The adoption of such a policy assumes that the accuracy of duplex scanning in that particular centre has been validated against angiography and that the reports issued contain an appropriate statement about the reliability of the study. Cardiac arrhythmias, calcification and arterial coiling make a duplex examination unreliable. If angiography is considered mandatory in symptomatic patients prior to surgery, carotid duplex is used to select those patients who are likely to have a 70–99% stenosis.

2. Vertebrobasilar territory

Symptoms suggestive of vertebrobasilar insufficiency including dizziness, vertigo, diplopia or drop attacks are an indication for colour duplex imaging of the vertebral vessels to determine whether there is evidence of intrinsic disease which occurs most commonly at the origin of the vertebral arteries.[20] Vertebral duplex sonography is of particular value in diagnosing the subclavian steal syndrome when reverse flow may be demonstrated in the vertebral artery due to a stenosis or occlusion of the proximal subclavian artery. Blood flows in a retrograde direction form the basilar circulation and down the ipsilateral vertebral artery to supply an ischaemic arm often resulting in symptoms of posterior circulation ischaemia during exercise of the affected limb.[20]

Asymptomatic patients

There is evidence from North America that patients with asymptomatic carotid artery stenosis (>60%) have a reduced incidence of subsequent stroke following carotid endarterectomy compared with medically treated controls.[14] In the UK clinical trials are underway to further assess the benefit of carotid endarterectomy in asymptomatic patients with critical stenoses. If these studies confirm that surgery is beneficial then duplex scanning will be a valuable screening test for the detection of occult carotid bifurcation disease in high risk groups. One of the most common indications for a duplex scan is the presence of a carotid bruit on routine clinical examination but scans are also frequently requested in asymptomatic patients with coronary artery disease, peripheral vascular disease, diabetes, hypertension and hyperlipidaemia. In such patients the finding of a severe stenosis is a warning to the surgeon and anaesthetist to maintain a high blood pressure and adjust preoperative medication accordingly. In such patients we often do not allow the patient to take their antihypertensive medication on the morning of operation.

Preoperative

When a symptomatic patient has been selected for carotid endarterectomy there is occasionally a delay between the initial duplex scan and surgery. It is wise in such a case to repeat the carotid duplex prior to surgery to make sure that the stenosis has not progressed to an occlusion which would no longer require surgical intervention. Carotid duplex scanning is being performed with an increasing frequency, in asymptomatic patients with atherosclerosis who are to undergo major surgery, which may be associated with intraoperative hypotension. In our institution duplex scanning of the carotids is routinely performed prior to coronary artery bypass grafting. In those patients with evidence of haemodynamically significant lesions in the carotid vessels (unilateral occlusion or bilateral stenoses (>80%) intracerebral flow velocities are measured under baseline conditions and following CO_2 inhalation with transcranial Doppler. Patients with poor collateralization or markedly decreased cerebral reactivity are considered for prophylactic carotid surgery prior to cardiac surgery, to prevent the development of a haemodynamic stroke during the relative hypotension which occurs during cardiopulmonary bypass. In patients undergoing coronary bypass surgery it is relatively easy to maintain a high perfusion pressure whilst on cardiopulmonary bypass.

Intraoperative

Carotid duplex may be used following the completion of the carotid endarterectomy to exclude technical error such as intimal dissection.[26] Monitoring the middle cerebral artery mean velocity during carotid endarterectomy using transcranial Doppler can provide useful haemodynamic information.[27] Serious cerebral ischaemia may be detected when the carotid artery is clamped especially in patients with contralateral carotid occlusion. This is one of the methods used to determine whether to shunt.[27] Transcranial Doppler monitoring during carotid surgery does pose technical problems and may not be possible at all in some patients with a thick skull.

Postoperative

Carotid duplex is of value in the immediate postoperative period following endarterectomy in patients who develop hemispheric symptoms or signs. In a patient who wakes up from the anaesthetic and moves all four limbs and subsequently develops a neurological deficit duplex scanning is indicated. The finding of an occluded internal carotid artery is an indication to return to theatre for exploration.

VENOUS DISEASE

Duplex scanning for deep venous thrombosis

Duplex scanning has been used since the early 1980s for the diagnosis of deep venous thrombosis (DVT).[28,29] Colour flow duplex imaging which provides instant visualization of blood flow and its direction has speeded up the examination and improved its accuracy. The exact anatomical site and extent of acute DVT can be visualized with a high degree of accuracy by both conventional and colour coded duplex scanning. Colour duplex imaging has an overall accuracy of 96-100% in detecting symptomatic DVT in the femoropopliteal veins.[31] The detection of isolated calf DVT is less accurate but nevertheless still approaches 90% in experienced hands.[31] Patient factors such as obesity, tissue oedema and collateral veins result in difficulties in diagnosing tibioperoneal DVT. Visualization of the iliac veins is often impaired by overlying bowel gas and the patency of the iliac veins often has to be inferred from the flow pattern in the common femoral veins. Continuous, non-phasic flow in a patent common femoral vein associated with poor augmentation implies obstruction of the iliac vein or vena cava.[31]

Indications

Symptomatic patients
Colour-coded duplex scanning is indicated in any patient with acute symptoms (limb swelling, pain, erythema) and signs (oedema, tenderness, warm skin) suggestive of DVT. Almost all proximal thrombi in symptomatic patients can be detected by this method and a positive scan is sufficiently accurate to justify anticoagulation. Similarly a negative above- and below-knee scan virtually excludes significant DVT and those patients (about 50% of total number scanned) are spared an unnecessary hospital admission and/or venography. Because the cost of duplex scanning is only a fraction of the cost of the contrast media used in venography the use of this test results in major savings not only in bed usage but also in real terms (pharmacy and radiology budget). Duplex scanning is also of value in identifying other pathology (haematomas, popliteal cysts, tumour masses and enlarged lymph nodes) which may be confused with acute DVT.

Asymptomatic patients
Certain groups of postoperative patients are at appreciable risk of DVT. Although prophylactic measures significantly reduce the incidence of venous thrombosis after abdominal surgery they are less effective following orthopaedic operations.[30] There is, therefore, a strong argument for postoperative duplex surveillance in high risk patients to detect occult DVT. However, at the moment in asymptomatic patients duplex scanning as a screening test is a research tool.

Duplex scanning for chronic venous dysfunction

Colour-coded duplex scanning can detect the presence and anatomic extent of chronic venous obstruction and/or reflux.[31-34] It has become a practical and accurate tool in identifying the sites of deep to superficial reflux (saphenofemoral, saphenopopliteal and perforating vein reflux), and has virtually replaced venography in the preoperative assessment of recurrent varicose veins. It is also an invaluable investigation in the diagnosis and assessment of the post-thrombotic syndrome.

Duplex scanning is superior to continuous wave Doppler ultrasound because not only can it detect more accurately the presence of venous reflux or obstruction, it can also define the anatomical site and extent. In normal veins, cephalad flow, phasic with respiration is indicated by a blue colour in the vein lumen which is enhanced by distal calf or thigh compression. On release of the compression, reflux or reverse flow is shown as a red colour. Significant reflux is defined as that lasting more than one second in the standing position.[35] It is important to appreciate that although duplex scanning can accurately identify all the sites of venous incompetence, the total amount of reflux within a limb cannot be easily quantified. Furthermore the relative contributions of deep and superficial reflux in a patient with chronic venous insufficiency cannot be measured with duplex scanning. Finally colour duplex is a very sensitive test and small amounts of reflux are often present in asymptomatic individuals. The value is not in the demonstration of presence or absence of reflux but in the determination of the anatomic extent.

Indications

In patients with varicose veins
The sites of reflux in patients with primary varicose veins can usually be assessed accurately by a careful clinical examination and the use of continuous wave Doppler ultrasound. A small proportion of patients will need further investigation with colour flow duplex imaging (see below).

1. To determine the sites of deep to superficial reflux in patients with recurrent varicose veins
Duplex scanning will accurately define the anatomy at the long and short saphenous junctions as well as documenting perforator or deep venous incompetence. This information will ensure that the correct operation is performed and will also enable the surgeon to predict the results of further surgery so that the patient can be fully informed.

2. Preoperative marking of the saphenopopliteal junction
The anatomy of the saphenopopliteal junction is variable and preoperative marking of the skin with duplex enables the skin incision to be sited accurately.[36] In addition a drawing showing the anatomic relationship of the short saphenous, gastrocnemial, and Giacomini veins, and their junctions in relation to the popliteal vein will enable the surgeon to plan the appropriate procedure.

3. Preoperative marking of incompetent perforating veins
Incompetent calf perforators may be visualized and ligated under direct vision using a subfascial endoscope which is inserted through a small incision in the upper calf.[37] Preoperative skin marking of the sites of the incompetent perforating veins using duplex scanning is particularly helpful during this procedure.

4. To exclude significant reflux or occlusion in the deep veins

Superficial venous reflux may occur in association with obstruction or marked reflux in the deep veins. Deep venous pathology should be suspected in patients with a prior history of DVT, and those with evidence of chronic skin changes and venous collaterals. Such patients should have their deep veins imaged with duplex ultrasound prior to surgical treatment of the superficial varicosities. The presence of deep venous obstruction is a contraindication to ligation of the superficial veins. In the presence of reflux in the deep veins an operation for incompetent superficial veins is less likely to be successful and patients should be warned that symptoms may persist following surgical intervention.

5. To determine the diagnosis of post-thrombotic syndrome

Duplex scanning has virtually replaced venography in the diagnosis and investigation of the post-thrombotic limb (patients presenting with swelling, skin changes and/or ulceration). Accurate information with regard to the sites and extent of obstruction and/or reflux are obtained which enable appropriate treatment to be planned.

6. Duplex preoperative skin marking in patients scheduled to have femoropopliteal or femorocrural vein bypass[38]

This test provides information on the size (suitability), position in relation to the skin and integrity of the long saphenous or cephalic vein prior to surgery. The skin markings prevent undermining which may result in skin necrosis and marked prolongation of hospital stay.

Air-plethysmography[39]

Venous hypertension is the result of impaired venous return. The latter is often due to the combined effect of venous reflux, obstruction and poor calf muscle function. Duplex scanning goes a long way towards defining the anatomic extent of reflux and obstruction, whereas air-plethysmography has the ability to quantify each of these components and has contributed to our better understanding of venous pathophysiology. The air-plethysmograph consists of a tubular air cylinder which surrounds the whole leg. It is inflated with air to a low pressure and is connected by a transducer to a pen recorder or computer. Changes in the volume of the leg as a result of filling or emptying of the veins produces corresponding changes in the pressure of the air-chamber. Thus leg volume can be measured in ml according to calibration. Various calculations can be made using air-plethymography which provide quantitative information about the severity of venous obstruction and/or reflux. These include the rate of venous filling of the leg, evaluation of venous outflow following release of a proximal tourniquet and the change in volume of the leg following contraction of the calf muscles. Pressure may be applied over the long saphenous vein and the measurements repeated to assess the contribution of long saphenous reflux to the various measurements. The reduction in limb volume following a single calf muscle contraction provides information about the function of the calf muscle pump (ejection fraction) which may be impaired because of either deep venous obstruction or poor muscle contractility. The residual volume fraction is the percentage of the total dependent limb volume which remains following a series of ten tip-toe movements. A high residual volume fraction reflects the combined effects of venous reflux, obstruction and ejection fraction and correlates closely with the ambulatory venous pressure and the subsequent risk of leg ulceration in post-thrombotic limbs.

Indications

1. To predict the risk of ulceration in limbs with chronic venous dysfunction (prognostic value)

A high residual volume, rapid venous refilling, reduced venous outflow, poor ejection fraction and high residual volume fraction are all associated with an increased risk of leg ulceration in patients with symptoms and signs of chronic venous disease (Table 1). Air-plethysmography enables the aetiology of the venous dysfunction to be elucidated. Patients with evidence of deep venous obstruction or significant deep venous reflux should be advised to wear compression hosiery on a permanent basis. If there is a significant reflux component in the long saphenous system then surgical ligation may be recommended.

Table 1. The incidence of leg ulceration in relation to the residual volume fraction (RVF) in 175 limbs with venous disease

n	RVF (%)	Incidence of ulceration (%)
20	<30	0
24	31–40	8
48	41–50	18
43	51–60	42
32	61–80	72
8	>80	88

(Reproduced from ref 41, with permission.)

2. To determine whether a leg ulcer of unknown or doubtful aetiology is likely to be the result of a hidden venous abnormality

Air-plethysmography provides a rapid, well tolerated and accurate assessment of venous haemodynamics which can detect the contribution of different components (reflux or obstruction) to the aetiology of a chronic leg ulcer. This test used in combination with duplex avoids the need for venography and ambulatory venous pressure measurements.

3. To quantify reflux and exclude obstruction in patients in whom deep venous reconstruction is contemplated

This test enables the identification of patients with chronic venous insufficiency which is likely to be due to gross deep venous reflux rather than obstruction. Patients who show evidence of deep venous obstruction can be spared venography and treated conservatively whereas in those patients without obstruction valve reconstruction may be considered. In this subgroup descending venography will be required to determine whether reflux is a result of post-thrombotic changes or due to primary leaky valves. The latter are amenable to valvuloplasty.[40]

4. To exclude any suspected deep venous obstruction in patients for varicose vein surgery
As discussed earlier, varicose vein surgery should be avoided in patients with deep venous obstruction which may be identified with air-plethysmography (low outflow fraction) and duplex scanning.

CONCLUSION

This chapter has focused on common vascular disorders and the methods of non-invasive investigation which are performed routinely in the clinical setting. It can be clearly seen from this discussion that the first investigation to be perfomed in almost all patients with vascular disorders is non-invasive, and in many instances the results of these tests will provide enough accurate clinical information to allow the surgeon to plan management. Further technological advances are likely to broaden the clinical indications for these tests so that they enter the interventional arena. Balloon angioplasty under ultrasound control has already been performed in several centres. Other tests now being used as research tools may enter the clinical arena when it can be demonstrated as a result of such research that appropriate clinical decisions can be made.

REFERENCES

1. Yao JST: Hemodynamic studies in peripheral arterial disease. *Br J Surg* **57**: 761–4, 1970
2. Strandness DE Jr, Bell JW: Peripheral vascular disease: diagnosis and objective evaluation using a mercury strain gauge. *Ann Surg* **161**(Suppl): 1–9, 1965
3. Sumner DS, Strandness DE Jr: The relationship between calf blood flow and ankle blood pressure in patients with intermittent claudication. *Surgery* **65**: 783–87, 1969
4. Pemberton M, London NJM: Colour flow duplex imaging of occlusive arterial disease of the lower limb. *Br J Surg* **84**: 912–19, 1997
5. Kohler TR, Nance DR, Cramer MM *et al.*: Duplex scanning for diagnosis of aortoiliac and femoropopliteal disease: a prospective study. *Circulation* **76**: 1074–80, 1987
6. Moneta GL, Yeager RA, Antonovic R *et al.*: Accuracy of lower extremity arterial duplex mapping. *J Vasc Surg* **15**: 275–83, 1992
7. Koelemay MJW, den Hartog D, Prins MH *et al.*: Diagnosis of arterial disease of the lower extremities with duplex ultrasonography. *Br J Surg* **83**: 404–09, 1996
8. Legemate DA, Teeuwen C, Hoeneveld H, Eikelboom BC: Value of duplex scanning compared with angiography and pressure measurement in the assessment of aortoiliac arterial lesions. *Br J Surg* **78**: 1003–8, 1991
9. Moneta GL, Yeager RA, Antonovic R *et al.*: Accuracy of lower extremity arterial duplex mapping. *J Vasc Surg* **17**: 578–82, 1993
10. Hatsukami TS, Primozich JF, Zeirler RE *et al.*: Colour doppler imaging of infrainguinal arterial occlusive disease. *J Vasc Surg* **16**: 527–31, 1992
11. Pemberton M, Nydahl S, Hartshorne T *et al.*: Can lower limb vascular reconstruction be based on colour duplex imaging alone? *Eur J Vasc Endovasc Surg* **12**: 452–54, 1996
12. North American Symptomatic Carotid Endarterectomy Trial Collaborators: Beneficial

effect of carotid endarterectomy in symptomatic patients with high-grade carotid stenosis. *New Engl J Med* **325**: 445–53, 1991

13. European Carotid Surgery Trialists Collaborative Group: MRC European carotid surgery trial: Interim results for symptomatic patients with severe (70–99%) or with mild (0–29%) carotid stenosis. *Lancet* **337**: 1235–43, 1991

14. Executive Committe for the Asymptomatic Carotid Atherosclerosis Study: Endarterectomy for asymptomatic cartoid artery stenosis. *J Am Med Ass* **73**: 1421–28, 1995.

15. Polak JF: Noninvasive carotid evaluation: Carpe diem. *Radiology* **186**: 329–31, 1993

16. Nicolaides AN, Shifrin EG, Bradbury A *et al.*: Angiographic and duplex grading of internal carotid stenosis: Can we overcome the confusion? *J Endovasc Surg* **3**: 158–65, 1996

17. Moneta GL, Edwards JM, Chitwood RW *et al.*: Correlation of North American Symptomatic Carotid Endarterectomy Trial (NASCET) angiographic definition of 70% to 99% internal carotid artery stenosis with duplex scanning. *J Vasc Surg* **17**: 152–59, 1993

18. Steinke W, Hennerici M, Rautenberg W, *et al.*: Symptomatic and asymptomatic high grade carotid stenosis in Doppler colour flow imaging. *Neurology* **42**: 131–7, 1992

19. De Bray JM, Galland F, Lhoste P *et al.*: Color Doppler imaging duplex sonography and angiography of carotid bifurcations. Prospective and double blind study. *Neuroradiology* **37**: 219–24, 1995

20. Bartels E: Vertebral sonography. In: Tegeler CH, Babikian VL, Gomez CR (Eds). *Neurosonology*, pp. 83–100. St Louis, Missouri: Mosby, 1996

21. Byrd SM: An overview of transcranial color flow imaging: A technique comparison. *Ultrasound Quart* **13**: 197–210, 1996

22. Otis SM, Ringelstein EB: Transcranial Doppler examination: Principles and applications of transcranial Doppler sonography. In: Tegeler CH, Babikain VL, Gomez CR (Eds) *Neurosonology*, pp. 113–28. St Louis, Missouri: Mosby, 1996

23. Bragoni M, Feldmann E: Transcranial Doppler indeces of intracranial haemodynamics. In: Tegeler CH, Babikain VL, Gomez CR (Eds) *Neurosonology*, pp. 129–39. St Louis, Missouri: Mosby, 1996

24. Babikain VL, Schwarze JJ: Cerebral blood flow and cerebrovascular physiology. In: Tegeler CH, Babikain VL, Gomez CR (Eds) *Neurosonology*, pp. 140–55. St Louis, Missouri: Mosby, 1996

25. Ringelstein EB, Otis SM: Physiological testing of vasomotor reserve. In: Newell DW, Aaslid R (Eds) *Transcranial Doppler*, pp. 83–99. New York: Raven Press, 1992

26. Bandyk DF: Intraoperative assessment of cartoid endarterectomy. In: Bernstein EF (Ed) *Vascular Diagnosis* pp. 452–6. St Louis, Missouri: Mosby, 1993

27. Halsey JH Jr: Transcranial doppler monitoring of carotid endarterectomy. In: Tegeler CH, Babikian VL, Gomez CR (Eds) *Neurosonology*, pp. 439–42. St Louis, Missouri: Mosby, 1996

28. Talbot SR: Use of real-time imaging in identifying deep venous obstruction: a preliminary report. *Bruit* 1982; **6**: 41–8, 1982

29. Flanagan LD, Sullivan ED, Cranley JJ: Venous imaging of the extremities using real-time B-mode ultrasound. In: Bergan JJ, Yao JST (Eds) *Surgery of the Veins*, Orlando, Florida: Grune and Stratton, 1985

30. Sumner DS, Mattos MA: Diagnosis of deep vein thrombosis with real-time color and duplex scanning. In: Bernstein EF (Ed) *Vascular Diagnosis*, pp. 785-800. St Louis, Missouri: Mosby, 1985

31. Sadager G, Williams LR, McCarthy WR *et al.*: Assessment of venous valve function by duplex scan. *Bruit* **10**: 238-46, 1986

32. Semrow C, Ryan TJ, Buchbinder D *et al.*: Assessment of valve function using real-time B-mode ultrasound. In: Negus D, Jantet G (Eds) *Phlebology '85*, pp. 352–5. London: John Libbey & Co, 1986

33. Rollins DL, Semrow C, Buchbinder D *et al.*: Diagnosis of recurrent deep vein thrombosis using B-Mode ultrasonic imaging. *Phlebology* **1**: 181–8, 1986

34. Szendro G, Nicolaides AN, Zukowski AJ *et al.*: Duplex scanning in the assessment of deep venous incompetence. *J Vasc Surg* **4**: 237–42, 1986

35. Van Bemmelen PS, Bedford G, Beach K, Strandness DE Jr: Quantitative segmental evaluation of venous valvular reflux with duplex ultrasound. *J Vasc Surg* **10**: 425–31, 1989

36. Vasdekis SN, Clark H, Hobbs JT, Nicolaides AN: Evaluation of noninvasive methods in the assessment of short saphenous vein termination. *Br J Surg* **76**: 929–32, 1989
37. Paraskeva PA, Cheshire N, Stansby G, Darzi AW: Endoscopic subfascial ligation of incompetent perforating calf veins. *Br J Surg* **83**: 1105–6, 1996
38. Kupinski AM, Leather RP, Chang BB, Shah DM: Preoperative mapping of the saphenous vein. In: Bernstein EF (Ed) *Vascular Diagnosis*, pp. 897–901. St Louis, Missouri: Mosby, 1993
39. Belcaro G, Nicolaides AN, Veller M: Assessment of the venous and lymphatic systems. In: Belcaro G, Nicolaides A, Veller M (Eds) *Venous Disorders: A Manual of Diagnosis and Treatment*, pp. 31–52. London: WB Saunders Co, 1995
40. Belcaro G, Nicolaides AN, Veller M: Chronic venous insufficiency and postphlebitic syndrome. In: Belcaro G, Nicoloides A, Veller M (Eds) *Venous Disorders: A Manual of Diagnosis and Treatment* pp. 124–42. London: WB Saunders Co, 1995
41. Nicolaides AN, Sumner DS (Eds): *Investigation of Patients with Deep Vein Thrombosis and Chronic Venous Insufficiency*, pp. 39–43. London: Med-Orion.

Editorial comments by R.M. Greenhalgh

This is a most comprehensive description of indications for non-invasive vascular investigations in an excellent laboratory. The authors' definition of a vascular technologist is interesting: 'a specialist who when confronted with questions posed by the clinician, performs a series of observations and measurements which he/she interprets and provides the 'answers'. Many of the indications are unspoken. It is a matter of very great importance whether a non-invasive laboratory such as this should have an open access. If it does, non-vascular specialists could easily abuse vascular technologists and give them enormous work. A vascular technologist has emerged alongside vascular surgeons. In practice it is the vascular surgeon with the technologist who determine the indications for tests in a vascular laboratory. It would be very easy for a non-specialist to ask for very inappropriate tests. The established partnership of vascular technologist and surgeon works and is supported. This chapter explains very accurately what the tests of today can do.

AUDIT AFFECTING INDICATIONS

Can Endovascular National Audit Affect Indications for Intervention?

J.R. Rochester and J.D. Beard

INTRODUCTION

Audit has become an integral part of surgical practice and a compulsory part of surgical training. However, audit can be interpreted in many ways, both within the profession and by health care administrators. This has led to different methods being applied to audit with variable results. Broadly, audit is a method of reviewing practice, comparing outcome with a standard, and implementing change to improve practice. A repeat audit is required to monitor the effect of the change. This is the audit cycle (Fig. 1).

To some authors, audit is a retrospective analysis of clinical outcome data, others confine it to prospective data collection which is to be analysed 'in the future'. It can also be used to study new, rapidly developing methods of treatment such as endovascular aneurysm repair. Whichever method of audit is applied, the reason for it has to be carefully considered as this will determine the choice of data collected. Prospective audit allows appropriate and accurate data collection which is more likely to achieve a meaningful result than a retrospective review.

Endovascular exclusion of abdominal aortic aneurysms using a graft placed via the femoral artery was first described in 1991[1] and has now been shown to be technically feasible in several centres.[2-7] The concept of minimally invasive aneurysm repair has excited vascular surgeons and radiologists worldwide. There was a risk that this enthusiasm would lead to a widespread adoption of the technique before it had been properly developed and evaluated. Fortunately, we have learnt from the negative publicity that surrounded the rapid, and unsupervised introduction of laparoscopic cholecystectomy and are able to take a more sober approach to the introduction of endovascular aneurysm repair.

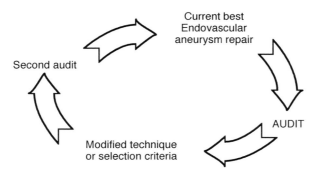

Fig. 1. The audit cycle.

There are many aspects to new endovascular treatments which need monitoring and these include, the prosthesis, indications, deployment technique and outcome, both in the short and long term.

MONITORING NEW SURGICAL TECHNOLOGY

Currently all commercially available devices require a European Community (CE) mark which indicates the device meets a level of safety and performance specified by the Medical Devices Directive. The CE mark is awarded by a competent authority, which in the UK is the Medical Devices Agency (MDA). However, the MDA is only responsible for safety and performance and is not concerned with indications for use or efficacy.[8] The Safety and Efficacy Register of New Interventional Procedures (SERNIP) which has been established by the Academy of Medical Royal Colleges in the UK is a voluntary 'intelligence centre' for new interventional procedures. Its purpose is to work closely with the Standing Group on Health Technology to evaluate new procedures where research is felt to be an important requirement in determining whether a new interventional procedure should be introduced into Health Service Practice. At present, endovascular grafting of abdominal aortic aneurysms is classified as 'safety and efficacy not yet established; procedure requires a fully controlled evaluation and may only be used as part of systematic research, comprising either an observational study or a randomized controlled trial'.

THE REGISTRY FOR ENDOVASCULAR TREATMENT OF ANEURYSMS

The Joint Working Party of the Vascular Surgical Society of Great Britain and Ireland and the British Society of Interventional Radiologists agreed on principles for the introduction of endovascular grafting of abdominal aortic aneurysms in 1995.[9] These principles included a centralized prospective audit to be maintained by the Joint Working Party; the Registry for Endovascular Treatment of Aneurysms (RETA), which would report to SERNIP and make the audit data available to all centres involved in endovascular aneurysm exclusion.

The RETA registry is voluntary although it is expected that all members of the Vascular Surgical Society of Great Britain and Ireland and the British Society of Interventional Radiologists will submit their data. Data is collected on a machine readable proforma which records details of the indications for the procedure, suitability for conventional repair, co-morbidity and anaesthetic risk factors, aneurysm morphology, the type of device used, operative procedure and the immediate and 30-day outcome. The register commenced on 1 January 1996 and the results of the first year's audit were presented at the eleventh meeting of the European Society for Vascular Surgery[10] and are reported below. A European registry (Eurostar) also commenced at about the same time as RETA. This registry concentrates on commercially available systems (see chapter by Harris and Brennan pp. 27–36).

THE FIRST YEAR'S RESULTS

A total of 139 patients were entered from 12 centres (median of nine procedures per centre: range 1–32). In all, 116 procedures were performed electively for asymptomatic aneurysms, 19 electively for symptoms, two acutely for non-ruptured aneurysms and two acutely for contained ruptures. Three different graft configurations were used (Fig. 2).

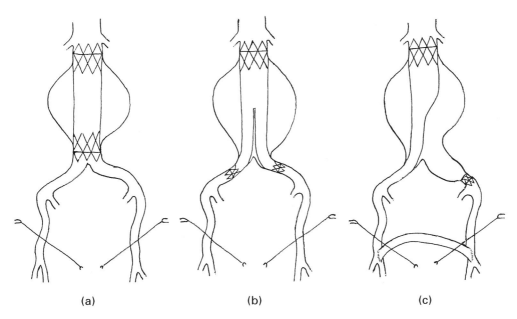

(a)   (b)   (c)

Fig. 2. Type of prosthesis. (a) Aortic tube (n=12): Bard (4), Stentor (3), Vanguard (3), Gianturco/Dacron (1), Palmaz/PTFE (1). (b) Aorto-bi-iliac (n=63): Stentor (32), Vanguard (20), Talent (5), EVT (3), Perth (3). (c) Aorto-uni-iliac and crossover (n=64): Palmaz/PTFE (33), Gianturco/Dacron (31).

Although 91 patients (65%) were considered fit for conventional repair (American Society of Anesthesiologists: ASA grades I to III), 48 (35%) were considered unfit for the reasons detailed in Table 1. Two of 12 patients (17%) undergoing aortic tube grafting were unfit for conventional repair, compared with 13 of 63 (21%) aorto-bi-iliac grafts, 15 of 31 (48%) Gianturco/Dacron and 18 of 33 (55%) Palmaz/polytetrafluroethylene (PTFE) grafts.

The median aneurysm diameter was 5.8cm (range 3.6–12cm) with a median infrarenal neck of 2.6cm (range 1.0–6cm). The age and aneurysm diameter were similar for all procedures. Aneurysms less than 5cm in diameter were mostly saccular.

Vascular access was gained by surgical cutdown to the femoral artery in all cases, with a contralateral percutaneous femoral puncture for most aorto-bi-iliac devices. An iliac conduit was used for access in 18 (53%) of the Palmaz/PTFE grafts because

Table 1.   Fitness for conventional repair

*48 patients (35%) were considered unfit for the following
reasons (one or more):*

No.	Reason
12	Poor left ventricular function
10	Severe ischaemic heart disease/angina
4	Other cardiac
4	Previous conventional repair abandoned
2	Inflammatory abdominal aortic aneurysms
6	Hostile abdomen
4	Poor respiratory function
8	Renal failure
3	Refused conventional repair
1	Paraplegia

of the large calibre of the delivery system. The median duration of the procedure was
150 minutes (range 35–695 min) and was related to the type of procedure. All centres
used general anaesthesia except for one that used epidurals. There was a median
blood loss of 700ml (range 50–8000+ml) and blood loss was also related to the type of
procedure.

In 101 cases (73%) the aneurysm was excluded by the primary procedure with no
peroperative complications. Nine patients required immediate conversion to a
conventional repair, five because of distal displacement of the proximal stent, one for
rupture of the neck by the stent, two for a large persistent proximal leak and one for
macroembolization. Conversion was not possible in another patient, where the stent
had ruptured the neck, because of dense intra-abdominal adhesions. Thirty-eight
patients had other immediate complications which are detailed in Table 2.

Postoperative complications within 30 days, or before discharge from hospital,
occurred in 37 patients. There were technical problems with the graft in eight cases.
Four graft limb occlusions were treated by two bypass grafts, one stent and one
thrombectomy. Five persistent endoleaks were treated by further stent placement on
two occasions, embolization coils in two and delayed conversion to an open repair in
one patient. Four patients developed groin haematomas, three a minor wound
infection, nine a persistent postoperative pyrexia (all Stentor devices), three renal
failure and there was one case each of left ventricular failure, pulmonary embolus,
stroke, confusion, colonic ischaemia, ureteric obstruction and small bowel perforation.

One hundred and eighteen aneurysms (85%) were successfully excluded from the
circulation, including five conventional repairs, at 30 days, or at discharge if sooner.
Eight patients (5.7%) had persistent endoleaks which were mainly from patent
lumbar vessels or the inferior mesenteric artery. There were 13 deaths (9.4%) and one
major amputation was required because of microembolization (Table 3).

The death rate was related to the type of procedure with a mortality of only 4.1%
for entirely endovascular aortic tube or aorto-bi-iliac devices compared with 15.6%
for aorto-uni-iliac devices combined with conventional crossover grafts. However,
fitness for conventional repair was also a factor, (6.6% if fit compared with 14.6% if
unfit). The need for immediate conversion to conventional repair carried a high

Table 2. Immediate outcome

Aneurysm excluded, no complications 101 (73%)	
Additional endovascular procedures	10
Leak – second stent	4
Kinking/stenosis – angioplasty/stent	4
Leak – coil embolization	2
Additional surgical procedures	4
Femoral aneurysm – repair	2
Displaced limb of Stentor – repair	2
Limb of Talent too long – crossover	1
Conversion to open repair	9
Stent slipped out of neck	5
Palmaz stent ruptured neck	1
Persistent proximal leak	2
Macroembolization	1
Other technical problems	14
Leak but no action taken	7
Difficulty with 2nd limb of Stentor	4
Microembolization	2
Bard stent too small (removed)	1

Table 3. 30-day/discharge outcome

Aneurysm excluded/repaired	118	(85%)
Persistent leak	8	(5.7%)
Aorto-bi-iliac	5/63	(7.9%)
Aorto-uni-iliac and crossover	2/65	(3.1%)
Aortic tube	1/10	(10%)
Major amputation	1	
Deaths	13	(9.4%)
Palmaz/PTFE	6/34	(17.5%)
Gianturco/Dacron	4/31	(12.9%)
Aorto-bi-iliac	2/63	(3.2%)
Aortic tubes	1/10	(10%)
Immediate conversion	5/9	(55%)
Deaths per centre	0–4	(5.5–20%)
Deaths in fit patients	6/91	(6.6%)
Deaths in unfit patients	7/48	(14.6%)

mortality of 55%. The death rate per centre varied from 5.5 to 20%. The median hospital stay was 6 days (range 1-30+ days). Hospital stay was also related to the type of procedure, being a median 5 days (range 2 –12) for aortic tubes, 5 days (1–30+) for aorto-bi-iliac, 7 days (4–24) for Palmaz/PTFE and 8 days (2–17) for Gianturco/Dacron grafts.

DISCUSSION

The first year of the national audit confirms that endovascular repair of abdominal aortic aneurysms is now undertaken by a considerable number of centres. Although the Registry is voluntary, the Working Party is not aware of any centre failing to submit its results. At present, all centres are teaching hospitals that are likely to conform to the agreed principles of specific training in endovascular grafting, an adequate workload in terms of elective conventional aneurysm repairs and high quality angiographic imaging facilities. All procedures involved a vascular surgeon and interventional radiologist as agreed by the two societies.[9]

Most repairs were performed for asymptomatic aneurysms with a diameter that would be considered appropriate for conventional repair (> 5cm). At present there is no evidence that conventional or endovascular repair of smaller aneurysms is justified.[11] The choice of procedure depends on two factors, the anatomy of the aneurysm and the fitness for conventional surgery and this is shown by the audit. Many centres prefer to offer conventional repair to fit patients who are unsuitable for a pure endovascular technique. This has resulted in a smaller number of unfit patients in the aorto-aortic and aorto-bi-iliac prosthesis groups. Conversely, unfit patients who cannot be offered conventional repair, and whose aneurysm morphology is unsuitable for existing commercial devices, are being offered more complex combined repairs. This selection would appear to be appropriate as the death rate for fit patients of 6.6% is similar to conventional repair. The mortality for unfit patients of 14.6% may be lower than conservative aneurysm management provided endovascular repair is durable in the long term.

The immediate outcome of 73% of aneurysms successfully excluded without complication is encouraging but ten patients required conversion to open repair and 21 needed additional endovascular or surgical procedures. The complexity of the repair, preoperative co-morbidity, incomplete exclusion requiring additional procedures and conversion to conventional repair all increased the complication rate.

The choice of aneurysm repair, which is directly related to the anatomy of the aneurysm, had the largest impact on outcome variables. Death rate, duration of operation, blood loss and duration of hospital stay, although not truly independent variables, were all higher with aorto-uni-iliac grafts and a conventional crossover than with entirely endovascular repairs. Evidence of a learning curve was also apparent with lower mortality rates in centres with a large experience of a particular technique.

Overall the results show marked heterogeneity in choice of procedure, complications and outcome and it is only by combining the data from a large number of patients in national or international audits that there will be sufficient information to be of clinical value. The audit does affect indications for intervention in a number of ways. It has given a clearer view of which patients should be offered endovascular repair considering both their general fitness for surgery and the anatomy of the aneurysm and indicates that two groups should be considered separately – fit patients whose results should be compared with conventional repair and unfit patients whose results must be compared with conservative management. It has also demonstrated the technical demands that this new technology makes on the surgeon and radiologist and supports the view of the Joint Working Party that the RETA database should be maintained and the technique limited to a number of dedicated centres until it has proved to be effective in the short and long term.

CONCLUSION

Endovascular repair of abdominal aortic aneurysms remains an experimental technique with an overall, immediate and 30-day complication rate which is above that expected for conventional repair. The procedure is constantly evolving and many of the complications continue to test the ingenuity of the radiologist and surgeon. Only by continuous audit, both within individual units, nationally and internationally can maximal advantage be taken of advances in technology and technique for the benefit of the 'aneurysm population' and the attending physician. The RETA reporting forms have been updated, 1-year follow-up forms are being issued and the second year results are now being analysed.

REFERENCES

1. Parodi JC, Palmaz JC, Barone HD: Trans femoral intraluminal graft implantation for abdominal aortic aneurysms. *Ann Vasc Surg* **5**: 491–9, 1991
2. Parodi JC: Endovascular repair of abdominal aortic aneurysms and other arterial lesions. *J Vasc Surg* **21**: 549–55, 1995
3. White GH, Jay J, McGahan T *et al.*: Historical control comparison of outcome for matched groups of patients undergoing endoluminal versus open repair of abdominal aortic aneurysms. *J Vasc Surg* **23**: 201–12, 1996
4. Stelter W: 1.5 year experience with the 'Stentor' device for repair of abdominal aortic aneurysm. *J Endovasc Surg* **3**: 121–2, 1996
5. Thompson MM, Sayers RD, Bell PRF: Endovascular aneurysm repair. *Br Med J*, **314**: 1139–40, 1997
6. Kretschmer G, Holzenbein T, Lammer J *et al.*: The first 15 months of transluminal aortic aneurysm management: a single centre experience. *Eur J Vasc Endovasc Surg* **14**: 24–32, 1997
7. Yusef SW, Whitaker SC, Chuter TAM, Hopkinson B: Early results of endovascular abdominal aortic aneurysm repair with aorto-uni-iliac graft and femoro-femoral bypass. *J Vasc Surg* **25**: 165–72, 1997
8. Eikelboom BC, Duijst P: Regulatory requirements for medical devices in the European Union. *Eur J Vasc Endovasc Surg* **12**: 3–4, 1996
9. Harris PL: Endovascular grafting for abdominal aortic aneurysms. *Ann R Coll Surg Eng* **78** (Suppl): 23–4, 1996
10. Beard JD: Registry of endovascular treatment of aneurysms (RETA): Preliminary results. Abstract presented at the XI meeting of the ESVS Lisbon, Portugal, 19 Sept 1997
11. May J, White GH, Yu W *et al.*: Concurrent comparison of endoluminal repair vs no treatment for small abdominal aortic aneurysms. *Eur J Vasc Endovasc Surg* **13**: 472–6, 1997

Editorial comments by R.M. Greenhalgh

The authors have taken the challenge and attempted to answer the question posed. Indeed they say the audit does affect the indications for intervention in a number of ways. The value of RETA is that it is a national audit. The authors believe it to be a comprehensive audit of 1 year of British endovascular experience for stent graft repair of aortic aneurysm. This is much more than a report of a subset of results by an enthusiastic group. It is also much more than a report of a single company product at a number of centres. Importantly, they report the result in those patients fit and unfit for open repair. Mortalities are given for both groups. This is the best evidence we have presently for the expected mortality for endovascular repair of aortic aneurysm for fit and unfit patients on a national basis.

The authors seem to think they know what the mortality for fit patients is nationally and in this they have more confidence than I, as I would choose to await the outcome of the UK Small Aneurysm Trial due to report in the autumn of 1998. From data then it would be possible to calculate exactly how many patients would be required in the random allocation trial to compare open repair with endovascular stent graft repair in patients fit for both. The working party and these authors are to be congratulated on this most valuable audit and its report here. Many never realised just how many patients being treated by stent graft are unfit for open repair. This implies that centres offering stent graft repair for aortic aneurysm are under immense pressure to accept patients not fit for open repair. With the known national mortality figures quoted here, this can only affect indications for stent graft repair as the authors claim. There will surely need to be a random allocation study in patients deemed unfit for open repair. This could be, for example, between a group treated with the best medical practice and stent graft repair against best medical practice alone. All surgeons wish to see a random allocation study comparing stent graft repair and open repair. The trials will need to be kept quite separate.

Is There a Case For Limiting Endovascular Repair of Abdominal Aortic Aneurysms to Commercially Available Devices?

P.L. Harris and J. Brennan

INTRODUCTION

The technical feasibility of exclusion of an infrarenal aortic aneurysm from the circulation by endovascular placement of a stent graft is now well established.[1] This approach, carrying as it does the benefits of minimal surgical invasion of the patient, has understandably generated considerable interest amongst vascular surgeons and radiologists. However, a number of important questions concerning the proper role of this technique, and especially its long-term durability, remain unanswered.

Which system to use is an issue about which it is difficult to obtain unbiased guidance and as more products and newer concepts are developed, this decision may become even more difficult. Commercial companies have to recoup their investment in research and development and in this new field all commercial products are extremely expensive. One way of dealing with the problem of high cost is to make your own endograft. This approach could also carry additional benefits e.g. 'homemade' endografts can be made to measure so that patients whose aneurysms do not match conveniently the anatomical prerequisites of off the shelf commercial devices, can be catered for. Given the infinite number of combinations of sizing and configuration necessary to accommodate all aneurysms, the flexibility of homemade devices means that a greater proportion of patients can be treated.[2]

But is the homemade or DIY approach reasonable and safe, or should endovascular procedures for repair of aneurysms be restricted to commercially available products only? In this chapter we assess the scant evidence currently available for guidance on this question.

HISTORICAL PERSPECTIVE

Initially all stent grafts used for aneurysm repair were of necessity of the homemade variety since there were no commercial products available. The very first system described by Parodi was made using a Palmaz stent sutured to a poly-tetrafluoroethylene (PTFE) graft which had been stretched with an angioplasty balloon (see chapter by Parodi (pp. 199–210)). Others followed this lead and a number of combinations of different stents and graft materials have been described.[3–5]

Parodi's first attempt at endovascular aneurysm repair involved an aorto–aortic graft using a straight tube, the proximal end of which was held in place by a Palmaz stent and the distal end of which was left loose. It was soon realized that stents were required to fix and seal the graft at both proximal and distal ends. Subsequently it has become apparent that, with few exceptions, aorto–aortic endografts are inherently unstable because of problems with maintaining an effective seal at the distal fixation point.[6] Most present day homemade systems involve an aorto–uni–iliac endograft with endovascular occlusion of the opposite common iliac artery and a femorofemoral bypass to maintain perfusion of both legs.[7]

The first commercially available system came on the market in 1994. This was the modular Stentor system described by Claude Mialhe and marketed by MinTec (Freeport, Bahamas). This first-generation commercial product was not without its problems but the modular concept, whereby a bifurcated stent graft could be constructed *in situ* by wholly endovascular means obviating the need for a significant surgical component, was very attractive. The shortcomings of this product were related mostly to the poor quality of the fabric component and weakness at suture lines, which tended to be a source of leakage. In 1996 MinTec was acquired by the Boston Scientific Corporation (Watertown MA, USA) and the Stentor system was upgraded and renamed Vanguard. Superior, thin-wall Dacron fabric was used and the suture lines were eliminated. The Vanguard system can therefore be considered to be a second-generation device along with others more recently introduced onto the market. These include the Talent (World Medical, Sunrise FL, USA) and AneuRx (Medtronic, Cupertino CA, USA) systems, which are of the modular bifurcated design, and the EVT (Endovascular Technologies, Menlo Park CA, USA) which is a one-piece bifurcated graft. In addition, Bard (Murray Hill NJ, USA) and Baxter (Irvine CA, USA) have both entered the clinical evaluation stage with aorto–aortic tube devices.

THE RELATIVE MERITS OF COMMERCIAL AND HOMEMADE ENDOGRAFTS

The principal advantage of a commercially produced endograft is first, a guarantee that it has been developed, produced, sterilized and packaged under stringent conditions of safety and quality control imposed by national and international regulatory authorities. Second, commercial devices are marketed with clearly defined indications and product limitations to ensure their appropriate use. All manufacturers to date have adopted a highly responsible marketing policy of ensuring that the clinicians to whom they are willing to release their product have received some specific training in the deployment of their device. Furthermore, the commercial companies provide very valuable technical support to assist clinicians in the early part of their experience to select patients and devices properly and to offer guidance to overcome any technical problems encountered during the operative procedures. To date all commercial companies in this field have also taken considerable trouble to ensure adequate follow-up of their devices following implantation either independently or through organizations such as the Eurostar project.

The main disadvantage of the commercial systems is that they are of necessity manufactured in a limited range of sizes and combinations of aortic and limb diameters. Even with a modular system, the range is very limited. One reason for this is the laudable objective of all manufacturers to make the introducer systems as small as possible. The race is on to introduce onto the market the first truly percutaneous system for abdominal aortic aneurysm repair. The introduction of overlapping stents within stents, the 'trombone' concept (Fig. 1),[8,9] and tapered or flared stent grafts, are likely to allow many more patients with aneurysms to be treated with these products in the very near future.

The increased flexibility inherent in a made-to-measure approach is the principal advantage of using a homemade system. It is likely, however, that the standards of quality control during manufacture are considerably less demanding than those imposed upon commercial manufacturers by statutory regulation, therefore there is potential for error during manufacture which could well add to technical problems associated with the surgical procedures.

Most currently used homemade systems consist of an aorto–uni–iliac stent graft and a femorofemoral crossover.[7] The surgical procedure to implant the device therefore involves more surgical trauma than is associated with deployment of commercially available bifurcated systems. Proponents may argue that the additional surgical trauma is not clinically significant but there is underlying concern that a more invasive procedure is likely to be associated with a higher risk of complications, particularly in elderly patients, most of whom have serious co-morbidities. As far as fit patients are concerned there are reservations about employing an extra-anatomical bypass when systems are available to replace the diseased aorta with a bifurcated system.

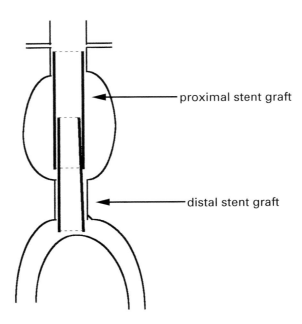

Fig. 1. The 'trombone' concept of stacked stent grafts developed at the Royal Prince Alfred Hospital, Sydney, Australia. Although the aorto–aortic tube format is not widely applicable the same principle can be adopted for aorto–uni–iliac grafts.

Homemade devices constructed from Dacron fabric involve a suture line and in commercial products leakage from suture lines was found to be a cause of late endoleaks. Where PTFE is used, conventional graft material is expanded with a balloon to three or four times its original diameter. There is to date little information about the durability of balloon-expanded PTFE.

While acceptable results with homemade devices have been achieved in a few centres, it appears to be the case that these techniques do not travel well. This is perhaps not surprising, since a homemade system developed in one institution is specific to that institution. In the absence of detailed protocols on manufacture and surgical deployment of these devices, it is to be expected that changes of methodology, either major or subtle, will occur in transfer to another unit. This is likely to increase the learning curve effect.

Because homemade systems are constructed from components which were never designed to be combined into one product, they tend to be relatively bulky. This results in introducer systems which are on average three or four French sizes larger than those necessary to introduce commercial devices.

Finally, in the present environment of ever dwindling health care resources a principal advantage of homemade systems is their cost. Whereas all commercial devices on the market are currently priced at around £4500, a homemade device can be put together for around £1000, including its introducer system. However, cost alone is not an appropriate criterion upon which to base the choice of device for aneurysm repair. Much more important are safety and clinical efficacy. Information about the performance of homemade devices is available from the published results of individual centres in the UK and from the UK Registry of Endovascular Treatment of Aneurysms (RETA) (see chapter by Beard and Rochester (pp. 19–26)). The most valuable source of data on commercial devices currently available is the Eurostar project.

THE EUROSTAR PROJECT

Uncertainty about the long-term durability of endovascular stent graft repair of abdominal aortic aneurysms signalled the need for very close monitoring of the outcome of aortic stent graft procedures over time.[10,11] The number of these procedures being undertaken in most individual vascular units is too small to allow relevant conclusions to be drawn from local audit. Collation of data from a large number of centres is therefore necessary in order to establish a useful database. The more centres, the sooner reliable answers will be obtained to the important questions.

The Eurostar (EUROpean collaborators on Stent graft Techniques for abdominal aortic Aneurysm Repair) project was established in Liverpool in February 1996 and a data registry centre in Eindhoven shortly afterwards. In July 1997 data from 430 patients submitted by 47 different vascular surgery units from 11 European countries had been entered onto the Eurostar database, with an average follow up of 10 months. It was made clear from the outset that the Eurostar project was to be an independent professional initiative without any allegiance to a single commercial company. However, there was a consensus amongst the Eurostar collaborators that entry onto the registry would be restricted to patients undergoing treatment with devices that qualified for a European Community (CE) mark. This is awarded by competent regulatory authorities in European Union countries to medical products which satisfy agreed standards of safety and quality control in manufacture.

Data contribution to the registry was invited from vascular units fulfilling the following criteria:

1. They should demonstrate close co-operation between vascular surgeons and radiologists with extensive experience of endovascular interventional techniques.
2. They should have received specific training with the type of aortic endograft they propose to deploy in their patients.
3. They should treat a minimum number of ten patients with aortic aneurysms by endovascular repair annually.
4. They should abide by the Eurostar protocol especially in respect of inclusion and exclusion and criteria and regular follow-up assessments.

The Eurostar registry provides information about the early results of endovascular grafting of aneurysms and procedural complications but its principal objective is to determine the efficacy of these techniques over time, and it is intended that follow-up will extend for a minimum of 5 years.

RESULTS OF ENDOVASCULAR ANEURYSM REPAIR WITH HOMEMADE AND COMMERCIAL DEVICES

Applicability

Neither the Eurostar nor the RETA databases include information about patients who were rejected for endovascular repair. Therefore, for information about device applicability, we have to turn to the reported experience of individual units. In Liverpool, of 155 patients with aneurysms assessed by spiral computed tomography (CT) scanning and measuring catheter angiography, 47 (30.3%) were found to be contenders for endovascular repair using the Vanguard bifurcated system (Fig. 2). The experience of other units using similar commercially available bifurcated devices has been similar with applicability in the range of 25–40%. The exclusion criteria for the 108 cases considered unsuitable for endovascular repair in the Liverpool series are seen in Fig. 3. For many of these there was more than one reason for exclusion.

In Nottingham, where homemade systems have been used almost exclusively, of 154 patients assessed, 15 (10%) were found to be suitable for an aortic tube graft and 85 (55%) for an aorto–uni–iliac endograft with femorofemoral crossover.[12] Using this system the surgeons in Nottingham were able to accommodate more patients with iliac artery disease and those with wider aortic necks. The upper limit of aortic diameter that can be accommodated by most commercially available devices is of the order of 25 mm. However, it is questionable whether an aortic diameter in excess of 25 mm at the level of the renal arteries can be considered to be healthy or showing evidence of aneurysmal dilatation. The long-term effects of implanting a stent graft into an aorta which is already subject to pathological dilatation at this level are likely

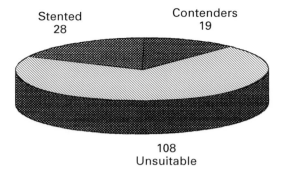

Stented
28

Contenders
19

108
Unsuitable

Fig. 2. Suitability for endovascular aneurysm repair using commercial modular systems. Patients from 155 consecutive cases were assessed with spiral CT initially, proceeding to calibrated aortography if the CT appearances were favourable. The majority (70%) were not suitable.

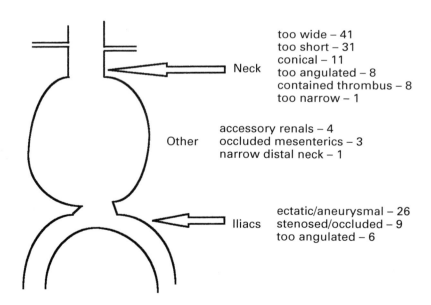

Neck

too wide – 41
too short – 31
conical – 11
too angulated – 8
contained thrombus – 8
too narrow – 1

Other

accessory renals – 4
occluded mesenterics – 3
narrow distal neck – 1

Iliacs

ectatic/aneurysmal – 26
stenosed/occluded – 9
too angulated – 6

Fig. 3. Principal exclusion criteria for endovascular aneurysm repair in 108 cases from a series of 155 assessed for modular commercial systems. For some cases there was more than one reason for exclusion.

to be disappointing; however, the available data supports the contention that homemade devices do have wider applicability than the current range of commercially available products.

Initial outcome of operation

Registration of patients onto the Eurostar database is made on an 'intention to treat' basis. This means that patients are identified on the database prior to treatment and accurate information is obtained about the failures as well as the successes. Of 430 patients registered, stent grafts were deployed successfully in 420, amounting to a technical success rate of 98%. Eight patients required conversion to open repair and in two cases the endovascular repair was supplemented by an extraanatomic bypass.

Bifurcated devices were deployed in the overwhelming majority, 376 (93%). Local arterial complications occurred in 37 (9%) and systemic complications in 80 (19%). These are listed in Table 1. In the whole series of 430 patients there were 14 (3.2%) deaths within 30 days. For patients with an American Society of Anesthesiologists ASA grade of III or lower the mortality rate was 2.8% but in 47 patients with an ASA grade of IV or V, the mortality rate was 9.3%.

Table 1. Local arterial and systemic complications reported to the Eurostar registry in 430 patients undergoing endovascular aneurysm repair with commercially produced devices

Local/arterial		Systemic (14 deaths)	
Haematoma/false aneurysm	24	Cardiac (MI, CCF, arrhythmia)	20
Iliofemoral trauma	6	Pulmonary	15
Thromboembolism	6	Renal	24
Wound infection	7	Cerebrovascular	5
		GI	9

MI: Myocardial infarct

The RETA study recorded data on 138 patients during the first year, 1996/7, from 11 centres. The duration of operation and the mean total blood loss was greater in patients having their aneurysms repaired with homemade aorto–uni–iliac devices with femorofemoral crossover than those who received commercial endografts. The technical success rate overall was 73% and the mortality rate was 10% (13/138). There was a difference between the mortality rate of patients receiving commercial devices, 3/73 (4.1%), and those receiving homemade aorto–uni–iliac devices with crossover, 10/64 (15.6%). However, this difference may be accounted for by a higher proportion of unfit patients in the group which were treated with homemade devices. Of 48 patients considered to be 'unfit', there were seven deaths (14.6%) compared with six of 91 (6.6%) who were 'fit'. Unfortunately, patients entered onto the RETA database have not been classified according to ASA grading.

Direct comparison between the immediate result and complication rates of commercially available and homemade endovascular devices is not possible because of the different indications and patient populations included. Only a randomized comparison would provide acceptable evidence of the superiority of one approach over the other. In the meantime, it is a matter of conjecture as to whether or not the higher mortality associated with homemade systems can be accounted for by a higher risk patient population, or whether other factors are also involved.

Longer term outcome

The Eurostar registry is providing valuable information about the impact of endovascular repair with commercial devices upon the subsequent morphological changes of successfully excluded aneurysms and late complications such as endoleak and graft limb occlusion. After 12 months 15% of aneurysms either remain unchanged or have actually increased in size, and presumably remain at risk from rupture. On discharge 15% of patients show evidence of an endoleak and during the next 12 months another 12% develop new endoleaks. The majority of these either seal spontaneously or are closed by a secondary endovascular procedure. Only a few have required conversion. There is a small incidence of graft limb occlusion but this complication seems to be increasing with time and there is evidence that it may be related to kinking of the stent graft caused by remodelling and shortening of the aneurysm sac.

No follow-up data are yet available from the RETA study. However, reports from UK centres that have used homemade devices indicate that a similar percentage of patients show continued expansion of their aneurysm following endovascular repair. Migration of the proximal stent has also been reported and is known to be a source of late endoleaks. It is to be expected that devices which are constructed from proximal and distal stents with unsupported graft material between will be susceptible to this complication. It has not been reported in any patient in the Eurostar database which relates almost exclusively to devices which are supported by stents throughout their length.

It must be anticipated that late device-related complications will occur in association with homemade systems as they do with commercial devices. The recent issue of suture breakage between the stent rings of the Boston Scientific Vanguard device has illustrated the importance of rigorous follow-up and the necessity of ready access to technical resources in order to evaluate and resolve such problems.

SUMMARY

Published evidence indicates that technically successful aneurysm exclusion is feasible with a variety of commercially produced and homemade devices. There are no randomized studies comparing these two approaches and each has clearly perceived advantages and disadvantages.

The Eurostar project has shown already that, although safe in the short term, endoleaks and other late complications occur following endovascular repair of aneurysms which are not associated with the conventional operation, and these problems have yet to be resolved. When making a choice between commercial and homemade products, clinicians must balance the lower cost and greater flexibility of homemade systems on the one hand against the rigorous standards of quality control in manufacture and high level of technical support of commercial systems on the other. Furthermore, commercial systems lend themselves more easily to the process of multicentre audit. Although higher mortality rates have been reported with homemade systems, this may be accounted for by different selection criteria which lead to the inclusion of a high proportion of 'compassionate' patients.

Currently there is no acceptable evidence available to justify the restriction of endovascular repair of abdominal aortic aneurysm to commercially available devices only. However, worldwide experience demonstrates very clearly that the majority of clinicians who have become involved in this new and exciting approach to aneurysmal disease feel more secure in offering their patients a commercially manufactured device rather than one they can make themselves despite the considerably higher cost.

REFERENCES

1. Parodi JC, Palmaz JC, Barone HD: Transfemoral intraluminal graft implantation for abdominal aortic aneurysms. *Ann Vasc Surg* **5**: 491–9, 1991
2. Armon MP, Yusuf SW, Whitaker SC *et al.*: The anatomy of abdominal aortic aneurysms: Implications for sizing of endovascular grafts. *Eur J Vasc Endovasc Surg* **13**: 398–402, 1997
3. Chuter TA, Green RM, Ouriel K *et al.*: Transfemoral endovascular aortic graft placement. *J Vasc Surg* **18**: 185–97, 1993
4. May J, White G, Waugh R *et al.*: Treatment of complex abdominal aortic aneurysms by a combination of endoluminal and extraluminal aortofemoral grafts. *J Vasc Surg* **19**: 924–33, 1994
5. Yusuf SW, Baker DM, Chuter TA *et al.*: Transfemoral endoluminal repair of abdominal aortic aneurysm with bifurcated graft. *Lancet* **344**: 650–1, 1994
6. May J, White GH, Yu W *et al.*: Importance of graft configuration in outcome of endoluminal abdominal aortic aneurysm repair. Presented at European Society for Vascular Surgery, Lisbon, September 1997
7. Yusuf SW, Baker DM, Hind RE *et al.*: Endoluminal transfemoral abdominal aortic aneurysm repair with aorto–uni–iliac graft and femorofemoral bypass. *Br J Surg* **82**: 916, 1995
8. Yu W, White GH, May J, Stephen MS: Endoluminal repair of abdominal aortic aneurysms using the trombone technique. *Asian J Surg* **19**: 37–40, 1996
9. Chuter TAM, Malina M, Brunkwall J *et al.*: A telescopic stent-graft for aorto-iliac implantation. *Eur J Vasc Endovasc Surg* **13**: 79–84, 1997
10. Harris PL: Endovascular grafting for abdominal aortic aneurysms. Principles agreed jointly by the Vascular Surgical Society of Great Britain and Ireland and the British Society of Interventional radiologists for assessment of endovascular grafting techniques and their introduction into clinical practice. *Ann R Coll Surg Engl* **78** (Suppl): 23–4, 1996
11. Veith FJ, Abbott WM, Yao JS *et al.*: Guidelines for development and use of transluminally placed endovascular prosthetic grafts in the arterial system. Endovascular Graft Committee. *J Vasc Surg* **21**: 670–85, 1995
12. Armon MP, Yusuf SW, Latief K *et al.*: Anatomical suitability of abdominal aortic aneurysms for endovascular repair. *Br J Surg* **84**: 178–80, 1997

Editorial comments by B.R. Hopkinson

This chapter gives a very good review of commercially available devices for endovascular repair of abdominal aortic aneurysm. It does point out the shortcomings in terms of the limited number of patients that they are able to fit and also the limited applications that are available for some of these devices. For instance some systems have FDA approval but only for patients fit for open surgery whereas other systems are only available for patients who are unfit for conventional surgery. Consequently, it may be somewhat unfair to compare the results of treatment using these different devices for differing indications.

The term 'homemade' or 'do-it-yourself' is slightly pejorative and I would prefer to use 'tailor-made' or 'custom-made' for the individual patient by the surgeons involved. Vascular surgeons have many years of experience of tailoring grafts to an appropriate shape and size for open repair of aneurysms and are not coming to the field as raw beginners or enthusiastic amateurs. They come as dedicated professionals using all their skills to put together what they believe to be the best combination for the individual patient. Custom-made devices, generally speaking, use standard components for the graft material and for the fixation devices, assembled around standard commercially available catheters, sheaths and introducers. One of the immediate and most obvious advantages for using a surgeon-made device is that if during the course of insertion difficulties are met, the surgeon who made the gadget is in the best position to modify it. The people using a commercial device made by a third party are to some extent employing a 'black box' and are not in a position to adjust things quite so readily.

The reason why most surgeon-made systems are of the aorto–uni–iliac stent–graft variety with a femorofemoral crossover is quite simply because there is not currently available a commercially manufactured aorto–uni–iliac device. I think we would all agree that a bifurcation device has a certain surgical nicety about it, particularly as it does not involve suture lines in the groins. Unfortunately it is only available for some 30% of patients so what are we to do with the other 70%?

The whole question of fit and unfit patients needs to be sorted out with some sort of risk stratification. It is a field for much future research. The ASA grading is not sufficiently accurate as a prognostic indicator.

It is essential for the future that we have trials comparing different endografts with open surgery in comparable risk cases. At the moment we have quite a hotch-potch with considerable confusion.

CAROTID ARTERY QUESTIONS AND INDICATIONS

Should We Use General or Local Anaesthesia for Carotid Artery Surgery?

Paolo Fiorani, Enrico Sbarigia, Francesco Speziale, Hadi Abi Rached,
Patrizio Sbraga, Alvaro Zaccaria, Carmine Dario Vizza,
and Mario Antonini

INTRODUCTION

Most vascular surgeons nowadays prefer to do carotid endarterectomy in patients under general anaesthesia.[1-4] Not only is this anaesthetic technique believed by many to provide better preservation of brain function, but it is also more practical, generally less time-consuming, and more comfortable for patients and surgeons alike. However, it has shortcomings, notably the poor reliability of the current standard intraoperative monitoring technique (carotid artery stump pressure measurements)[5,6] or some more sophisticated techniques (EEG, somatosensory evoked potentials, regional blood-flow measurement by xenon 133, or more recently transcranial Doppler sonography) provide a more accurate intraoperative assessment of brain function or of cerebral blood flow, but they all require elaborate equipment and necessitate the presence of specialized personnel during operation.[7-12]

It is not without concern that many authors, like ourselves, have met a consistent number of intraoperative complications that escape detection by intraoperative monitoring, becoming evident only when patients awaken from anaesthesia.[13-16] Many of these complications remain unexplained because of lack of positive intraoperative monitoring and normal patency of the arterial reconstruction. Because nowadays, surgeons face increasing demands for carotid endarterectomy in severely ill patients, carotid endarterectomy which is a relatively low-risk procedure, often poses a surgical challenge.

For this reason and to find a means of overcoming the problems related to general anaesthesia, in 1987 we started using local anaesthesia for carotid endarterectomy.

The results of a previous retrospective study[17] on 893 patients operated on for a total of 1020 carotid endarterectomies comparing general anaesthesia with cervical block (Tables 1, 2) showed a significant reduction of:

1. internal carotid artery shunting;
2. incidence of perioperative neurological morbidity and mortality;
3. incidence of perioperative cardiac morbidity and mortality.

Concerning the reduction of neurological morbidity and mortality an explanation was easily found (more reliable intraoperative cerebral monitoring; certainty of the cause of the complications, which determined some changes in operative technique). Recently,

Table 1.   Shunting

	General anaesthesia 337 cases n (%)	Cervical block 683 cases n (%)	
Shunt	75 (22.5)	93 (13.2)	p=0.0004

Table 2.   Perioperative results

	General anaesthesia 337 cases n (%)	Cervical block 683 cases n (%)	
Neurological morbidity	11 (3.24)	9 (1.31)	p=0.03
Neurological mortality	4 (1.18)	3 (0.44)	p=ns
Total neurological complications	15 (4.44)	12 (1.75)	p=0.01
Cardiac morbidity	2 (0.59)	2 (0.29)	
Cardiac mortality	2 (0.59)	2 (0.29)	
Total cardiac complications	4 (1.18)	4 (0.58)	p=ns
TOTAL	19 (5.64)	16 (2.34)	

p: by χ^2 contingency tables.

a systematic review of the literature has concluded that non-randomized published studies report significant benefits in terms of perioperative neurological morbidity and mortality rates after carotid endarterectomy using regional anaesthesia.[18]

Nevertheless, a detailed analysis of data in our patient population, failed to explain a 50% reduction in cardiac morbidity and mortality in those patients operated under cervical block anaesthesia with similar cardiac clinical conditions. An accurate review of the literature about perioperative cardiac complications in carotid surgery with special regard for the possible implications of the type of anaesthesia on cardiac outcome, failed to find any study on this specific argument.

This was the stimulus to start a small prospective monocentric randomized trial in our department to try to assess the possible role of anaesthetic techniques (general and local anaesthesia) in determining cardiac complications (intra- or perioperative cardiac ischaemia) during carotid endarterectomy. The following paragraphs briefly report the preliminary data of this study.

METHODS

Classification of the coronary artery disease and allocation to the type of anaesthesia

The cardiologist classified the patients enrolled in the study in two groups according to the New York Heart Association (NYHA) functional classification: cardiac (NYHA I, II, III): Group A; non-cardiac patients (NYHA 0): Group B. After approval of the study by the local ethics committees, a prospective randomization of the type of anaesthesia (general or locoregional) was prepared for each group of patients. Anaesthesia was induced by the same team of anaesthetists.

Both the anaesthetic techniques and intraoperative cardiovascular and cerebral monitoring, management and protection have been described elsewhere.[17]

Cardiac monitoring

In all patients, heart activity was monitored continuously throughout operation and for 24 h afterwards by computerized 12-lead electrocardiography (ECG) (STM Mortara Instruments Bologna, Italy). A 12-lead monitoring procedure guaranteed a highly reliable ECG. As perioperative symptomatic cardiac events are quite rare (0.5–1%), the primary ischaemic end-point was defined as ST-segment upsloping or downsloping of >2 mm.

The data on eligible patients were entered into a database and interpreted by a cardiologist who was unaware of the type of anaesthesia used for surgery.

Statistical analysis

Results were expressed by descriptive statistics: mean ± SD and percentiles. Differences between cardiac and non-cardiac groups and between local and general anaesthesia were assessed for statistical significance by χ^2 statistics, Student's t-test, and Wilcoxon test and ANOVA. A p value of equal to or more than <0.05 was considered to indicate statistical significance.

PATIENTS

From November 1995 to September 1997, 85 consecutive patients with carotid artery stenosis, scheduled for carotid surgery, were recruited for this study. Informed consent was obtained from all patients before entry. After randomization was applied, four (4.7%) patients were excluded because they declined cervical block anaesthesia; in another case (1.2%) local anaesthesia was converted to general anaesthesia because of patient anxiety and restlessness. Eighty subjects therefore remained in the study.

The 80 patients had the following clinical characteristics: 69 men (86.25%) and 11 women (13.75%), whose ages ranged from 50 to 85 years (mean age 69.8 years, median age 70 years). The following risk factors were present at entry: hypertension (65 patients, 81.25%), current smoking (54 cases, 67.5%), diabetes (30 cases, 37.5%) and high blood lipid levels (30 cases, 37.5%). Cardiovascular disorders were distributed as follows: 35 patients (43.75%) had obstructive arteriopathy of the lower limbs; seven (8.7%) had abdominal aortic aneurysms and three (3.7%) had renovascular hypertension. Nine patients (11.5%) had previously undergone surgery (seven endarterectomy of the carotid bifurcation plus two subclavian carotid artery bypass grafts). Five patients (6.25%) had undergone previous coronary artery revascularization; at the time of carotid endarterectomy three of the five patients had persisting symptoms of cardiac ischaemia. The indications for surgery were transient ischaemic attack (56 cases, 70%); >70% asymptomatic stenosis (16 cases, 20%); and previous cerebral stroke (eight cases, 10%). All patients underwent non-invasive preoperative assessment of carotid artery stenosis with echo-colour Doppler (Diasonics Spectra series F 7117). Twenty-nine patients (36.2%) were submitted to digital angiography by Seldinger technique. Computed tomographic (CT) cranial scans were obtained in 50 patients (69.4%).

RESULTS

Patients

Preoperative investigations demonstrated in 43 patients (53.7%) evidence of bilateral carotid stenosis; 32 (40%) had unilateral stenosis, and five (6.2%) patients had a unilateral carotid stenosis and a contralateral occlusion. In 29 patients (36.2%) the data from non-invasive haemodynamic investigations were confirmed by digital angiography according to Seldinger technique. Scans in 38 cases (65.5%) showed evidence of a cerebral infarction involving the territory supplied by the middle cerebral artery.

Classification of the coronary artery disease and allocation to the type of anaesthesia

The 80 patients recruited for the study were subdivided into two groups: 51 patients (63.7%) with coronary artery disease (NYHA classes I and II) and 29 patients (36.2%) without cardiac disorders (NYHA class 0). In the cardiac disease group 24 patients (47%) had surgery under local anaesthesia and 27 (53%) under general anaesthesia according to the randomization. In the non-cardiac disease group 18 patients (62%) received local anaesthesia and 11 (38%) general anaesthesia. There were no differences in risk factors between cardiac and non-cardiac patients and associated vascular disorders.

Type of anaesthesia and intraoperative management

Invasive continuous intraoperative pressure monitoring disclosed a statistically significant difference between the mean pressure in patients assigned to local and those receiving general anaesthesia (107 ± 4 mm Hg vs 95 ± 7 mm Hg) ($p=0.0001$) (Fig. 1).

This was the reason why more patients assigned to local than to general anaesthesia received intensive hypotensive medication (34/42 patients, 81% vs 7/38, 18%; $p=0.0001$). Conversely, administration of hypertensive agents did not differ significantly in the two groups of patients between the two techniques (7/35, 16% vs 1/38, 2.6%; $p=0.08$). A Sundt shunt was placed in four of 80 patients (5%): three of the four patients had been assigned to cervical-block anaesthesia and suffered neurological deficits at the clamping test. A shunt was also necessary in a patient receiving general anaesthesia, because intraoperative transcranial Doppler ultra-sonography detected a fall (<10 cm/s) in the mean middle cerebral artery blood-flow velocity.

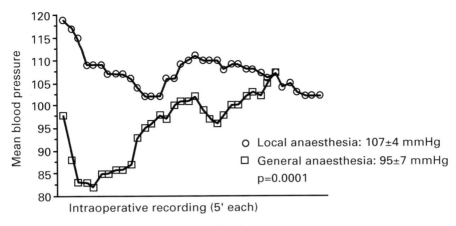

Fig. 1.

Neurologic perioperative results

None of the operations in this series led to neurologically related deaths. Permanent neurological morbidity was 1.25%: a patient who had internal carotid artery thrombosis. After immediate revision to clear the carotid axis the patient was transferred to intensive care and later discharged with sequelae of right hemiparesis. In three patients (3.75%) perioperative transient ischaemic attacks all regressed without sequelae.

Cardiac monitoring

In 13 patients (16.25%), all men, perioperative ECG monitoring showed the occurrence of ischaemia (Table 3). Of these events 11 (21.5%) involved the group with cardiac disease and two (6.8%) the group without cardiac disease. Comparison between the two anaesthetic groups showed that in the group with cardiac disorders six ischaemic events (22.2%) occurred in patients receiving general anaesthesia and five events (20.8%) in those receiving local anaesthesia.

In the group without cardiac disorders the two ischaemic events occurred in two patients (11.1%) receiving local anaesthesia. None of the nine patients without

Table 3. Perioperative cardiac events according to the type of anaesthesia

		New York Heart Association			
		Group A (1–2) 51 patients		Group B (0) 29 patients	
		Events	No events	Events	No events
Local anaesthetic	42	5	19	2	16
General anaesthetic	38	6	21	0	11
TOTAL	80	11	40	2	27

cardiac disease assigned to general anaesthesia had signs of cardiac ischaemia during monitoring.

DISCUSSION

Cardiac events (myocardial ischaemia, fatal or non-fatal myocardial infarction and sudden cardiac death) now account for half of all complications occurring during surgery or in the immediate postoperative period.[19-22] In the numerous case series reported in recent years, the incidence of clinically evident coronary artery disease in patients awaiting surgery for carotid surgery ranges from 30 to 49%.[13,23] In addition, an estimated 75–85% of all myocardial ischaemic events manifest without anginal chest pain. Patients with asymptomatic and symptomatic myocardial ischaemia nonetheless have a similar prognosis.[19,22] Hence, the problem of coronary disease in patients scheduled for carotid artery revascularization is of far greater importance than the clinical data alone would suggest.

Attention has focused also on the importance of anaesthetic techniques. Anaesthetic drugs could adversely impair intraoperative cardiac function through various mechanisms, for example by acting directly on myocardial kinetics or indirectly on the pattern of and response to drugs used for pressure control. The only two published studies addressing these questions have yielded unclear or contradictory results.[24,25]

The preliminary results of our prospective study show that most of the acute perioperative ischaemic events occurred in patients in NYHA classes I–II (patients with cardiac disease, 51 cases); but we found no differences related to the type of anaesthetic procedure the patient received (Table 3). At first sight of the specific results of this prospective study, the two anaesthetic techniques yielded equal outcomes in terms of the ischaemic end-point sought by monitoring during the immediate 24 h after surgery. In the non-cardiac group (29 cases, NYHA class 0), ischaemic events developed in two patients receiving local anaesthesia but in none of the patients receiving general anaesthesia. As expected, the non-cardiac group had fewer perioperative cardiac events, but this result may have been based by the chance initial enrollment of fewer non-cardiac than cardiac patients.

Among the cardiologic complications during hospitalization, at the end of 24-h monitoring, in two patients in the group with cardiac problems, both of whom underwent surgery with general anaesthesia, high-frequency atrial fibrillation developed. One of the two died of acute cardiac failure. Such complications, reasonably, cannot be assigned to the type of anaesthetic technique used.

Our additional data on intraoperative monitoring of systemic arterial pressure showed that patients who underwent local anaesthesia had significantly higher systemic blood pressures (regardless of whether they had cardiac disease) and therefore needed hypotensive or hypertensive medication significantly more frequently than patients treated under general anaesthesia.

As reported by others, the higher systemic blood pressure regimen during operation under local anaesthesia could represent a significant risk factor for cardiac complication.[26] At present, these suggestions still cannot be proved by our data.

Moreover, the strict control and manipulation of systemic arterial pressure in preventing perioperative myocardial ischaemic events, failed to change the incidence of perioperative myocardial infarction.[20]

CONCLUSION

Cervical block anaesthesia potentially helps to reduce neurologic complications because it is a simple technique for monitoring brain function. Patients needing an internal carotid artery shunt are detected and clamping ischaemia is *de facto* eliminated.

A prospective multicentre randomized study on the effect of these two anaesthesiological techniques could be useful to decide if one or other offers advantages in terms of neurological complications. We predict that local anaesthesia will demonstrate better results, when, after an initial phase of practice, the shortcomings raised by many (i.e. stress for patients and surgeon, uncomfortable and often hurried operations) are overcome.

Conversely, as the preliminary results of our monocentric prospective trial, at present, do not show any favourable or unfavourable effects of local or general anaesthetic on perioperative cardiac complications, a prospective multicentre study would demonstrate even a difference between the two anaesthesiological techniques in terms of cardiac complications.

REFERENCES

1. North American Symptomatic Carotid Endarterectomy Trial Collaboration: Beneficial effect of carotid endarterectomy in symptomatic patients with high grade stenosis. *New Engl J Med* **325**: 445–54, 1991
2. MRC European Carotid Surgery Trial: Interim results for symptomatic patients with severe (70–99%) or with mild (0–29%) carotid stenosis. *Lancet* **337**: 1235–43, 1991
3. Nunn DB: Carotid endarterectomy in patients with territorial ischemic attacks. *J Vasc Surg* **8**: 447–52, 1988
4. Whittemore AD, Mannik JA: Surgical treatment of carotid disease in patients with neurologic deficits. *J Vasc Surg* **5**: 910–13, 1987
5. Evans WE, Hayes JP, Waltke EA *et al.*: Optimal cerebral monitoring during carotid endarterectomy: neurologic response under local anaesthesia. *J Vasc Surg* **4**: 543–5, 1986
6. Hafner CD, Evans WE: Carotid endarterectomy with local anesthesia: results and advantages. *J Vasc Surg* **7**: 232–9, 1988
7. Sundt TM, Sharbrough FW, Marsh WR *et al.*: The risk-benefit ratio of intraoperative shunting during carotid endarterectomy. *Ann Surg* **203**: 196–204, 1986
8. Boysen G, Engell HC, Pistolese GR *et al.*: On the critical lower level of cerebral blood flow in man with particular reference to carotid surgery. *Circulation* **49**: 6, 1974
9. Markand ON, Dilley RS, Moorthy SS, Warren C: Monitoring of somatosensory evoked responses during carotid endarterectomy. *Arch Neurol* **41**: 375–87, 1984
10. Jorgensen LG, Schroeder TV: Transcranial Doppler for detection of cerebral ischemia during carotid endarterectomy. *Eur J Vasc Surg* **6**: 142–7, 1992
11. Ackerstaff RGA, Jansen C, Moll FL *et al.*: The significance of microemboli detection by means of transcranial Doppler ultrasonography monitoring in carotid endarterectomy. *J Vasc Surg* **21**: 963–9, 1995

12. Giannoni MF, Sbarigia E, Panica MA *et al.*: Intraoperative transcranial Doppler sonography monitoring during carotid surgery under locoregional anaesthesia. *Eur J Vasc Endovasc Surg* **12**: 407–11, 1996
13. Ennix Jr CL, Lawrie GM, Morris Jr GC: Improved results of carotid endarterectomy in patients with symptomatic coronary artery disease: an analysis of 1546 consecutive carotid operations. *Stroke* **43**: 122–5, 1979
14. Ferguson CC: Carotid endarterectomy: to shunt or not to shunt. *Arch Neurol* **43**: 615–7, 1986
15. Blackshear Jr Wm, Di Carlo SKB, Connar RG: Advantage of continuous electro-encephalografic monitoring during carotid artery surgery. *J Cardiovasc Surg* **27**: 146–53, 1986
16. Fiorani P, Pistolese GR, Ventura M *et al.*: Predictive value of CT scan evaluation in carotid surgery. In: Greenhalgh R (Ed), *Diagnostic Techniques and Assessment Procedures in Vascular Surgery* pp. 151–9. London: Grune & Stratton, 1985
17. Fiorani P, Sbarigia E, Speziale F *et al.*: General anaesthesia versus cervical block and perioperative complications in carotid artery surgery. *Eur J Endovasc Surg* **13**: 37–42, 1997
18. Tanganakul G, Counsell CE, Warlow CP: Local versus general anaesthesia in carotid endarterectomy: a systemic review of the evidence. *Eur J Vasc Endovasc Surg* **13**: 491–9, 1997
19. McCann RL, Clements FM: Silent miocardial ischemia in patients undergoing peripheral vascular surgery: incidence and association with perioperative cardiac morbidity and mortality. *J Vasc Surg* **9**: 583–7, 1989
20. Thomas S, Riles MD, Kopelman I, Imparato AM: Miocardial infarction following carotid endarterectomy: A review of 683 operations. *Surgery* **85**: 249–52, 1979
21. Goldman L: Assessment of the patient with known or suspected ischaemic heart disease for non-cardiac surgery. *Br J Anaesth* **61**: 38–43, 1988
22. Goldman L, Caldera DL, Nussbaum SR *et al.*: Multifactorial index or cardiac risk in non-cardiac surgical procedures. *New Engl J Med* **297**: 845–50, 1977
23. Hertzer NR, Beven EG, Young JR *et al.*: Coronary artery disease in peripheral vascular patients: a classification of 1000 coronary angiograms and results of surgical management. *Ann Surg* **199**: 223–33, 1984
24. Allen BT, Anderson CB, Rubin BG *et al.*: The influence of anesthetic technique on perioperative complication after carotid endarterectomy. *J Vasc Surg* **19**: 834–43, 1994
25. Corson JD, Chang BB, Shah DM *et al.*: The influence of anesthetic choice on carotid endarterectomy outcome. *Arch Surg* **122**: 807–12, 1987
26. Imparato AM, Ramirez A, Riles T, Minzer R: Cerebral protection in carotid surgery. *Arch Surg* **117**: 1073–8, 1982

Editorial comments by C.V. Ruckley

The safer carotid endarterectomy can be made, the greater the patient benefits and the stronger the case for overcoming the apparently continuing reluctance to refer patients with carotid occlusive disease to vascular surgeons. The question is how best to further improve the operation's safety? Is the mode of anaesthesia an important factor in the risk–benefit equation? Is it a controversy which may not be easily resolved. The authors of this chapter align themselves with the proponents of local anaesthesia, rightly pointing out that operating on the awake patient offers the optimal and least expensive means of cerebral monitoring. However, the implication is that the maintenance of cerebral perfusion is a key factor in the avoidance of perioperative neurological complications. In the majority of carotid operations this is not the case. Most complications arise as the result of technical imperfections at the endarterectomy site.

Proponents of general anaesthesia will argue that the best way of minimizing complications is to adopt an unhurried, meticulous technique. Any pressures to alter surgical technique by reducing operating time are to be eschewed. Stress on the part of the patient or the surgeon are better avoided. In this context it is interesting that the patients' blood pressures in the local anaesthesia group in this chapter were significantly higher throughout the operation. It would have been interesting to monitor the surgeon's blood pressure too.

It is my prejudice that the ideal end-product of the operation is a meticulously cleaned endarterectomy site, an accurately secured distal intima and a straight artery which, in most cases, has been widened by patching. The proof of the pudding, incidentally, will lie not merely in surviving the operation but also in the later follow-up. Thus, the anaesthesia debate becomes inextricably entwined with the other time-worn debates: whether or not to shunt, whether or not to patch, whether or not to apply shortening procedures and whether to favour eversion or conventional endarterectomy.

The authors of this chapter focus on the cardiac risk in this population of patients. The small single-centre trial they report showed no difference in cardiac events between the two types of anaesthesia. They advocate a larger trial in which the blood pressure findings and the general cardiovascular outcome events would be an important component.

Uncontrolled series of cases operated under local anaesthesia can carry little weight while an option remains for the surgeon or the patient to choose general anaesthesia. Case selection and case mix will continue to obscure the true picture unless a major trial can be performed. So the question is whether a major trial is worthwhile? Carotid endarterectomy is gradually becoming a safer operation as the effects of audit, trials, specialization, experience, training and consolidation of surgical and anaesthetic techniques all combine to raise standards. At the worst scenario, it is likely that a major trial would produce morbidity and mortality outcomes no worse than those in the European Carotid Surgery Trial (in which the great majority of patients were treated under general anaesthesia and probably substantially better. Thus a very large trial would be required sufficient in size to allow subgroup analysis to identify the impact of risk factors and technical variables which might interact with patient selection and choice of surgical technique and could influence outcome. A follow-up of many years would also be required if the impact of technical variations were also to be given due weight. A trial could only be undertaken after surgeons and anaesthetists who have no experience of local anaesthesia, i.e. the great majority, have worked through a learning curve of the local technique. There is virtue in a surgical team becoming practised in and adhering carefully to a particular technique shown to produce acceptable results. Introducing random variation into theatre routines may not be without risk. If resource for major multicentre trials is in short supply will patients benefit more from trials comparing details of anaesthetic or surgical technique or from trials designed to define the indications for intervention and the respective places for surgery and endovascular technology? The debate will no doubt continue.

Is Carotid Endarterectomy Indicated in the Very Elderly, and If So, Why?

Bertram L. Smith, Jesse E. Thompson, Brandy L. Noel,
C.M. Talkington, Wilson V. Garrett and Gregory J. Pearl

INTRODUCTION

Though efficacy of carotid endarterectomy for the prevention of stroke in patients under 80 years of age has been demonstrated in recent prospective randomized trials, this efficacy has not been proven in patients over 80. The mean age of patients in the North American Symptomatic Carotid Endarterectomy Trial (NASCET) was 64 years, and no patient over the age of 79 was included.[1] In the Asymptomatic Carotid Atherosclerosis Study (ACAS) no patient over 79 was admitted.[2] Reports of the other randomized trials did not discuss the matter of age as a factor in selection of patients for entry into the trials.[3-5] In an article entitled 'Carotid Endarterectomy: Practice Guidelines,' from the Joint Council of the Society for Vascular Surgery (SVS) and the North American Chapter of the International Society for Cardiovascular Surgery (ISCVS), the issue of age is not mentioned.[6] Similarly, in an article dealing with risk factors associated with carotid endarterectomy age is not considered.[7]

DEMOGRAPHICS

The population is aging. The number of Americans over 65 will double to 22% of the population by the year 2030. It is projected that 40% of the population will survive to the age of 80. In the USA, the average life expectancy for white women at age 80 is 9.1 years; for white men it is 7.0 years. In the UK, life expectancy is 8.1 years for women and 6.2 years for men.[8-12]

The incidence of cerebrovascular disease correlates closely with age. The overall incidence of stroke per 100 000 population is 262 for persons between the ages of 55 and 64, 582 for those aged 65 to 74, 1382 for persons aged 75 to 84, and a remarkable 1824 for persons over the age of 85. Approximately 60% of these strokes are the result of carotid bifurcation atherosclerosis, a disease well treated by carotid endarterectomy.[13]

The impact of stroke increases with age. While approximately 65% of patients under 75 years of age survive an initial stroke and are alive 6 months later, only 52% of patients between 75 and 84, and only 33% of patients over 85 survive to 6 months. Though survival rates are less, the large number of patients in the 80+ age group makes the financial burden, now estimated at three billion dollars annually in the USA, an even more significant health care expenditure in the future.[10,11,13]

Elderly patients constitute the fastest growing group in the population. It is imperative that age be considered as a factor in the selection of patients for carotid endarterectomy.

Since the publication of the results of the various randomized trials for both symptomatic and asymptomatic patients, the incidence of carotid endarterectomy is on the increase, especially among patients with tight, stenotic lesions who are asymptomatic. Many of these fall in the older age group, and this situation must be taken into account if these patients are to be treated properly and strokes are to be prevented.[11]

TREATMENT ALTERNATIVES

Treatment alternatives for patients with cerebrovascular insufficiency syndromes due to extracranial carotid occlusive disease at present include observation, anti-platelet therapy, anticoagulants, and carotid endarterectomy. Whether balloon angioplasty with or without stenting will become a viable alternative remains to be seen. We have chosen carotid endarterectomy as the preferred method of treatment in selected elderly patients. Carotid endarterectomy has proven efficacy in the prevention of stroke in patients under 80 years of age. It should be equally efficacious in patients over 80 if those octogenarians are chosen carefully.

In the past, several investigations have challenged the rationale for carotid endarterectomy in elderly patients on the basis of perceived increased operative risk. As an example, in a review of Medicare files in Massachusetts in 1984 for patients over the age of 80 undergoing carotid endarterectomy, the 30-day mortality was 4.7%.[14] In 1981, the Rand Corporation reviewed the performance of carotid endarterectomy on 1302 Medicare patients in three geographic areas and reported a 6.4% perioperative stroke rate and a 3.4% mortality. Both studies were from multiple centres, and in many hospitals the volume of procedures per surgeon was quite low.[11] A number of studies have appeared, however, that support the contention that advanced age alone is not necessarily a contraindication to carotid endarterectomy.[10,11,15,16]

PERSONAL EXPERIENCE

In order to elucidate further the rationale for carotid endarterectomy in octogenarian patients, we have recently reviewed in retrospect a series of patients in this age group who had carotid endarterectomy performed between 1 January and 31 December, 1996. In all, 43 patients underwent 51 carotid endarterectomies. Eight patients had bilateral procedures. Ages ranged from 80 to 94 years with an average of 84.3 years. Five patients were aged 90 years or older; 25 patients were male, and 18 were female.

Indications for operation included prior stroke in one patient (2.3%), recent stroke in one (2.3%), amaurosis fugax in six (14%), transient ischaemic attacks in 13 (30%), global ischaemia in three (7%), and asymptomatic critical stenosis in 19 (44%) patients.

Co-morbid conditions were consistent with this elderly group and included hypertension, diabetes mellitus, significant coronary artery and cardiac valvular disease, tobacco usage, carcinoma and hyperplasia of the prostate, chronic obstructive pulmonary disease, degenerative joint disease, carcinoma of the colon, previous radical neck dissection, peripheral vascular disease, hypothyroidism, remote abdominal aneurysm repair, remote deep venous thrombosis, and asthma. All of these co-morbid conditions were treated carefully and were under control prior to consideration for carotid endarterectomy.

In most cases angiography was performed on an outpatient basis the day prior to operation. The majority of patients had conventional digital subtraction angiogram studies. Others had duplex ultrasound combined with magnetic resonance angiography, while a few were operated upon following only duplex ultrasound. All stenoses were severe and were 70% or greater (Fig. 1) by NASCET criteria. In symptomatic patients with ulcerated plaques, lesser degrees of stenosis were accepted as an indication for operation.

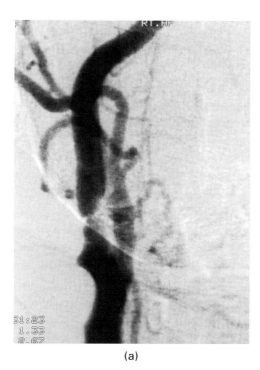
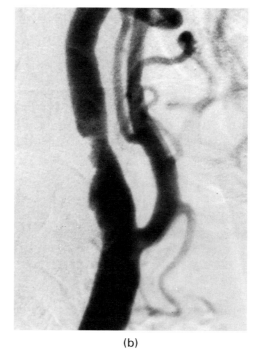

(a)   (b)

Fig. 1. Right anteroposterior (a) and lateral (b) carotid arteriogram of a 94-year-old female with prior aortic aneurysm repair and a mild right hemispheric stroke with minimal residual deficit in the left arm, showing a tight internal carotid stenosis. She was fully active and asymptomatic 18 months following right carotid endarterectomy.

TECHNIQUE

Operations were performed under general anaesthesia, using inlying shunts and arteriotomy closure with Dacron or polytetrafluoroethylene patch grafts in most cases. Heparin was given routinely and aspirin was administered preoperatively and postoperatively.

The patients were ambulated on the first postoperative day, and most were discharged on the third postoperative day. The average length of stay was 3.9 days.

RESULTS

No perioperative (30 days) death, strokes, or transient ischaemic attacks occurred in this series. Five postoperative complications occurred including pulmonary oedema in two, bradyarrhythmia in one, and palsy of the mandibular branch of the facial nerve in two patients. There were no perioperative or postoperative myocardial infarctions.

FOLLOW-UP STUDIES

Follow-up in this group of 43 patients has been 100% and ranges from 8 to 21 months, with an average of 13.2 months. Four deaths have occurred at intervals of 1 month, 13 months, 14 months, and 17 months following operation. Three deaths were cardiac in origin, and one was secondary to renal failure and congestive heart failure. One patient suffered a stroke 13 months postoperatively, but survived.

In a related study we compared the time of resumption of normal daily activities following carotid endarterectomy in 56 octogenarians with that of 50 younger patients (mean age 68): 78% of the octogenarians reported resumption within 3 weeks while 85% of the younger patients reported resuming their prior activities within 3 weeks.

DISCUSSION

Recent studies, both short-term and long-term, support the contention that advanced age alone is not a contraindication to carotid endarterectomy. No prospective randomized trials have been carried out to prove this contention. It is likely that such trials will not be done in view of the reports of previous trials and the clinical studies which have appeared dealing with elderly patients.

In a recent review of eight series in the literature, Perler found the operative mortality from carotid endarterectomy in patients over the age of 75 to range from 0% to 3.7% with an average of 1.75%. The perioperative stroke rate varied from 0% to 5.6% with an average 3.2%.[10] In our own series of 51 operations, the operative mortality was zero, and there were no strokes associated with operation.

In a report by Rosenthal *et al.* on a series of 90 operations, the perioperative mortality was 2.2%, and the operation-related stroke rate was 5.6%. During an 8-year follow-up, the incidence of late stroke in these patients was 2%. In a comparable series without carotid endarterectomy, the late stroke rate was 17%.[17]

In a recent study from the Cleveland Clinic of 173 carotid endarterectomies in patients over the age of 80, the perioperative stroke and transient ischaemic attack rate was 4%, and the operative mortality was 0.6%. Moreover, with follow-up of 98% at a mean interval of 2.7 years, the estimated 5-year survival was 46%, and the 5-year freedom-from-stroke rate was 42%.[18]

Perler has reported a series of patients from the Johns Hopkins Hospital. Over a 12-year period, 63 carotid endarterectomies on 59 octogenarians were carried out. There were no operative deaths and only three (4.8%) perioperative strokes. These patients were followed from 1 to 122 months (mean 27.4 months). During follow-up there were no fatal strokes; six deaths occurred, yielding a statistical survival of 80% for 5 years and 52% at 10 years. Two non-fatal strokes occurred at 23 and 50 months, yielding a stroke-free survival of 85% at 4 years and 68% at 5 years follow-up.[10] In our series of carotid endarterectomy patients with an average age of 65 years, 5-year survival was 71%.[19]

The number of elderly patients presenting for treatment of cerebrovascular disease is increasing.[11] The incidence of stroke increases with advancing age, and the impact on morbidity and death is devastating. Carotid endarterectomy should *a priori* improve the outlook for appropriate patients with extracranial cerebrovascular disease. The results of our study presented here and data from the literature tend to bear out the contention that there is a place for carotid endarterectomy in carefully selected elderly patients over the age of 80 years. Operative mortality is very low, comparable with that in younger patients. The perioperative stroke rate is also low and acceptable. Perioperative complications are reasonable for this group of patients with multiple co-morbid conditions. The length of stay, surprisingly, is about 3 days, about the same as that for younger patients. The time for resumption of prior normal activities of daily living is somewhat longer than that for the younger patients, but most patients resume their activities within 3 weeks. If the patients are chosen carefully, short-term death from other causes is quite low. The incidence of long-term strokes appears to be considerably lower than that of comparable patients not having endarterectomy but no prospective randomized data are available to document this claim. In the largest series of patients reported to date, the 5-year survival was 46% and the 5-year freedom-from-stroke or death was 42%.[18] Long-term deaths are largely cardiovascular with a low incidence of death from stroke. The economic consequences of reduction in stroke incidence can be enormous.

CONCLUSION

On the basis of non-randomized clinical reports, the indications for carotid endarterectomy are the same for elderly patients over 80 years of age as for younger patients. One must be judicious in selection of patients for operation, co-morbid conditions must be carefully treated and controlled, and the operation must be skillfully performed by experienced operators. Under these circumstances, operation appears justifiable; chronological age alone is not necessarily a contra-indication for carotid endarterectomy. The physiological age and clinical status of the patient are the important factors. Operation can be carried out safely in these elderly patients.

REFERENCES

1. North American Symptomatic Carotid Endarterectomy Trial Collaborators: Beneficial effect of carotid endarterectomy in symptomatic patients with high grade carotid stenosis. *New Engl J Med* **325**: 445–3, 1991
2. Executive Committee for the Asymptomatic Carotid Atherosclerosis Study: Endarterectomy for asymptomatic carotid stenosis. *J Am Med Ass* **273**: 1421–8, 1995
3. European Carotid Surgery Trialists' Group: MRC European Carotid Surgery Trial: Interim results for symptomatic patients with severe (70–99%) or with mild (0–29%) carotid stenosis. *Lancet* **337**: 1235–43, 1991
4. Mayberg MR, Wilson SE, Yatsu F and the Veterans Affairs Cooperative Program 309 Trialist Group: Carotid endarterectomy and prevention of cerebral ischemia in symptomatic carotid stenosis. *J Am Med Ass* **266**: 3289–94, 1991
5. Hobson RW, Weiss DG, Fields WS *et al.*: and the Veterans Affairs Cooperative Study Group: Efficacy of carotid endarterectomy for asymptomatic carotid stenosis. *New Engl J Med* **328**: 221–7, 1993
6. Moore WS, Mohr JP, Najafi H *et al.*: Carotid endarterectomy: Practice guidelines. *J Vasc Surg* **15**: 469–79, 1992
7. Beebe HG, Clagett GP, DeWeese JA *et al.*: Assessing risk associated with carotid endarterectomy. *Circulation* **79**: 472–3, 1989
8. Hamilton J O'C, Freundlich N: Can we end heart disease? *Business Week* 106–112: September 22, 1997
9. Treiman RL, Levine VA, Cohen JL *et al.*: Aneurysmectomy in the octogenerian: A study of morbidity and quality of survival. *Am J Surg* **144**: 194–7, 1982
10. Perler BA: Carotid endarterectomy in symptomatic and asymptomatic patients over 80 years of age: Indications and results. In Veith FJ (Ed), *Current Critical Problems in Vascular Surgery* Vol 7, pp. 312–7. St Louis: Quality Medical Publishing Inc., 1996
11. Perler BA: The impact of advanced age on the results of carotid endarterectomy: An outcome analysis. *J Am Coll Surg* **183**: 559–64, 1996
12. Manton KG, Vaupel JW: Survival after the age of 80 in the United States, Sweden, France, England and Japan. *New Engl J Med* **333**: 1232–5, 1995
13. Robins M, Baum HM: Natural survey of stroke incidence. *Stroke* **121**(Suppl 1): 45–47, 1981
14. Fisher ES, Malenka DJ, Solomon NA *et al.*: Risk of carotid endarterectomy in the elderly. *Am J Publ Hlth* **79**: 1617–20, 1989
15. Thompson JE, Austin DJ, Patman RD: Carotid endarterectomy for cerebrovascular insufficiency: Long-term results in 592 patients followed up to thirteen years. *Ann Surg* **172**: 663–79, 1970
16. Schultz RD, Sterpetti AV, Feldhaus RJ: Carotid endarterectomy in octogenarians and nonagenarians. *Surg Gynec Obst* **166**: 245–51, 1988
17. Rosenthal D, Ruddemann RH, Jones DH *et al.*: Carotid endarterectomy in the octogenarian: Is it appropriate? *J Vasc Surg* **3**: 782–7, 1986
18. O'Hara PJ, Hertzer NR, Mascha EJ *et al.*: Carotid endarterectomy in octogenarians: Early and late results. *J Vasc Surg* in press, 1998
19. Thompson JE: Carotid Surgery: The Past is Prologue. The John Homans Lecture. *J Vasc Surg* **25**: 131–40, 1997

Editorial comments by R.M. Greenhalgh

These authors clearly believe that carotid surgery is indicated in octogenarians. As the authors say, their views are on the basis of non-randomized clinical reports and their own retrospective audited data of a remarkable experience of 43 patients undergoing 51 carotid endarterectomies in a 12-month period. The results are outstanding. It would be difficult to imagine better results in any age group than these. The authors clearly feel so confident in the outcome and expect such low morbidity that they are able to offer this operation for asymptomatic critical stenosis. Indeed 44% of the series reported here are for asymptomatic disease. The authors have not pointed to any future trials which they would care to see. This implies that with such results, they feel that no further proof is necessary. The problem is perhaps that their results need not be representative of a wider population outcome.

What Are the Indications for Operation in Asymptomatic Carotid Stenosis?

Alison W. Halliday

INTRODUCTION

Stroke is the third commonest cause of death in Western societies. The major risk factors for stroke and myocardial infarction are smoking, hypertension, excessive alcohol consumption, heart disease, lack of exercise and diabetes. Risk factors which distinguish stroke from heart disease include a past history of transient ischaemic attack or stroke and the presence of carotid artery stenosis. As death from heart disease is much more common than stroke in patients with asymptomatic carotid stenosis, detection and effective treatment of coronary disease and non-rheumatic atrial fibrillation are vitally important.[1,2] Operation for carotid stenosis is a decision only to be taken after these measures have been completed.

IDENTIFYING PATIENTS WITH ASYMPTOMATIC CAROTID STENOSIS

Screening populations for carotid stenosis is not thought to be cost-effective as most stenoses detected are too mild to consider for operation.[3] The following groups continue to be screened by duplex ultrasound:

Patients with bruit

The Framingham study[4] showed that 7% of 65–79 year-olds had carotid bruits and that their stroke rate was more than twice that expected for age and sex. The bruit was regarded as a non-specific sign of advanced atherosclerotic disease rather than an indicator of focal stenosis preceding cerebral infarction. Ten years later in 1991, Norris et al.[5] found in follow-up of a population with bruits that a >75% carotid stenosis was associated with a stroke rate of 2.5% per year (ipsilateral in 75%).

Peripheral vascular disease

Peripheral vascular disease is a rich source of patients with asymptomatic carotid stenosis. Ahn[6] found that 45% of these patients over 68 years had more than 50% carotid stenosis on routine duplex scanning. An identical incidence was reported in 1996 by Marek et al.[7] who associated increasing likelihood of stenosis with decreasing ankle brachial pressure index. In considering which screened patients might be candidates for surgery, Alexandrova et al[8] found that 25% of the peripheral vascular disease group had stenoses of 60–99%, and 80% had no carotid symptoms.

Preoperative vascular procedures

Other vascular procedures (particularly coronary bypass grafting) may, if patients have carotid stenosis, be associated with increased stroke risk. Gerraty et al.[9] recently reported a prospective clinical and duplex ultrasound study of major coronary or vascular operations in which there was a moratorium on carotid endarterectomy for asymptomatic carotid stenosis. Fourteen percent of patients had >50% and 7% had >80% stenosis. No ipsilateral strokes occurred. In 1995 Schwarz et al.[10] studied a population of 582 patients undergoing cardiopulmonary bypass. Twenty-two percent had >50% stenosis, and 12% had >80% stenosis or occlusion. He found that unilateral >80% or bilateral 50–99% stenosis or occlusion was associated with a risk of hemispheric stroke of 3.8–5.3%.

Patients who have had carotid surgery for symptoms

Patients who have had carotid surgery for symptoms are always 'screened' at least once for contralateral disease. In the European Carotid Surgery Trial (ECST), 2295 patients were followed for a mean period of 4.5 years. Again there was an increased prevalence of heart disease and peripheral vascular disease with increasing contralateral asymptomatic carotid stenosis, but only 5.5% patients had 70–99% stenosis. The stroke rate in these patients was 5.7% at 3 years and the authors concluded that this group had too few outcome events to justify surgery outside the confines of a randomized controlled trial.[11] About 5–10% of patients in the last three groups will have severe (>75–80%) carotid stenosis; this is the patient population which is usually considered for surgery.

It seems unlikely that, in North America, screening will be funded by Medicare, as federal legislation has banned screening except for specifically designated tests such as cervical smears or mammography. In Canada, the Canadian Stroke Consortium[12] also recommended that screening should not be routine for asymptomatic carotid stenosis, on the basis that there was insufficient evidence that prophylactic carotid endarterectomy was an effective means of stroke prevention.

AUTHOR'S CHOICE

I prefer to use conventional carotid endarterectomy (rather than the eversion technique), selective shunting and patching with intraoperative transcranial Doppler monitoring and completion duplex scanning, whilst the patient receives general anaesthesia.

However, at present I would not consider that surgery should be performed on patients with asymptomatic carotid stenosis unless:

(a) there is a strong likelihood that the patient is substantially at risk from stroke;
(b) the patient is fully aware of the risks of operation;
(c) the patient has been evaluated for cardiac disease (including exercise testing, and cardiac echo) and has been fully and appropriately treated for other risk factors such as diabetes and hypercholesteraemia.

If all these criteria are met, patients should be considered for surgery only within the context of the ongoing Asymptomatic Carotid Surgery Trial[13] (see below).

EVIDENCE SUPPORTING AUTHOR'S CHOICE

There is now good evidence to support the view that screening patients with bruits is neither cost effective for detection of disease or, more importantly, for prevention of stroke.

However, once tight stenosis has been detected, patients and physicians may feel bound to treat it as the fear of stroke may, although small, be difficult to live with. Often other factors will sway decisions towards surgery. Extra 'risk' factors such as contralateral occlusion and CT scan infarction are commonly cited as reasons to operate. In 1992 Norris and Zhu[14] found that CT scan infarction was commoner in tight (>75%) asymptomatic carotid stenosis with two-thirds of lesions ipsilateral to the stenosis. However the following year Brott et al.[15], reported some baseline data from the ongoing Asymptomatic Carotid Atherosclerosis Study (ACAS). He found that for completely asymptomatic patients with more than 80% stenosis (one-quarter of the study group), and also the smaller groups with bilateral >80% stenosis or contralateral occlusion, there was no association between CT infarction and category of stenosis.

Describing an association between tight asymptomatic carotid stenosis and contralateral occlusion Faught et al.[16] reported that stenosis of 80–99% contralateral to an occlusion was associated with future stroke and advocated surgery for this group. Recent American Heart Association Guidelines for carotid endarterectomy[17] list as an acceptable (though not proven) indication for surgery, ipsilateral >75% stenosis with contralateral 75–100% disease. These guidelines were modified when the results of the ACAS became available that year.

TRIALS SUPPORTING THE AUTHOR'S VIEW

Several trials have now been completed and to date only one, the ACAS trial[18] has shown that carotid endarterectomy may, under certain circumstances reduce the risk of subsequent stroke, but not disabling stroke. A total of 1662 patients were randomized to receive appropriate medical treatment (100%) and operation (50%). Operation was carried out by a carefully selected group of surgeons who had submitted track records of their previous 50 operations for carotid endarterectomy. They had an overall 30-day mortality and morbidity (death and stroke) rate of less than 3%. Patients were entered by using ultrasound screening, but only the surgical group were required to have preoperative angiography. After a mean follow-up of 2.7 years, ACAS reported that there was a positive result favouring surgery in men.

The estimated 5-year differences between surgical and medical groups suggested that, providing the beneficial trend continued, surgery would reduce the stroke rate in this group from 2% to 1% per year. Operation results were dependent on surgeons having less than 3% morbidity and mortality and on careful patient selection (careful screening for cardiac disease was mandatory). Despite these stringent precautions, there was no significant reduction in disabling stroke. Although surgical patients all had angiograms (1.2% suffered a stroke as a result of this investigation) there were not enough events in the study group to subdivide stenosis to identify a group with greater benefit.

The consequence of ACAS has been that surgery is now 'indicated' in millions of patients in North America and Europe, but the cost is enormous and the benefit very small.[19] The principal investigators of both North American (NASCET) and ECST symptomatic trials delivered strong criticisms of ACAS.[20,21] These were based on the large populations that would need operation to achieve small, and doubtful benefit. Screening has been discounted as too expensive, surgeons do not all have less than 3% complication rate for carotid endarterectomy in asymptomatic carotid stenosis, and probably the biggest disappointment of all, angiography is too dangerous to use for routine measurement of asymptomatic carotid stenosis.

Following ACAS, routine angiography is now much less common and there is considerable confusion about the assessment of stenosis by duplex scanning alone. The scanners used to select patients for ACAS have largely been superceded by more sophisticated equipment, but the criteria for selecting appropriate patients are very varied and, because of operator-dependence, inaccuracies may occur.

MEASURING ASYMPTOMATIC CAROTID STENOSIS WITH DUPLEX ALONE

There are many criteria for estimating carotid stenosis and none has been universally adopted. Huge and important differences are apparently ignored as one laboratory may report an area reduction, while others report diameter (closer to angiographic) stenosis. Whilst angiography was confusing when ECST and NASCET reported differing methods of measurement and apparently different surgical results, these were resolved when an equivalent stenosis of 70% in NASCET and 82% in ECST were shown to yield the same surgical benefit.

The measurements used in ACAS have led to much confusion. Ultrasound peak systolic (and sometimes end diastolic) frequency was used to recruit patients who, if treated surgically, all had angiograms. Thus although the American Heart Association guidelines now apparently recommend surgery for symptomatic 70–99% and, paradoxically, for asymptomatic carotid stenosis of 60–99%, the measurement techniques are different. In ACAS, 60% is meant to reflect a conversion to diameter stenosis by a comparison of peak frequencies on Doppler with arteriographic diameter measurements. These measurements were validated within ACAS. This means that, unless a laboratory continues to update its correlation of angiography with ultrasound, there will be no up-to-date method of ensuring that future surgical patients fall within ACAS guidelines.

For the future it will be necessary to adopt a much more uniform and stringent set of ultrasound guidelines, with interobserver agreement and duplex machine testing which assures clinicians that patients really have tight asymptomatic carotid stenosis. Angiography, computed tomography or magnetic resonance will be necessary in some cases where duplex cannot be relied on.

FUTURE TRIALS NEEDED

There are two patient areas which require clarification; patients with asymptomatic carotid stenosis alone , and patients with asymptomatic carotid stenosis who need to undergo major surgery. The second group, in particular patients requiring coronary bypass grafting face potential stroke risks from neck lines, hypotension, aortic cross-clamping, bypass tubing insertion and use of an extracorporeal circulation. The stroke risk from heart bypass is usually estimated as 1–2% but may be much higher in patients with asymptomatic carotid stenosis. Although a prospective randomized trial in this area would be of great importance, none has yet been reported.

Table 1. Baseline entry characteristics of patients in the ongoing ACST (October 1997)

Total patients	1665
Percent males	67.7%
Percent females	32.3%
Age range	41–89 years (mean 67.7)
Number of patients randomized to surgery and BMT	833
Number of patients randomized to BMT only	832
Number of months trial has been running	54
Mean period between randomization and surgery	42 days
Total number of patient-years of follow-up	2256
Mean follow-up per patient	1.36 years
Percentage that are diabetic	19.6%
Percentage with definite coronary artery disease	33.8%
Mean plasma cholesterol	6.09 mmol/l
Percentage taking lipid-lowering therapy	17.9%
Percentage taking antihypertensive therapy	61.1%
Percentage taking antiplatelet and/or anticoagulant therapy	93.2%
Percentage having a previous contralateral CEA	25.1%
Percentage of those having a contralateral CEA who had contralateral symptoms	65.6%
Percentage with contralateral occlusion	8%
Median ipsilateral stenosis	80%
Number answering on echolucent plaque	1024
Percentage of respondents with ipsilateral echolucent plaque	48.4%
Number who had a CT scan	1129
Percentage of respondents with an ipsilateral CT infarct only	6.9%
Percentage of respondents with a contralateral CT infarct only	12.9%
Percentage of respondents with a bilateral CT infarct	6.4%

BMT: best medical treatment
CEA: carotid endarterectomy

Table 2. The CONSORT (Consolidated Standards of Reporting Trials) statement

Heading	Subheading	Descriptor
Title		Identify the study as a randomized trial
Abstract		Use a structured format
Introduction		State prospectively defined hypothesis, clinical objectives, and planned subgroup or covariate analyses
Methods	Protocol	Describe
		Planned study population, together with inclusion or exclusion criteria
		Planned interventions and their timing
		Primary and secondary outcome measure(s) and the minimum important difference(s), and indicate how the target sample size was projected
		Rationale and methods for statistical analyses, detailing main comparative analyses and whether they were completed on an intention to treat basis
		Prospectively defined stopping rules (if warranted)
	Assignment	Describe
		Unit of randomization (for example, individual, cluster, geographical)
		Method used to generate the allocation schedule
		Method of allocation concealment and timing of assignment
		Method to separate the generator from the executor of assignment
	Masking (blinding)	Describe
		Mechanism (for example, capsules, tablets)
		Similarity of treatment characteristics (for example, appearance, taste)
		Allocation schedule control (location of code during trial and when broken)
		Evidence for successful blinding among participants, person during intervention, outcome assessors and data analysts
Results	Participant flow and follow-up	Provide a trial profile (a) summarizing participant flow, numbers and timing of randomization assignment, interventions, and measurements on each randomized group
	Analysis	State estimated effect of intervention on primary and secondary outcome measures, including a point estimate and measure of precision (confidence interval)
		State results in absolute numbers when feasible (for example, 10 of 20 not 50 per cent)
		Present summary data and appropriate descriptive and interferential statistics in sufficient detail to permit alternative analyses and replication
		Describe prognostic variables by treatment group and any attempt to adjust for them
		Describe protocol deviations from the study as planned, together with any reasons
Discussion		State specific interpretation of study findings, including sources of bias and imprecision (internal validity) and discussion of external validity, including appropriate quantitative measures when possible
		State general interpretation of the data in light of the totality of the available evidence

One large ongoing trial is still recruiting patients with asymptomatic carotid stenosis alone.

The Asymptomatic Carotid Surgery Trial is entering patients prospectively for randomization to medical treatment (100%) and carotid endarterectomy (50%). Surgeons and neurologists, as in ECST, must be substantially uncertain as to whether the patient will benefit from operation, and the patient must be fit for and willing to undergo surgery if indicated. The details of this trial have been described in a previous volume in this series.[22] Patients may be entered after ultrasound alone, and an assessment of plaque composition. This risk factor has not been studied in a randomized controlled trial and the ACST may help to determine whether soft, or heterogeneous plaques with more than 25% echolucent material may be important in determining stroke risk.

To date (October 1997) the ACST has recruited 1700 patients and has over 100 collaborators from 25 countries, making it the largest trial of asymptomatic carotid stenosis in the world. The patient characteristics are shown in Table 1. Mean follow-up per patient is, however, just over 16 months. The last data monitoring committee report urged that recruiting continue, and that collaborators should randomize patients with tight stenosis. The trial end-points, like ACAS, are death and stroke, but it is now vitally important to continue to recruit to ACST as, unless there is a clear indication that disabling stroke is preventable by carotid endarterectomy, operation will continue to be performed with little measurable patient benefit

In a series of recent articles on surgical research, the standards for reporting clinical trials have been idealized into the CONSORT (Consolidated Standards of Reporting Trials) statement[23] (Table 2). Although carotid surgical trials have been remarkably successful in changing clinical practice, they have also led to statistically significant confusion. Even though they have conformed to most of the CONSORT requirements, the ACAS fell foul of a common miscalculation; their carefully planned numbers and power calculations (helpful and advocated by CONSORT) had failed to provide a clinically meaningful result. Perhaps trials should only be stopped when an outside independent group of clinical assessors agree that the result has been achieved or that, despite statistical significance, that a result cannot be obtained. For asymptomatic carotid stenosis, the ongoing ACST may be the last chance of obtaining an affordable answer to the question 'what are the indications for operating on asymptomatic carotid stenosis?'. It is vitally important that more patients with tight stenosis are entered to obtain that answer.

REFERENCES

1. Love BB, Grover-McKay M, Biller J *et al*.: Coronary artery disease and cardiac events with asymptomatic and symptomatic cerebrovascular disease. *Stroke* **23**: 939–45, 1992
2. Chimowitz MI, Weiss DG, Cohen SL *et al*.: Veterans Affairs Cooperative Study Group 167. Cardiac prognosis of patients with carotid stenosis and no history of coronary artery disease. *Stroke* **25**: 759–65, 1994
3. Lee TT, Solomon NA, Heidenreich PA *et al*.: Cost-effectiveness of screening for carotid stenosis in asymptomatic patients. *Ann Int Med* **126**: 337–46, 1997
4. Wolf, PA, Kannel WB, Sorlie P, McNamara P: Asymptomatic carotid bruit and risk of stroke. *J Am Med Ass* **245**: 1442–5, 1981
5. Norris JW, Zhu CZ, Bornstein NM, Chambers BR: Vascular risks of asymptomatic carotid stenosis. *Stroke* **22**: 1485–90, 1991

6. Ahn SS, Baker JD, Walden K, Moore WS: Which asymptomatic patients should undergo routine screening duplex scan? *Am J Surg*; **162**: 180–4, 1991
7. Marek J, Mills, JL, Harvich J *et al*.: Utility of routine duplex screening in patients who have claudication. *J Vasc Surg* **24**: 572–9, 1996
8. Alexandrova NA, Gibson WC, Norris JW, Maggisano R: Carotid artery stenosis in peripheral vascular disease. *J Vasc Surg* **23**: 645–9, 1996
9. Gerraty RP, Gates PC, Doyle JC: Carotid stenosis and perioperative stroke risk in symptomatic and asymptomatic patients undergoing vascular or coronary surgery. *Stroke* **24**: 1115–8, 1993
10. Schwarz LB, Bridgeman AH, Kieffer RW: Asymptomatic carotid artery stenosis and stroke in patients undergoing cardiopulmonary bypass. *J Vasc Surg* **21**: 146–53, 1995
11. The European Carotid Surgery Triallists Collaborative Group: Risk of stroke in the distribution of an asymptomatic carotid artery. *Lancet* **35**: 209–12, 1995
12. Perry JR, Szalai JP, Norris JW for the Canadian Stroke Consortium: Consensus against both endarterectomy and routine screening for asymptomatic carotid artery stenosis. *Arch Neurol* **54**: 25–8, 1997
13. Halliday AW: The asymptomatic carotid surgery trial (ACST); rationale and design. *Eur J Vasc Surg* **8**: 703–10, 1994
14. Norris JW, Zhu CZ: Silent stroke and carotid stenosis. *Stroke* **23**: 483–5, 1992
15. Brott T, Tomsick T, Feinberg W *et al*.: Baseline silent cerebral infarction in the Asymptomatic Carotid Atherosclerosis Study. *Stroke* **25**: 1122–1129, 1994
16. Faught WE, vab Bemmelen PS, Mattos MA *et al*.: Presentation and natural history of internal carotid occlusion. *J Vasc Surg* **18**: 512–24, 1993
17. Moore WS, Barnett HJM, Beebe HG *et al*.: Guidelines for carotid endarterectomy. A multidisciplinary consensus statement from the Ad Hoc Committee, American Heart Association. *Circulation* **91**: 566–79, 1995
18. Executive committee for the Asymptomatic Carotid Atherosclerosis Study: Endarterectomy for asymptomatic carotid artery stenosis. *J Am Med Ass* **273**: 1421–8, 1995
19. Cronenwett JL, Birkmeyer JD, Nackman GB *et al*.: Cost-effectiveness of carotid endarterectomy in asymptomatic patients. *J Vasc Surg* **25**: 298–309, 1997
20. Barnett HJ, Meldrum HE, Eliasziw M: The dilemna of surgical treatment for patients with asymptomatic carotid disease. *Ann Int Med* **123**: 723–5, 1995
21. Warlow CP: Endarterectomy for asymptomatic carotid stenosis? *Lancet* **345**: 1254–5, 1995
22. Halliday AW. Has the definitive study been done to determine the place of carotid endarterectomy in the asymptomatic patient? The ACST Study. In: Greenhalgh RM, Fowkes FGR (Eds), *Trials and Tribulations in Vascular Surgery*, pp. 65–76. London: WB Saunders, 1996
23. Begg C, Cho M, Eastwood S *et al*.: Improving the quality of reporting of randomised controlled trials. The CONSORT statement. *J Am Med Ass* **276**: 637–9, 1996

Editorial comments by R.M. Greenhalgh

The author has answered the question in a number of ways. The review of the ACAS Trial is interpreted by the author as showing that carotid endarterectomy may reduce the risk of subsequent stroke but not disabling stroke. Nevertheless it is plain that the author's personal view is that she is unsure and wishes to know the answer to this question and the best way to do so is to encourage recruitment into the present ACST Trial. In short the author has given us her preference and what trials support her view and she is to be commended for conducting the very future trial which could settle the matter once and for all.

When is Cerebral Hypoperfusion an Indication for Carotid Surgery?

Torben V. Schroeder

INTRODUCTION

Transient ischaemic attacks and strokes in patients with carotid artery disease are generally considered to be due to embolism from thrombogenic atheromatous plaques at the origin of the internal carotid artery (ICA). However, in a subset of patients, symptoms may be caused by haemodynamic failure. The existence of an ischaemic penumbra, i.e. a Sleeping Beauty, in which cerebral blood flow is insufficient for normal tissue function, but sufficient for cellular viability, has been assigned varying importance over the years.[1] Evidence in favour of this concept is accumulating, but also indicates this to be an infrequent occurrence.[2,3]

HYPOPERFUSION AND CEREBRAL HAEMODYNAMIC FAILURE

The pathophysiological events behind haemodynamic failure are initiated by a reduced perfusion pressure. By dilating the resistance vessels cerebral perfusion may be maintained at an unchanged level, the process known as autoregulation.[4] At a certain level vasodilatation may no longer compensate for the decreasing perfusion pressure, and cerebral blood flow falls. In cases of focal reduction of perfusion pressure, flow may even decrease due to a steal phenomenon.[5] Also a reduction of systemic blood pressure, that normally has no effect on cerebral perfusion, may further reduce cerebral blood flow. However, metabolism may still be maintained below the lower limit of autoregulation by compensatory increase of oxygen extraction fraction. If perfusion pressure continues to fall the energy demands of the brain may no longer be fulfilled and clinical evidence of dysfunction will occur. Unless the circulation is restored rapidly, permanent tissue damage may result.

An arterial stenosis is considered to be of haemodynamical significance when the diameter reduction exceeds 50%, corresponding to a 75% reduction of lumen. While a stenosis greater than 50% is necessary for haemodynamic compromise, it is not sufficient. The decreased flow contributed through the one carotid artery may be fully compensated by collateral circulatory pathways. This is illustrated in Fig. 1 displaying the intraoperatively measured ratio of the internal to common carotid artery (CCA) pressures, (cerebral perfusion pressure index) related to the degree of carotid artery stenosis.[6] Although a significant inverse relationship was found between perfusion pressure and degree of stenosis, a considerable scatter was also noted. Thus, some 90% of stenoses were accompanied by a major pressure drop across the stenosis, while in others hardly any pressure gradient was detected. A

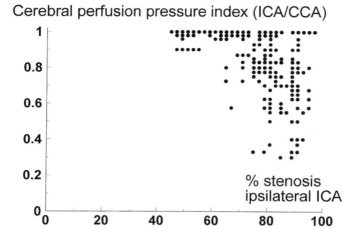

Fig. 1. Internal to common carotid artery pressure ratio, measured before cross-clamping, related to degree of ipsilateral internal carotid artery stenosis in 153 patients undergoing carotid endarterectomy. (Data reproduced from Nielsen *et al.*[6])

reduction of perfusion pressure of 25 and 50% was observed in 55 (47%) and 12 (10%) patients with 70–99% stenoses, respectively, compared with two (6%) and zero patients with 30–69% stenosis (p<0.0005). These figures are somewhat higher than previously published data from our institution in which 17% of patients presented with a 25% reduction of perfusion pressure.[7] This change probably reflects today's consensus of only operating on severe stenoses, as opposed to the situation before 1991 when stenosis criteria were less strict.[8,9] A 50% reduction of cerebral perfusion pressure may be expected in approximately 10% of those patients considered candidates for carotid surgery by today's standard, i.e. more than 70% stenosis. This figure is similar to the generally held view, that symptoms are caused by hypoperfusion in 10–15% of patients.

NATURAL HISTORY OF CEREBRAL HYPOPERFUSION

A state of hypoperfusion will manifest itself as a decreased vasoreactivity or an increased sensitivity to a drop in systemic perfusion pressure. Though an immediate adverse effect of an impaired perfusion reserve is not apparent in most cases, it has generally been assumed that an exhausted perfusion reserve makes the brain tissue more susceptible to the effect of embolism or reduction of systemic perfusion pressure. In this context it should be realized, that the two pathophysiologic causes of cerebral ischaemia, are not mutually exclusive. Minor embolic events, which in a normal cerebral circulation would be of no consequence, may cause ischaemia when the haemodynamic reserves are already exhausted. Retrospective observations have revealed larger infarcts occurring between neighbouring territories in the so-called watershed areas, or more severe symptoms in patients with poor collateral circulation.[10–12] A relationship has also been identified between an impaired CO_2 reactivity, measured by transcranial Doppler, and the incidence of ipsilateral ischaemic stroke.[13,14] Also comparison of patterns of infarction in CT scans and the cerebral reserve capacity has shown a significant relation between low-flow infarct and an exhausted CO_2 reactivity.[14]

This issue has also been addressed in an animal model.[15] Middle cerebral artery ligature was performed in two groups of rats, in the one preceded by ICA occlusion, simulating the effect of extracranial arterial disease (Fig. 2). In the examined rats ICA occlusion lowered the distal ICA pressure by 50%. Infarct size, measured 4 days later, was significantly larger in those rats that had ICA occlusion prior to middle cerebral artery occlusion.

Only few clinical data exist: two small longitudinal studies have not been able to demonstrate a relationship between cerebral haemodynamics, assessed with position emission tomography and the subsequent occurrence of stroke.[16,17] In a 1-year follow-up study none of 21 patients, with symptomatic severe occlusive carotid disease causing abnormal haemodynamics, developed relevant stroke.[16] In another study of 23 similar patients who underwent extracranial–intracranial (EC–IC) bypass surgery, three suffered ipsilateral ischaemic stroke during the first postoperative year, giving

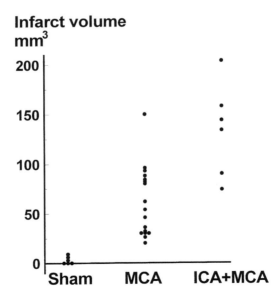

Fig. 2. Size of infarcted brain areas in three groups of animals (rats): Sham (n=6), sham-operated animals; MCA (n=17), middle cerebral artery occlusion; ICA+MCA (n=6), internal carotid artery and middle cerebral artery occlusion. (Data reproduced from Sillesen *et al.*[15])

little evidence to suggest that haemodynamic evaluation can identify a group of patients who would benefit from EC–IC bypass.[17,18] However, more recently two larger clinical studies have indicated an increased risk. Kleiser and Widder[19] followed 85 patients with angiographically proven ICA occlusion for an average of 38 months. In the group with sufficient CO_2 reactivity, determined with transcranial Doppler, four of 48 (8%) patients developed ipsilateral transient neurological symptoms, none a stroke. In cases with diminished or exhausted cerebrovascular reserve capacity, 12 of 37 (32%) patients suffered an ipsilateral event (four transient cerebral ischaemia and eight strokes) (p<0.01). The other study from Pittsburgh[20] included 95 patients with symptomatic occlusion (64 patients) or greater than 70% stenosis (31 patients) followed for an average of 20 months. Cerebral blood flow was measured by the stable xenon-CT technique at baseline and after vasodilatory challenge with intravenous acetazolamide. In the group of patients with sufficient vasodilatory capacity only one of 43 (2%) patients had a new stroke, but 15 of 52 (29%) patients with impaired reactivity did (p=0.0005). Though existing data are at variance, the more convincing studies indicate that this subset of patients with carotid artery disease and hypoperfusion, is at greater risk of stroke – in accordance with common sense.

PERIOPERATIVE COURSE AND HYPERPERFUSION SYNDROME

While data regarding the relationship of cerebral haemodynamics to stroke risk may be limited, there is much evidence that these patients run a greater risk of perioperative complications, first of all due to postendarterectomy hyperperfusion. This phenomenon, first acknowledged by Sundt et al.,[21] relates to the correction of a chronic low perfusion pressure, by carotid endarterectomy, which may result in a pronounced hyperaemia, thought to be related to temporary failure or readjustment of cerebral autoregulation.[22–26] This sequence of events has also been described following resection of cerebral arteriovenous malformations[27] and more recently following carotid percutaneous transluminal angioplasty (PTA).[28]

Cerebral blood flow studies, documented mainly with transcranial Doppler sonography[25,29,30] suggest that most patients will have some degree of hyperaemia following carotid surgery.[25,28,31,32] The hyperaemia may be short-lived, for example after clamp release or may develop over the first postoperative days. The majority will remain asymptomatic. Some of the patients, up to 10% will develop ipsilateral intense, throbbing unilateral pain in the head, face or eye, with or without nausea, transient or permanent focal cerebral deficits, focal epileptic seizures, or epileptic activity on the electroencephalogram.[6,32] Only between half and 2% will progress towards intracerebral haemorrhage.[26] In this context brain oedema should be considered a serious, but reversible component of the postoperative hyperperfusion syndrome.[33]

Patients developing hyperperfusion, who face the risk of intracerebral haemorrhage, are exclusively patients with the combination of severe carotid stenosis and poor collaterals, resulting in cerebral hypoperfusion. Based on intraoperative pressure studies, we have shown that haemorrhage, developing in eight of 622 consecutive cases, occurred only among patients who had a reduction of ICA/CCA pressure ratio of at least 20%.[7] In a more recent study we reported postendarterectomy seizures in five of 151 patients, and all five had a pressure reduction of 25% or more.[6] Though the ICA/CCA pressure ratio may not represent the haemodynamic conditions in the peripheral brain tissue, it may still be considered an indicator of high or low perfusion pressure. If the risk of intracerebral haemorrhage and other serious hyperperfusion related complications is around 1–2% in the general endarterectomy population, how high is then the risk among patients with cerebral hypoperfusion? No randomized or controlled data are available, but figures in the order of magnitude of 5–10% could be anticipated, in addition to which the risk of other cerebral complications should be added.

CONCLUSION

The question is then, whether the increased perioperative risk in patients with cerebral hypoperfusion is counterbalanced by the higher natural history risk? Again no randomized data are available – and will probably never be available. In a retrospective study we compared the outcome of a group of patients who had proven low cerebral perfusion pressure with that of a matched control group.[34] The results indicated a higher complication rate in the former group, though numbers were too small to obtain statistical significance. In view of the lack of solid evidence one might conclude that cerebral hypoperfusion is an indication for carotid surgery when conditions according to the large multicentre studies are fulfilled, i.e. a severe stenosis and relevant transitory symptoms.[8,9]

REFERENCES

1. Astrup J, Siesjö BK, Symon L: Thresholds in cerebral ischemia – the ischemic penumbra. *Stroke* **12**: 723–5, 1981
2. Baron JC, Bousser MG, Rey A *et al.*: Reversal of focal 'misery-perfusion syndrome' by extra-intracranial arterial bypass in hemodynamic cerebral ischemia. *Stroke* **12**: 454–9, 1981
3. Vorstrup S, Engell HC, Lindewald H, Lassen NA: Hemodynamically significant stenosis of the internal carotid artery treated with endarterectomy. *J Neurosurg* **60**: 1070–5, 1984
4. Paulson OB, Strandgaard S, Edvinsson L: Cerebral autoregulation. *Cerebrovasc Brain Metabol Rev* **2**: 161–92, 1990
5. Powers WJ, Press GA, Grubb RL *et al.*: The effect of hemodynamically significant carotid artery disease on the hemodynamic status of the cerebral circulation. *Ann Int Med* **106**: 27–35, 1987
6. Nielsen TG, Sillesen H, Schroeder TV: Seizures following carotid endarterectomy in patients with severely compromised cerebral circulation. *Eur J Vasc Endovasc Surg* **9**: 53–7, 1995
7. Schroeder T, Sillesen H, Boesen J *et al.*: Intracerebral hemorrhage after carotid endarterectomy. *Eur J Vasc Surg* **1**: 51–60, 1987
8. European Carotid Surgery Trialist' Collaborative Group: MCR European carotid trial: interim results for symptomatic patients with severe (70–99%) or with mild (0–29%) carotid stenosis. *Lancet* **337**: 1235–43, 1991
9. European Carotid Surgery Trialists' Group: MRC European Carotid Surgery Trial. Endarterectomy for moderate symptomatic carotid stenosis. Interim results. *Lancet* **347**: 1591–3, 1996

10. Norrving B, Nielsson B, Risberg J: rCBF in patients with carotid occlusion. Resting and hypercapnic flow related to collateral pattern. *Stroke* **13**: 154–62, 1982

11. Carpenter DA, Grubb RL, Powers WJ: Borderzone hemodynamics in cerebrovascular disease. *Neurology* **40**: 1587–92, 1990

12. Weiller C, Ringelstein EB, Reiche W, Buell U: Clinical and hemodynamic aspects of low-flow infarcts. *Stroke* **22**: 1117–23, 1991

13. Widder B, Paulat K, Hackspacher J, Mayr E: Transcranial Doppler CO2-test for the detection of hemodynamically critical carotid artery stenoses and occlusions. *Eur Arch Psychiat Neurol Sci* **236**: 162–8, 1986

14. Ringelstein EB, Sievers C, Ecker S *et al.*: Non-invasive assessment of CO2 induced cerebral vasomotor response in normal individuals and patients with internal carotid artery occlusions. *Stroke* **19**: 963–9, 1988

15. Sillesen H, Nedergaard M, Schroeder T *et al.*: Middle cerebral artery occlusion in presence of low perfusion pressure increases infarct size in rats. *Neurol Res* **10**: 61–3, 1988

16. Powers WJ, Tempel LW, Grubb RL: Influence of cerebral hemodynamics on stroke risk: One-year follow-up of 30 medically treated patients. *Ann Neurol* **25**: 325–30, 1989

17. Powers WJ, Grubb RL, Raichle ME: Clinical results of extracranial–intracranial bypass surgery in patients with hemodynamic cerebrovascular disease. *J Neurosurg* **70**: 61–7, 1989

18. EC/IC Bypass Group: Failure of extracranial–intracranial arterial bypass to reduce the risk of ischemic stroke. Results of an international randomized trial. *New Engl J Med* **313**: 1191–200, 1985

19. Kleiser B, Widder B: Course of carotid artery occlusions with impaired cerebrovascular reactivity. *Stroke* **23**: 171–4, 1992

20. Webster MW, Makaroun MS, Steed DL *et al.*: Compromised cerebral blood flow reactivity is a predictor of stroke in patients with symptomatic carotid artery occlusive disease. *J Vasc Surg* **21**: 338–45, 1995

21. Sundt TM, Sandok BA, Whisnant JP: Carotid endarterectomy: Complications and preoperative assessment of risk. *Mayo Clin Proc* **50**: 301–6, 1975

22. Bernstein M, Flemming JFR, Deck JHN: Cerebral hyperperfusion after carotid endarterectomy: A cause of cerebral hemorrhage. *Neurosurgery* **15**: 50–56, 1984

23. Schroeder T, Sillesen H, Sørensen O, Engell HC: Cerebral hyperperfusion following carotid endarterectomy. *J Neurosurg* **66**: 824–9, 1987

24. Schroeder T, Sillesen H, Engell HC: Hemodynamic effect of carotid endarterectomy. *Stroke* **18**: 204–9, 1987

25. Jørgensen LG, Schroeder TV: Defective cerebrovascular autoregulation after carotid endarterectomy. *Eur J Vasc Surg* **7**: 370–9, 1993

26. Naylor AR, Ruckley CV: The post-carotid endarterectomy hyperperfusion syndrome. *Eur J Vasc Endovasc Surg* **9**: 365–7, 1995

27. Spetzler RF, Wilson CB, Weinstein P *et al.*: Normal perfusion pressure breakthrough theory. *Clin Neurosurg* **25**: 651–72, 1978

28. Schoser BG, Heesen C, Eckert B, Thie A: Cerebral hyperperfusion injury after percutaneous transluminal angioplasty of extracranial arteries. *J Neurol* **244**: 101–4, 1997

29. Magee TR, Davies AH, Horrocks M: Transcranial Doppler evaluation of cerebral hyperperfusion syndrome after carotid endarterectomy. *Eur J Vasc Surg* **8**: 104–6, 1994

30. Barzó P, Vörös E, Bodosi M: Use of transcranial Doppler sonography and acetazolamide test to demonstrate changes in cerebrovascular reserve capacity following carotid endarterectomy. *Eur J Vasc Endovasc Surg* **11**: 83–9, 1996

31. Naylor AR, Whyman M, Wildsmith JAW *et al.*: Immediate effects of carotid clamp release on middle cerebral artery blood flow velocity during carotid endarterectomy. *Eur J Vasc Surg* **7**: 308–16, 1993

32. Jansen C, Sprengers AM, Moll FL *et al.*: Prediction of intracranial hemorrhage after carotid endarterectomy by clinical and intraoperative transcranial Doppler monitoring: Results of 233 operations. *Eur J Vasc Surg* **8**: 220–5, 1994

33. Breen JC, Caplan LR, DeWitt LD *et al.*: Brain edema after carotid surgery. *Neurology* **46**: 175–81, 1996

34. Schroeder T, Utzon NP, Aabech J *et al.*: Carotid artery disease and low cerebral perfusion pressure: symptomatology, operative risk and outcome. *Neurol Res* **12**: 35–40, 1990

Editorial comments by R.M. Greenhalgh

The author has addressed the question posed and even admits that no randomized data are available and that there probably never will be. There emerges a suspicion that there is a higher complication rate for patients undergoing carotid endarterectomy for proven low cerebral perfusion pressure, compared with a matched group. This would be the opposite of what many would predict. However, my own personal observations coincide with this author's findings that complications during carotid surgery can be higher in patients with poor cerebral perfusion. Our own worst results were in patients with symptoms of cerebral instability, particularly crescendo transient ischaemic attack, and many of these patients had bilateral very severe carotid stenosis. These are the patients that have the highest complication rate. The author does not say that patients with low cerebral perfusion should not have carotid surgery but draws attention to the possibility that the risks and complications of the procedure are greater than for patients in whom, for example the operation is being performed to reduce embolization. There are few centres in the world that are looking for reduced cerebral reserve to the extent that this has been achieved in Copenhagen.

This report is extremely welcome.

Should the Type of Carotid Plaque Determine the Carotid Procedure: Conventional or Endovascular?

G.M. Biasi and P.M. Mingazzini

INTRODUCTION

The endarterectomy surgical procedure has proved to be effective in the treatment of carotid artery disease through several trials with long follow-ups.

The validity of carotid endarterectomy and its superiority versus medical treatment has been documented in symptomatic patients with haemodynamic stenoses exceeding 70%, by the North American Symptomatic Carotid Endarterectomy Trial (NASCET),[1] the Veterans' Administration Symptomatic Endarterectomy Trial[2] and the European Carotid Surgery Trial.[3]

The efficacy of endarterectomy, compared with the best medical treatment in the prevention of stroke is supported also for asymptomatic patients in the Asymptomatic Veterans' Administration Trial and in the Asymptomatic Carotid Atherosclerosis Study, for carotid stenoses exceeding 50% (VA) and 60% (ACAS).[4,5]

The results of the symptomatic trials have certainly provided the guidelines for the indication of carotid endarterectomy. This is not the case as far as the carotid endovascular procedure is concerned. The number of articles dealing with balloon angioplasty of the carotid artery is rapidly increasing but most of these report only limited series of non-homogeneous cases so it is difficult to extract specific criteria for selection of patients and indications for the procedure.

ENDOVASCULAR TREATMENT

The great interest in and enthusiasm for endovascular treatment of the carotid bifurcation plaque is certainly due to the minimum invasiveness and reduction of risk connected with cross-clamping of carotid vessels. The arrest of blood flow in endovascular procedures is only a matter of seconds during the ballooning of the lesion. Nevertheless carotid ballooning may cause the most threatening complication of carotid angioplasty, which is cerebral embolization.

The question arises as to whether a direct relationship between the morphology of plaque and the risk of cerebral embolization can be predicted.

Some morphological characteristics of the carotid lesion are acknowledged to represent contraindication to endovascular procedures, for example in the case of heavily calcified plaques which cannot be dilated by balloon or even by stent. Irregular and complex atherosclerotic lesions extending from the common carotid artery through the bifurcation to the internal vessel are also not suitable for angioplasty and problems may arise in the correct positioning of the stent. In these cases the open surgical approach still seems to be the treatment of choice.

Experience acquired with balloon angioplasty of atherosclerotic lesions in vascular districts other than carotids, has demonstrated that some plaques are more at risk of embolization.[6] This is the case with soft plaques with high cholesterol content with a thin cap or with friable necrotic core, especially when there is ulceration of the plaque surface with soft thrombus apposition. Primary stenting in these cases does not guarantee full protection against possible embolization.

Primary stenting is our preference with carotid angioplasty, since positioning of the stent against the arterial wall during dilation can prevent carotid dissection, arterial recoil and considerably reduce the risk of fragmentation of the plaque, which ultimately can embolize to the brain. The primary stenting approach, adopted in the CAST study, showed a considerable reduction in the ischaemic events compared with balloon angioplasty alone.[7]

A favourable experience using coaxial occlusion balloons during angioplasty to protect against embolization of fragments in the distal stream has been reported by some authors. The device proposed also allows aspiration of eventual particles before deflating the distal balloon in the internal carotid artery.[8,9]

Other instruments are being developed in order to capture and remove embolic fragments. The rationale for these devices is evident, but unfortunately they are not able to protect from the eventual dislodgement of emboli during the preliminary passage of the guide-wire.

As already mentioned some plaques are thought to be more at risk than others, whereas there are also plaques, such as dense fibrous atherosclerotic plaques with a regular surface and also the restenotic lesions caused by intimal hyperplasia, which are not expected to fragment when ballooned. We therefore assume that there are both 'safe' and 'dangerous' plaques for balloon dilation.

ENDARTERECTOMY

The identification of the morphological type of the carotid plaque should consequently suggest the indication to endovascular procedures vs open endarterectomy. Duplex scan diagnostic techniques can precisely define the morphology of the plaque in a non-invasive manner. In order to improve efficacy of the ultrasound technique in evaluation of different pathological components of atherosclerotic plaque, we have devised an original method of computerized elaboration of the echographic image of the plaque.[10]

The scan of the plaque is transferred to a computer, outlined and elaborated through a software program obtaining a new image in the three different colours, which demonstrate the three principal components of the plaque: soft (lipidic, haemorragic or colliquated) fibrotic and calcific (Fig. 1). The gross and microscopic examination of the surgical carotid endarterectomy specimen is related and adjusted to the three components in the grey scale (Fig. 2). The echographic image of the carotid plaque (Fig. 3) is transferred into a computer where a new three-colour computerized image is developed (Fig. 4). This program provides the median

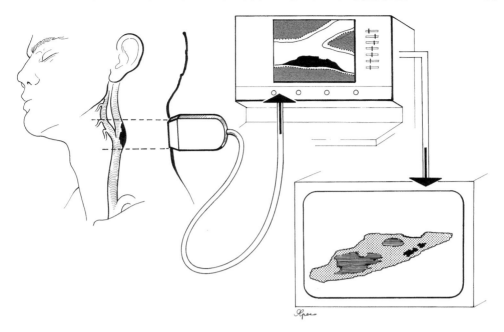

Fig. 1. The sonographer chooses the best image of the carotid plaque: a longitudinal section crossing the point of maximum stenosis. The echographic image of the plaque is then transferred to the computer and elaborated by a software program, which gives a new image of the plaque in three different colours, showing the principal morphologic components with different echodensity: soft (lipidic, haemorrhagic or colliquated) fibrotic and calcific.

echogenicity of the plaque and the densimetric histogram, which defines the three main pathological constituents quantitatively.

In a series of 206 patients utilizing this method we found a correlation between plaques 'at risk' and previous strokes documented with CT brain scan.[11] Nicolaides elaborated independently a similar method of computerized analysis showing correlation between echogenicity of the plaque and CT infarction.[12] A series of 95 of our patients were then analysed using Nicolaides' method. There was a correlation with previous CT infarction; CT infarction correlated more with grey scale median than with the percentage of stenosis[13] (Fig. 5). If these findings are confirmed by prospective studies, the echogenicity of the plaque would be the most relevant method to stratify patients at risk of stroke, rather than percentage of carotid stenosis. This computerized method is now part of The Asymptomatic Carotid Stenosis and Risk of Stroke (ACSRS) prospective trial, which will hopefully validate the effectiveness of this method.[14]

The computerized characterization of the carotid plaque should be useful also in recognizing the so-called 'safe' and 'dangerous' plaques for carotid balloon angioplasty. We recently started a multicentre trial, using this method of imaging in carotid angioplasty, to assess the risk of stroke (ICAROS). The aim of the study is to

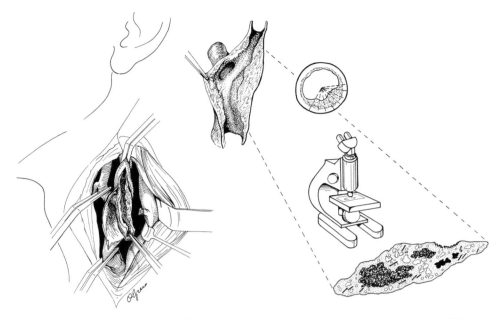

Fig. 2. Gross and microscopic examination of the surgical specimen verifies the echodensity of the different pathological constituents of the plaque.

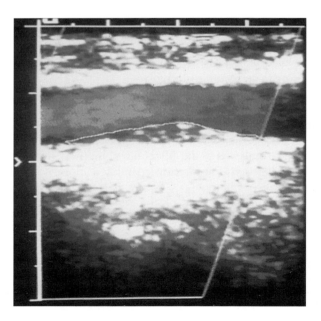

Fig. 3. The carotid plaque is outlined by the computer in the duplex scan image.

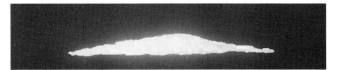

Percentage of echogenicity Low = 12%; Mid = 62%; High = 26%

Fig. 4. The computer elaboration of the echographic image of the carotid plaque differentiates the pathological components of different echodensity, giving the densimetric histogram and the median echogenicity.

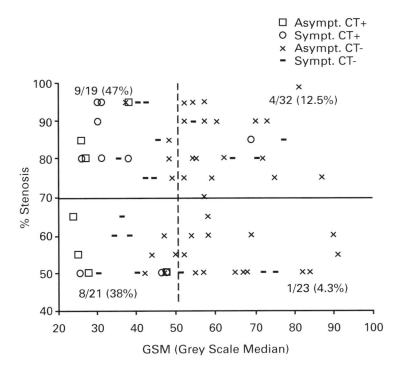

Fig. 5. Symptomatic and asymptomatic patients with positive or negative CT brain scan are reported in the graph according to the percentage of stenoses and to the echodensity of the plaque. Brain CT were more correlated with grey scale median than with the percentage of stenosis.

correlate the grey scale median echographic index of the plaque with the outcome of carotid angioplasty. A randomized trial of carotid endarterectomy versus stent angioplasty can perhaps be envisaged, in which grey scale median index will be used to determine groups to be studied.

REFERENCES

1. North American Symptomatic Carotid Endarterectomy Trial Collaborators: Beneficial effect of carotid endarterectomy in symptomatic patients with high grade carotid stenosis. *New Engl J Med* **325**: 445, 1991
2. Mayberg MR, Wilson SE, Yatsu F *et al*.: Carotid endarterectomy and prevention of cerebral schemia in symptomatic carotid stenosis: Veterans' Affairs Cooperative Study Program 309 Trialist Group. *J Am Med Assoc* **266**: 3289–94, 1991
3. European Carotid Surgery Trialists' Collaborative Group MRC: European Carotid Surgery Trial: Interim results for symptomatic patients with severe (70–99%) or with mild (0–29%) carotid stenosis. *Lancet* **337:** 1235–43, 1991
4. Hobson RW II, Weiss DG, Fields WS *et al*.: Efficacy of carotid endarterectomy for asymptomatic carotid artery stenosis. *New Engl J Med* **328**: 221–7, 1993
5. Executive Committee for the Asymptomatic Carotid Atherosclerosis Study: Endarterectomy for asymptomatic carotid artery stenosis. *J Am Med Assoc* **273**: 1421–8, 1995
6. Becquemin JP, Quarforolt P, Castler Y, Helliere D: Carotid angioplasty: Is it safe? *J Endovasc Surg* **3**: 35–41, 1996
7. Bergeron P: Carotid angioplasty and stenting: Is endovascular treatment of cerebrovascular disease justified? *J Endovasc Surg* **3**: 128–31, 1996
8. Kachel R: Results of balloon angioplasty in the carotid arteries. *J Endovasc Surg* **3**: 22–30, 1996
9. Theron J, Guimareaens L, Rogopoulos A: Carotid artery angioplasty – Evolving concepts. *Endovasc Impact* **2**: 15–8, 1997
10. Biasi GM, Albizzati MG, Maugeri G, Mingazzini PM: Analysis of preoperative diagnostic procedures for assessment of patients candidates for carotid endarterectomy. In: Honorary Volume P. Balas, Athens: Iatrikos Ed. 386–91, 1993
11. Biasi GM, Mingazzini PM, Sampaolo A, Ferrari SA: Echographic characterization of the carotid plaque and risk for cerebral ischemia. In: Castellani LD (Ed), *Progress in Angiology and Vascular Surgery* Vol V, p. 59. Torino: Minerva Medica, 1995
12. El-Barghouty N, Geroulakos G, Nicolaides AN *et al*.: Computer-assisted carotid plaque characterization. *Eur J Vasc Endovasc Surg* **9**: 389, 1995
13. Biasi GM, Sampaolo A, Mingazzini P *et al*.: Computer analysis of ultrasonic plaque echolucency in identifying high risk carotid bifurcation lesions. *Eur J Vasc Endovasc Surg* (in press)
14. Nicolaides AN: Asymptomatic Carotid Stenosis and Risk of Stroke (ACSRS) prospective trial. Identification of a high risk group. A natural history study.

Editorial comments by P.R.F. Bell

This chapter looks at a difficult area: endovascular procedures in the carotid artery which are known to cause embolization and have a significantly higher chance of causing a stroke than surgery in a specialized centre. It may be that if plaques at risk can be identified they can be operated on whereas those which are not too risky could be dealt with by angioplasty with or without a stent. The authors discuss the lesions using their own criteria of risk and correlate these with CT evidence. At present there is no foolproof way of labelling a plaque as risky or otherwise. Until this is done it will be difficult to justify using stenting and angioplasty in every patient with a severely stenosed artery. It may be that a metabolic or biological marker will be the best way forward. Echogenicity or echolucency has been looked at many times without any real success and this paper does not really take us much further in that direction.

Should Carotid Plaque be Removed Surgically or Stented?

P.R.F. Bell and M.M. Thompson

INTRODUCTION

Carotid endarterectomy has been practised for many years and the results have improved progressively.[1] The establishment of quality control during surgery and the use of early postoperative monitoring have ensured that results have reached the point where, in specialized centres a stroke and death rate of <1% can be regularly achieved.[2] If patching is used routinely a restenosis rate of <5% is also possible.[3] With these excellent results available the question really should be: is dilatation and stenting of the carotid worth contemplating? Into the equation, however, comes patient preference which is understandable, complication rates, costs and the long-term problems with plaque morphology.

COST

There is at present an increasing movement to reduce hospital costs by limiting inpatient stay. It used to be the case that patients stayed in hospital for 10 days after carotid endarterectomy but progressively this period has been reduced to the point where overnight stay is now regularly practised[4] with 2 days stay at the most being required. The patient does not need to stay in the intensive therapy unit and costs are now therefore very similar to angioplasty and stenting. There is, therefore, no benefit to be gained on the cost argument from angioplasty.

PATIENT PREFERENCE

Clearly patients would rather have a catheter inserted and a stent used to dilate their carotid artery than an operation which requires an incision. Patients should, however, be fully informed about the complications of both procedures properly by agreed written protocols rather than by enthusiasts for either procedure. At present there is no easy way of preventing embolization but complication rates published for angioplasty are of the order of 6–7% in specialized centres doing angioplasty regularly[4] and the risk of stroke and death from surgery is less than 1% in similar specialized centres.[5] These figures need to be put to the patient when the question of patient preference is being discussed.

WHAT IS A DANGEROUS PLAQUE?

Various clinical trials have shown that 30% of patients with symptomatic carotid disease will have a stroke in the next 3 years.[6] This of course means that 70% will not have a stroke and the challenge is to pick out those who need treatment and those who do not. At present there is no foolproof method of judging which is a dangerous plaque. In the past attempts to classify the plaque into those which are more likely to embolize have not been uniformly successful.[7] More recently studies have suggested that certain plaque characteristics such as echolucency can be associated with computed tomography (CT) pictures of silent emboli.[8] It may be that a biochemical approach to deciding whether a plaque is unstable and therefore dangerous will be possible in future. Measurement of metalloproteinase in plaques may give an indication of their likelihood to embolize but will only be useful if measurements of the same type can be carried out on tissue available before surgery, such as blood or white cells. At present the very fact that we do not know which plaques are dangerous and which plaques are not means that control of embolization from them is essential. In this uncertain situation stenting would be dangerous in a straight-forward case.

DEGREE OF STENOSIS

It seems reasonable to suppose that the insertion of a wire or a balloon covered by a stent about 2mm in diameter, can lead to pieces of atheroma or thrombus being loosened from the plaque and passing into the brain. It therefore would seem equally reasonable to avoid stenting any lesion which has a diameter of less than 2mm for the simple reason that pushing the stent and graft through this with or without pre-dilatation will cause a problem (Fig. 1). Attempts to avoid embolization by placing a balloon distally has been claimed to result in a better overall outcome.[9] The very act of passing anything, including a wire, through the severe stenosis leads to embolization.

THE PLAQUE AND ITS LONG-TERM EVOLUTION

We know that removal of the plaque from a carotid artery stenosis in the long term leads to good results with a low recurrence and stroke rate, particularly if a patch is applied.[3] The simple compression of a plaque by angioplasty with or without a stent leads to a situation where the plaque is intact and the possibility in the long term is that restenosis will occur. We know, for example, that in patients who have angioplasty in other areas restenosis occurs in 30% of cases.[10] The insertion of a stent into small blood vessels often produces intimal hyperplasia, particularly in the lower leg and this will lead to restenosis of the vessel. The insertion of a stent over a plaque which is often soft (Fig. 2), can lead to extrusion of material through the intestices of the stent which can embolize distally. If restenosis occurs and this cannot be dealt with by angioplasty, an operation at that point will cause great difficulty and lead to serious problems. We need to know in the long term, therefore, what happens to the

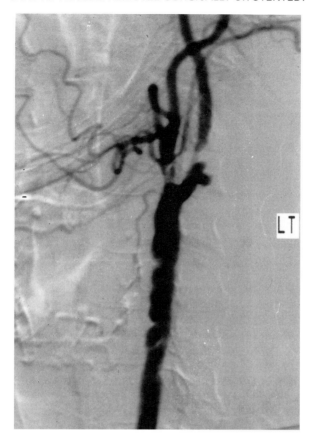

Fig. 1.   Severe carotid stenosis.

plaque, whether it actually diminishes or increases, whether the hyperplasia returns and what would be the consequences of operating on these patients with stents in place. It has been shown in other areas that operations in this situation can be a serious problem.

EMBOLIZATION

The majority of transient ischaemic attacks are due to embolic episodes from carotid plaque.[11] Embolization occurs regularly and can be detected and for this reason has been thought to be inconsequential. However, studies looking at embolization of solid material in the perioperative period have shown that emboli are far from being inconsequential in that they can cause strokes.[12] Quite apart from strokes, psychometric changes also occur. Embolization can occur during an operation when a simple skin incision is made and certainly can occur during mobilization of the

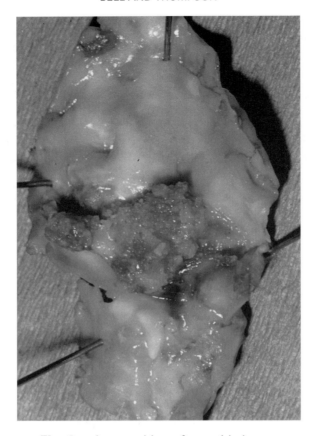

Fig. 2.   An unstable, soft carotid plaque.

vessels. However, during surgery this can be controlled by rapid clamping of the vessel and the insertion of a shunt.

In contrast, embolization from a carotid plaque during angioplasty cannot be controlled because the passage of a wire let alone the device through the stenosis will lead to embolization (Fig. 3). The emboli produced are dose-related in terms of stroke, the higher the number, the more likely that a stroke will occur. The big problem with angioplasty and stent insertion is embolization and unless this can be controlled, and it is hard to see how it can be because of the introduction of the device, particularly in cases where treatment is required, it cannot compare with surgical treatment where control is very much simpler. Apart from embolization the insertion of a stent and a balloon can lead to carotid occlusion and a stroke. When embolization prior to occlusion occurs there is no solution to the problem as there is no easy way of getting back the embolus once it has gone into the brain. Thrombolysis has so far not been found to be effective in doing this. Attempts to prevent embolization by the inflation of a distal balloon (Fig. 4) ignore the problem that the introduction of the device causes embolization not necessarily the angioplasty itself.

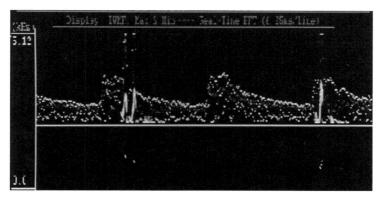

Fig. 3. Wire manipulation: emboli produced on a transcranial Doppler trace by the passage of a guide-wire.

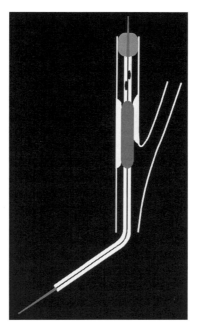

Fig. 4. The inflation of a distal balloon during angioplasty may reduce embolization.

CRANIAL NERVE COMPLICATIONS

These are often quoted as a cause for avoiding operations. Cranial nerve lesions to the 12th nerve in particular are relatively common at about 5% but are transitory and the majority recover within a few days.[13] The other problem is numbness over the lower face due to severing of the cutaneous nerves, this also recovers and does not cause long-term problems.

RESULTS

At present the justification for angioplasty is usually that the stroke rate during the European Carotid Surgery Trial (ECST) and the American trial was about 7%.[6] This of course is correct but is historical data from multicentre trials. The actual stroke and death rate in specialized centres is <1%. Angioplasty has been shown in published results to cause stroke rates of 6.4% in selected patients.[14] At present only one trial, done by us but not yet published, has proceeded on the basis of intention to treat and in this study 20 patients were randomized, ten to surgery and ten to angioplasty. Of the surgical series none had problems, in the angioplasty series five had strokes. In the CAVATAS study[14] the patients are not strictly randomized. Any patient that the investigator thinks should not be treated by angioplasty is not treated and stenoses as low as 50% are dealt with by stenting.

THE FUTURE

There is no question that certain patients do well from angioplasty and stenting and these are patients where there is a hostile neck, i.e. previous radiotherapy, where there is a recurrence of the lesion or there is fibromuscular hyperplasia. In other words those lesions where there is a smooth plaque with little chance of embolization. There is every reason to expect that in future once plaque morphology can be properly defined and diagnosed, there may well be cases where angioplasty and stenting is appropriate. It may also be that those cases with smooth stenoses do not need any treatment at all and may represent the 70% or so of patients in the ECST trial who would never have a problem. It seems unlikely at present that those patients who have ulcerated plaques, intraplaque haemorrhage or the kind of lesions that are frequently seen can be treated by angioplasty with comparable results to those seen surgically. In the latter situation control is complete, in the former the situation cannot be controlled properly or safely.

REFERENCES

1. Bergeron P: Carotid angioplasty and stenting: Is endovascular treatment for cerebrovascular disease justified? *J Endovasc Surg* **3**: 129–31, 1996
2. Naylor AR, Merrick MV, Ruckley CV: Risk factors for intraoperative neurological deficit during carotid endarterectomy. *Eur J Vasc Surg* **5**: 33–9, 1991
3. Eikelboom BC, Ackerstaff RGA, Hoeneveld H *et al.*: Benefits of carotid patching: a randomised study. *J Vasc Surg* **7**: 240–7, 1988
4. Ammar AD: Cost efficient carotid surgery: a comprehensive evaluation. *J Vasc Surg* **24**: 1051–6, 1996
5. Dietrich EB, Mohamadon N, Reid DB: Stenting the carotid artery: initial experience in 110 patients. *J Endovasc Surg* **3**: 42–62, 1996
6. North American Symptomatic Carotid Endarterectomy Trial Collaborators: Beneficial effect of carotid endarterectomy in symptomatic patients with high grade carotid stenosis. *New Engl J Med* **325**: 445–53, 1991

7. Gaunt ME, Brown T, Hartshorne T *et al.*: Unstable carotid plaques: preoperative identification and association with intraoperative embolisation detected by transcranial Doppler. *Eur J Vasc Endovasc Surg* **11**: 78–83, 1996
8. Meagher E, Grace PA, Bouchier-Hayes P: Are CT infarcts a separate risk factor in patients with transient cerebral ischaemic episodes? *Eur J Vasc Surg* **5**: 165–7, 1991
9. Theron J, Courtheoux P, Alachkar F *et al.*: New triple coaxial catheter system for carotid angioplasty with cerebral protection. *Am J Neur* **11**: 869–74, 1990
10. Blackshear JL, O'Callaghan WG, Califf RM: Medical approaches to prevention of restenosis after coronary angioplasty. *J Am Coll Cardiol* **9**: 834–8, 1987
11. Hayward JK, Davies AH, Lamont PM: Carotid plaque morphology: a review. *Eur J Vasc Endovasc Surg* **9**: 368–75, 1995
12. Ackerstaff RGA, Jansen C, Moll FL *et al.*: The significance of microemboli detection by means of transcranial doppler ultrasonography monitoring in carotid endarterectomy. *J Vasc Surg* **21**: 963–70, 1995
13. Rosenbloom M, Friedman SG, Lamparello PJ: Glossopharyngeal nerve injury complicating carotid endarterectomy. *J Vasc Surg* **5**: 469–73, 1987
14. Sivazuru A, Venables GS, Beard JD *et al.*: European Carotid Angioplasty Trial. *J Endovasc Surg* **3**: 16–20, 1996

Editorial comments by R.M. Greenhalgh

The authors have posed their question and also shown that it is simply not possible to answer it at present. They imply that in the future, by plaque analysis, it will not be necessary to operate upon so many patients as at present. They also draw attention to the fact that angioplasty with stent is a good idea in some patients. They have not pointed to the precise trial which needs to be performed for any comparison between carotid endarterectomy and angioplasty with stenting. In this sense, they have not answered the question nor pointed to the way forward but they have given us a number of interesting issues to be thinking about.

RENAL ARTERY QUESTIONS AND INDICATIONS

When is Transaortic Renal Endarterectomy Indicated?

Daniel Clair, Michael Belkin, Anthony D. Whittemore,
Magruder C. Donaldson and John A. Mannick

INTRODUCTION

Arteriosclerotic renovascular disease is commonly present in patients over 50 years of age who have atherosclerosis of the aorto–iliac and infrainguinal arterial systems.[1] In addition to its contribution to hypertension in many of these patients, arteriosclerotic renovascular disease is increasingly recognized as an important cause of kidney failure.[2-5] Recent reports on the natural history of renovascular disease strongly suggest that arteriosclerotic stenoses progress inexorably to occlusion.[2,6,7] These findings appear to justify a relatively aggressive stance toward renal revascularization in patients with arteriosclerotic renal artery disease particularly when the major arteries supplying both kidneys are involved. Because arteriosclerotic renal artery disease usually results from extension of aortic plaque into the proximal portions of the renal arteries, eversion endarterectomy is a convenient and expeditious technique for combined aortic and renal artery reconstruction. This has been the chief indication for transaortic renal endarterectomy in the authors' department over the past decade. The technique has also proved useful in a few patients who have symptomatic arteriosclerotic renal artery disease involving more than one renal artery where the aortic plaque is relatively well localized to the region of the renal artery orifices and who do not require infrarenal aortic replacement.

The chief alternative to transaortic renal endarterectomy in patients requiring combined aortic and renal artery reconstruction is aortorenal bypass grafting, usually performed with side limbs arising from the aortic graft. A further alternative in patients requiring repair of both aortic and renal artery disease would be balloon angioplasty of the renal artery lesions combined with stent insertion, either before or after repair of the aortic disease. While balloon angioplasty alone in a number of reports[8] has proven unsatisfactory as a treatment for arteriosclerotic renal artery disease involving the renal ostia, results of renal artery stenting are more encouraging in some but not all series.[8-11]

The major advantage of renal artery stenting, in theory at least, is the safety of the procedure itself. This has not always proved true in published reports, however.[8,10] While renal artery reconstruction is in general a low risk procedure when performed by experienced surgeons, combined aortic and renal artery reconstruction has been associated with a high postoperative mortality rate in a number of reported series in the 1980s and early 1990s.[12-15] Mortality rates of 8.3–24% were described while low mortality rates were reported for either aortic or renal artery surgery performed alone. However, more recent series have demonstrated lower mortality rates of 1–5.6% in series of combined aortic and renal artery reconstruction,[16-20] though in most of the latter reports aortorenal bypass has been the predominant technique.

Because of its technical simplicity and short operating time, transaortic renal endarterectomy appears to offer advantages over bypass techniques in patients who require renal revascularization in addition to operative repair of severe aorto-iliac occlusive disease or infrarenal abdominal aortic aneurysms.

REVIEW OF AUTHORS' EXPERIENCE

In order to assess the efficacy and safety of transaortic renal endarterectomy in our hands we recently reviewed our experience with this technique from 1985 to 1994. During this time we applied the technique to 78 renal arteries in 43 patients. During the same period an additional 56 patients underwent renal artery bypass grafting. Most of the latter individuals did not require concomitant aortic surgery. The clinical characteristics of the 43 patients undergoing transaortic renal endarterectomy are summarized in Table 1. It is apparent that the majority of patients were operated upon for hypertension or renal failure or both. The mean number of antihypertensive medications in the 38 patients operated upon for this indication was 2.5. The mean preoperative serum creatinine in the 28 patients with renal dysfunction was 3.0 mg/dl. Two individuals underwent bilateral renal endarterectomy prophylactically for high grade renal artery stenoses in the absence of severe hypertension or renal failure. The procedures were elective in 41 of the patients and urgent in two patients; one with recent onset of dialysis-dependent renal failure and one with malignant hypertension.

Table 1. Clinical characteristics and surgical indications for 43 patients undergoing transaortic renal endarterectomy between 1985 and 1994

Mean age	68 years (46–81)
Male: Female	25:18
Coronary artery disease	25 (58.1%)
Smoking	18 (41.9%)
Diabetes mellitus	2 (4.7%)
Hypertension	13 (30.2%)
Renal insufficiency	3 (7.0%)
Hypertension and renal insufficiency	25 (58.1%)
Aortic disease	39 (90.7%)
Infrarenal aneurysm	30 (69.8%)
Occlusive disease	9 (20.9%)
Isolated atherosclerotic kidney disease	4 (9.3%)

Reprinted with permission of the *Journal of Vascular Surgery*.

Renal artery endarterectomy was performed concomitantly with aortic bypass grafting for occlusive disease or aneurysm in 39 of the 43 patients. In four individuals renal endarterectomy was performed as the treatment for isolated bilateral disease involving multiple renal arteries. Patients who underwent combined visceral and renal endarterectomy and patients who underwent renal endarterectomy in concert with thoracoabdominal aneurysm repair were not included in this review.

The operative approach was transabdominal through a midline incision in 32 patients and left retroperitoneal in 11 depending upon the preference of the surgeon, the patient's habitus, and a history of prior intra-abdominal surgery. In the transabdominal approach, as described by Stoney and associates,[16] the perirenal artery was freed up with wide mobilization of the left renal vein and division of the crus of the diaphragm posterolaterally. Both renal arteries were freed up for at least 1 cm beyond the extent of palpable arteriosclerotic disease. Dissection was continued superiorly to the origin of the superior mesenteric artery. When the aorta just below the superior mesenteric was unsuitable for clamping because of the presence of calcific disease, supracoeliac aortic exposure was obtained through the gastrohepatic ligament.

The left retroperitoneal approach allowed easy assessment of the appropriate area for aortic clamp placement after division of the crus of the diaphragm. However, exposure of a sufficient length of right renal artery to determine the technical success of the endarterectomy was more difficult by this exposure.

After systemic administration of heparin and infusion of 12.5 g mannitol, the renal arteries were occluded with padded bulldog clamps followed by aortic outflow and suprarenal proximal aortic clamping. The aorta was opened longitudinally to a point proximal to the renal arteries and in cases of associated aortic disease, a partial transverse cuff was fashioned for graft insertion (Fig. 1). In most instances, the aortic plaque was divided at a point below the renal arteries and endarterectomy of the aortic plaque including the orificial disease in the renal arteries was carried out by eversion technique. If there was any doubt concerning the end-point of the endarterectomy in the renal arteries, a Fogarty balloon catheter was introduced into the renal artery, gently inflated and retracted into the aortic lumen allowing prolapse of the artery into the aorta for direct visualization of the end-point. In the four cases of isolated renal endarterectomy, the aortotomy was closed primarily. In the combined procedure the aortic prosthesis was sutured to the aortic cuff at or below the renal arteries as shown in Fig. 2. In a few instances where the aortic plaque was not prominent, endarterectomy of the renal artery orifices was carried out by the technique illustrated in Fig. 3 with incision of the aortic intima and media around the renal artery orifice and eversion endarterectomy of the orificial disease.

In all instances, the aorta was flushed vigorously before release of renal artery occlusion. The continuous wave Doppler probe was used routinely to assess adequacy of flow in the renal arteries upon completion of the procedure. In more recent cases, duplex ultrasonography was utilized for this purpose.

Aortic clamping was below the level of the superior mesenteric artery in 37 of the 43 patients and above the coeliac axis in six. Of the 78 endarterectomized arteries, 10 were totally occluded. Thirty patients underwent bilateral renal endarterectomies including accessory renal arteries in three. Nine had unilateral endarterectomies, two had unilateral endarterectomy with contralateral bypass to an occluded artery in one

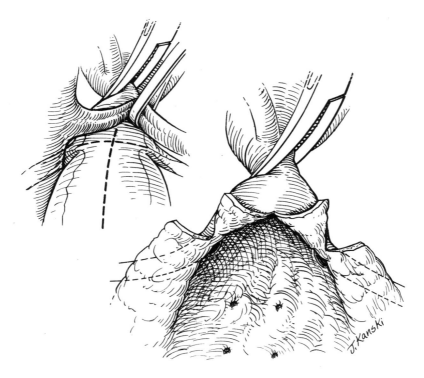

Fig. 1. Exposure for transaortic renal endarterectomy by the anterior approach. The perirenal aorta has been freed up sufficiently for application of a clamp just below the superior mesenteric artery. The incision in the aortic aneurysm has been carried up to above the level of the renal arteries and a partial proximal cuff is fashioned just below the renal artery orifices. An endarterectomy of the aortic plaque including the orifices of the renal arteries will next be carried out. (Reprinted with permission of the *Journal of Vascular Surgery*.)

case and to an artery with a more distal stenosis in another. Two patients had unilateral endarterectomy with contralateral therapeutic nephrectomy of small ischaemic kidneys. The mean renal ischaemia time was 35 minutes (range 12–60 min). Five (6%) of the 78 renal endarterectomies required intraoperative revision by implantation into the aortic graft (two) or a bypass originating from the graft (three). Two implantations were deemed necessary because of fragility of the orifices of the renal arteries after completion of the endarterectomy. The other two revisions were required when reduced pulsations and damped Doppler signals demonstrated inadequate flow upon completion of the endarterectomy. All revascularized renal arteries were patent by Doppler ultrasonography at the completion of surgery.

Major postoperative morbidity occurred in six patients (14%). This included renal failure requiring dialysis in two patients and myocardial infarction in two. There were two deaths within 30 days of operation. One patient had a fatal myocardial

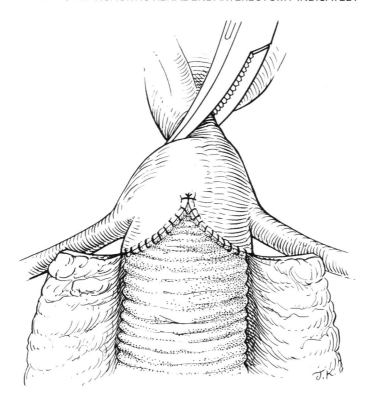

Fig. 2. A bifurcation graft has been sutured to the proximal aortic cuff just prior to restoration of circulation to the renal arteries following completion of the transaortic endarterectomy. The aortic graft will be clamped below the proximal anastomosis and circulation will be restored to the renal arteries. (Reprinted with permission of the *Journal of Vascular Surgery*.)

infarction with cardiac arrest on the first postoperative day after an apparently uneventful operative procedure. The other patient also died on the first postoperative day of complications related to bleeding and coagulopathy after an ill-advised attempt at bilateral renal endarterectomy in aneurysmal perirenal aorta.

Of the 26 surviving patients with preoperative renal dysfunction, six experienced postoperative elevation of serum creatinine of 1 mg/dl or greater above baseline levels. Four of the six have done well without dialysis in follow-up ranging from 14 to 45 months. Two patients in this group required institution of dialysis postoperatively. In one of the patients, dialysis was discontinued with recovery of renal function after 1 week, serum creatinine was below the preoperative level at 26 months follow-up. The other patient has required chronic dialysis. This individual was operated on urgently for a symptomatic abdominal aortic aneurysm and bilateral renal artery disease with a preoperative creatinine of 10.2 mg/dl.

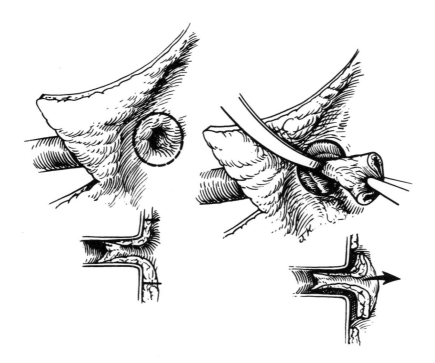

Fig. 3. Illustrates the technique of eversion endarterectomy in instances where atherosclerosis of the entire perirenal aorta is not prominent. The intima is incised around the renal artery orifice and an eversion endarterectomy is carried out without performing a complete aortic endarterectomy. (Reprinted with permission of the *Journal of Vascular Surgery.*)

In one of two patients undergoing dialysis preoperatively, dialysis could be discontinued after surgery. Among the four patients who required intraoperative revision after renal endarterectomy, only one had a significant postoperative serum creatinine elevation. This individual did not require dialysis. No patient with normal preoperative renal function experienced postoperative renal insufficiency. Among the patients with preoperative serum creatinine of 1.5 mg/dl or greater, 20% had a reduction of serum creatinine of 1 mg/dl or greater by 30 days postoperatively. At late follow-up mean serum creatinine among surviving patients with preoperative renal insufficiency was 3.0 mg/dl. Two patients required late institution of dialysis for progressive kidney failure. Both of these patients had preoperative serum creatinine levels of 5 mg/dl or greater and did not experience significant change in their creatinine in the early postoperative period.

At early follow-up at 30 days postoperatively, 11% of patients with preoperative hypertension were cured, 72% were improved, and 16% were unchanged, according to criteria previously published Dean and co-workers.[21] These results did not change significantly at late follow-up. At both early and late follow-up, the mean number of antihypertensive medications among the patients with preoperative hypertension was 1.3 per patient.

Only 27% of the patients and 22% of the renal arteries were evaluated for patency in the postoperative period. The reasons for evaluation were increasing antihypertensive medication requirements or significant elevation of serum creatinine. Renal scintigraphy was performed in ten arteries, arteriography in six arteries and duplex ultrasonography in one artery. An occlusion was found at 21 months in a small accessory artery that had been occluded preoperatively. A stenosis was found in a main renal artery at 8 months and corrected by balloon angioplasty. All other arteries were reported widely patent (Fig. 4).

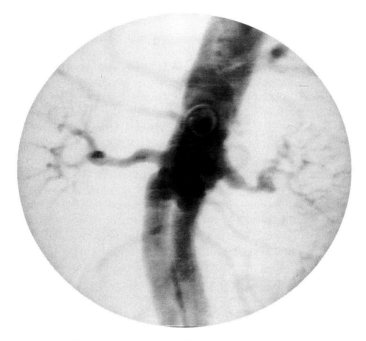

Fig. 4. Follow-up arteriogram on a patient in the authors' series 1 year after transaortic bilateral renal endarterectomy and insertion of an aortic bifurcation prosthesis for an abdominal aortic aneurysm. Both endarterectomized renal arteries remain widely patent. (Reprinted with permission of the *Journal of Vascular Surgery*.)

DISCUSSION

In the authors' series summarized above, the technical reliability of producing a satisfactory result after transaortic eversion endarterectomy was 96% as judged by palpation and continuous wave Doppler. Using operative duplex ultrasonography, Stoney *et al.*[16] found moderate or major defects in 12% of the 75 arteries they operated upon and only three arteries (4%) required operative revision. With colour assisted duplex ultrasonography, Dougherty *et al.*[22] found lesions requiring revision in six (10.7%) of 56 renal arteries treated by transaortic endarterectomy and one (12.5%) of eight aorto-renal bypass grafts. It thus appears that transaortic eversion endarterectomy with the methods used in our Service and in other recent series[16,20,22] is an acceptably reliable method of establishing renal artery patency. The durability of renal artery endarterectomy is well established since it has been used to treat renovascular disease since 1952.[23] While late angiographic follow-up is not complete in most series, published results suggest that late occlusions or haemodynamic stenoses occur in approximately 5% of renal arteries treated by transaortic endarterectomy. Interestingly, the reported postoperative occlusions have occurred in arteries that were occluded preoperatively. In the future more complete objective assessment of the results of renal artery reconstruction will almost certainly be possible with modern duplex ultrasound.[11]

The operative mortality in the present series of 4.7% is roughly twice as high as that in patients undergoing infrarenal aortic aneurysm repair at the Brigham and Women's Hospital in the same time period. However, an ill-advised attempt to endarterectomize a weakened and aneurysmal perirenal aorta was clearly responsible for one of the deaths. The use of bypass rather than endarterectomy in this individual may very well have avoided a mortality. The 30-day mortality rate was only 2.3% in the comparable series reported by Stoney *et al.*,[16] and 1% in a recent series of McNeil *et al.*[20] indicating that combined aortic and renal artery surgery can be performed using the transaortic endarterectomy technique without adding additional operative risk to that already inherent in the aortic surgical procedure itself.

Thus, the currently available evidence suggests that transaortic renal endarterectomy, particularly when combined with occlusive or aneurysmal disease of the infrarenal aorta, produces results which are at least as good as those reported for renal artery bypass grafting in similar groups of patients.[14,15,17,18] We doubt that a prospective randomized study comparing the two techniques in a sizeable series of patients will ever be initiated in this era of burgeoning endovascular surgery. For the present we continue to favour the use of transaortic endarterectomy in such individuals because it is technically easy to perform in most patients and adds very little additional operating time. In the future this operative approach in many patients may be supplanted by endovascular repair of infrarenal aortic aneurysms or occlusive disease combined with angioplasty and stenting of renal orificial stenoses. Whether or not these less invasive techniques replace open surgery clearly depends upon reliable assessment of their long-term efficacy in a substantial number of patients.

REFERENCES

1. Olin JW, Melia M, Young JR *et al.*: Prevalence of atherosclerotic renal artery stenosis in patients with atherosclerosis elsewhere. *Am J Med* **88**: 46N–51N, 1990
2. Schreiber MJ, Pohl MA, Novick AC: The natural history of atherosclerotic and fibrous renal artery disease. *Urol Clin N Am* **11**: 383–92, 1984

3. Jacobson HR: Ischemic renal disease: an overlooked clinical entity. *Kidney Int* **34**: 729–43, 1988
4. Mailloux LU, Bellucci AG, Mossey RT *et al.*: Predictors of survival in patients undergoing dialysis. *Am J Med* **84**: 855–62, 1988
5. Dean RH, Tribble RW, Hansen KJ *et al.*: Evolution of renal insufficiency in ischemic nephropathy. *Ann Surg* **213**: 446–56, 1991
6. Tollefson DFJ, Ernst CB: Natural history of atherosclerotic renal artery stenosis associated with aortic disease. *J Vasc Surg* **14**: 327–31, 1991
7. Zierler RE, Bergelin RO, Isaacson JA *et al.*: Natural history of atherosclerotic renal artery stenosis: A prospective study with duplex ultrasonography. *J Vasc Surg* **19**: 250–8, 1994
8. Novick AC: Percutaneous transluminal angioplasty and surgery of the renal artery. *Eur J Vasc Surg* **8**: 1–9, 1994
9. Blum U, Krumme B, Flugel P *et al.*: Treatment of ostial renal-artery stenoses with vascular endoprostheses after unsuccessful balloon angioplasty. *New Engl J Med* **336**: 459–65, 1997
10. Harden PN, MacLeod MJ, Rodger RSC *et al.*: Effect of renal-artery stenting on progression of renovascular renal failure. *Lancet* **349**: 1133–6, 1997
11. Tullis MJ, Zierler RE, Glickerman DJ *et al.*: Results of percutaneous transluminal angioplasty for atherosclerotic renal artery stenosis: A follow-up study with duplex ultrasonography. *J Vasc Surg* **25**: 46–54, 1997
12. Shahian DM, Najafi H, Javid H *et al.*: Simultaneous aortic and renal artery reconstruction. *Arch Surg* **115**: 1491–7, 1980
13. Diehl JT, Cali RF, Hertzer NR *et al.*: Complications of abdominal aortic reconstruction. An analysis of perioperative risk factors in 557 patients. *Ann Surg* **197**: 49–56, 1983
14. Dean RH, Keyser JE, DuPont WD *et al.*: Aortic and renal vascular disease: factors affecting the value of combined procedures. *Ann Surg* **200**: 336–44, 1984
15. Cambria RP, Brewster DC, L'Italien GJ *et al.*: The durability of different reconstructive techniques for atherosclerotic renal artery disease. *J Vasc Surg* **20**: 76–87, 1994
16. Stoney RJ, Messina LM, Goldstone J *et al.*: Renal endarterectomy through the transected aorta: A new technique for combined aortorenal atherosclerosis – a preliminary report. *J Vasc Surg* **9**: 224–33, 1989
17. O'Mara CS, Maples MD, Kilfore TL *et al.*: Simultaneous aortic reconstruction and bilateral renal revascularization: Is this a safe and effective procedure? *J Vasc Surg* **8**: 357–66, 1988
18. Chaikof EL, Smith RB, Salam AA *et al.*: Ischemic nephropathy and concomitant aortic disease: a ten year experience. *J Vasc Surg* **19**: 135–48, 1994
19. Mason RA, Newton GB, Kvilekval K *et al.*: Transaortic endarterectomy of renal visceral artery lesions in association with infrarenal aortic surgery. *J Vasc Surg* **12**: 697–704, 1990
20. McNeil JW, String ST, Pfeiffer RO: Concomitant renal endarterectomy and aortic reconstruction. *J Vasc Surg* **20**: 331–7, 1994
21. Dean RH, Krueger TC, Whiteneck JM *et al.*: Operative management of renovascular hypertension: results after a follow-up of fifteen to twenty-three years. *J Vasc Surg* **1**: 234–42, 1984
22. Dougherty MJ, Hallett JW, Naessens JM *et al.*: Optimizing technical success of renal revascularization: the impact of intraoperative color-flow duplex ultrasonography. *J Vasc Surg*, **17**: 849–57, 1993
23. Wylie EJ, Perloff DL, Stoney RJ: Autogenous tissue revascularization techniques in surgery for renovascular hypertension. *Ann Surg* **170**: 416–28, 1969

Editorial comments by C.V. Ruckley

Renal artery stenosis is a remarkably common radiological finding prior to reconstructive aortic surgery. Whether it should be treated and if so by what means is one of the most commonly recurring debates at combined surgical and radiological meetings. Conventional surgical wisdom has it that the addition of renal artery reconstruction to aortic surgery adds a dimension of risk which is frequently unacceptable. The temptation to treat radiological lesions should be resisted. Clair *et al.* limited renal reconstruction to patients with hypertension and/or renal failure in patients also requiring aortic reconstruction and achieved a mortality of 5%. Two patients developed renal failure, one of whom required long-term dialysis while two others survived myocardial infarcts. Allowing for the fact that the long-term results of percutaneous angioplasty and renal artery stenting have not been shown to be better than surgery, these excellent results, in an extremely high risk patient group, adjust and keep open a potentially important therapeutic option.

Should Severity of Renal Artery Disease Determine the Procedure Preferred?

Mohammed S. Sobeh and George Hamilton

INTRODUCTION

The treatment of renal artery disease is an area of medical and surgical therapy spectacularly devoid of good comparative data of various treatment modalities. There is only one prospective randomized comparison of interventional treatment but a host of publications from many centres, each describing their experience with the variety of treatments. Consequently this is an area of medicine where local expertise frequently formulates the bias towards preferred procedure. This chapter will therefore review the available evidence for assessment, investigation and treatment of renal artery stenosis before the authors' own bias for choice of treatment will be explored.

Renal artery disease remains an underdiagnosed condition. This is because it remains completely asymptomatic until the development of haemodynamically significant stenosis (usually defined as stenosis that reduces the vessel diameter by ≥ 60%) when hypertension and then renal failure supervene. The true incidence of renal artery stenosis is unknown, as there are no population-based studies that have measured the frequency of this disease. However, early autopsy studies and later angiographic and duplex ultrasonography studies have consistently reported a prevalence of between 30 and 50% amongst patients who have evidence of cardiovascular disease elsewhere.[1] Holley et al.[2] reported a prevalence of 56% in 256 autopsies of hypertensive patients. Using preoperative angiography Olin et al.[3] reported significant (> 50%) renal artery stenosis in 38% of patients with abdominal aortic aneurysms, 33% of patients with occlusive aorto–iliac disease and 39% of patients with infrainguinal occlusive disease. Sawiki et al.[4] reported a threefold increase of renal artery stenosis in patients with type II diabetes and many authors found a prevalence of 11–23% of severe renal artery stenosis during routine cardiac catheterization.[5-7] Harding et al.[5] found that old age, cardiac disease and peripheral vascular disease were the most important predictors of the presence of renal artery stenosis.

The natural history of renal artery stenosis, particularly atherosclerotic, is of progression of severity. This tendency was reported more than 30 years ago by Dustan[8] and by Wollenweber[9] who showed significant progression (> 50%) after a mean of 4–6 years of angiographic follow-up. More recently, precise figures of progression of renal artery stenosis became available from longitudinal follow-up studies. Using duplex ultrasonography, Zierler et al.,[10] reported the rate of progression in 76 patients screened for renal artery stenosis over a mean period of 32 months. In 132 arteries (20 arteries were excluded) an average progression rate of 7%

per year was found for all categories of baseline disease. However, when the groups were examined separately, the rate of significant progression in stenoses >60% was 30% at 1 year, 44% at 2 years, and 48% at 3 years. All four renal arteries in this study that progressed to occlusion had severe stenoses (>60%) at the initial visit. Most important, in those arteries with a severe stenosis at presentation, the cumulative incidence of progression to occlusion was 15% at 3 years. Similarly the Cleveland group[11] performed serial angiograms in 85 patients with renal artery stenosis over a 52-month period and found progression in 44% of patients. From these and other similar studies[12,13] it is clear that the degree of the initial stenosis best predicts rate of progression.

Atherosclerosis is the most common cause of renal artery disease responsible for 60–90% of all cases undergoing renal revascularization procedures.[14] This wide variability in its incidence is due to predominance of an ageing cohort of patients in some studies[15] compared with others.[16] The disease may be limited to the renal arteries (15–20% of cases) but is more often a manifestation of diffuse atherosclerosis involving the abdominal aorta, coronary, cerebral, or lower extremity vessels (80–85% of cases).[17] The lesion tends to be osteal or in the proximal third of the artery and is bilateral in approximately 50% of cases (own observation). The pathology of these lesions is similar to atherosclerosis elsewhere with intimal thickening, cholesterol deposition and sclerosis. There is a predominance of this disease in males older than 50 years. Another and more subtle form of atherosclerotic renal artery disease is atheroembolism. This manifestation, identified on renal biopsy specimens, is often associated with renal artery stenosis and systemic atherosclerosis. The cholesterol emboli are usually precipitated by anticoagulation, angiography, angioplasty, surgery or thrombolysis.[18,19]

Fibromuscular dysplasia represents the second most common cause of renal artery disease. Patients with fibromuscular dysplasia are usually female, less than 40 years old and stigmata of generalized vascular disease are absent. The lesions of fibromuscular dysplasia are often characterized by heavy deposition of collagen in the intima, media and/or the adventitia of the main renal artery or its segmental branches and can cause aneurysms as well as stenoses.

Arteritides such as Takayasu's, Kawasaki's, and polyarteritis nodosum are rare causes of renal artery disease as are aortic and renal artery dissection. Traumatic injuries of the renal vessels on the other hand are becoming more frequent and present an increasing therapeutic challenge.

The clinical manifestations of renal artery disease are usually hypertension and loss of renal function. Hypertension can be caused by stenosis of one or both renal arteries. This manifestation has been studied extensively since the advent of the two-kidney, one-clip model of renovascular hypertension[20] well over 60 years ago. The basic physiological events are reduction of blood flow by the stenotic lesion which leads to increased secretion of renin by the juxtaglomelular cells and causes the conversion of circulating angiotensinogen to angiotensin I then II with subsequent vasoconstriction, fluid retention and hypertension. Although renal artery disease is quite common in hypertensive patients,[20] it is generally held that renal artery stenosis is the cause in 5% of all cases.[21]

In contrast, loss of renal function or ischaemic nephropathy occurs only in the presence of high-grade (>75%) stenosis affecting the entire renal mass, i.e. bilateral renal artery stenosis or renal artery stenosis of a solitary kidney. There is increasing data documenting the true prevalence of ischaemic nephropathy as a cause of end stage renal failure. Mailloux *et al.*[22] in a retrospective study identified ischaemic nephropathy as the primary cause of end stage renal failure in 6.7% of patients between 1970 and 1981 and in 16.5% of patients between 1982 and 1985. In a prospective study at the Royal Free Hospital renal angiography was performed in all new patients with end stage renal failure during an 18-month period.[23] Ischaemic nephropathy was found to be the cause of end stage renal failure in 6% of all patients, and in 14% of patients older than 50 years of age. The pathophysiological events leading to ischaemic nephropathy are complex and ill-understood. It frequently co-exists with hypertension, and the current hypothesis suggest that chronic parenchymal ischaemia combined with adenosine triphosphate (ATP) depletion, alteration in intracellular calcium, oxygen radicals and apoptotic cell death results in fibrosis and tubular atrophy.[24]

ASSESSMENT OF RENOVASCULAR DISEASE

Renovascular disease is a progressive disorder with serious sequela if appropriate therapy is not instituted. The majority of patients will have generalized atherosclerosis and a multidisciplinary team approach involving renal physician, cardiologist, vascular interventional radiologist and surgeon is necessary for achieving optimal therapeutic results.

Assessment of renovascular hypertension

Accurate diagnosis of renovascular hypertension is very difficult and complex. The presence of renal artery stenosis on angiograms is not necessarily synonymous with renovascular hypertension because many patients with renal artery stenosis are normotensive or simply have essential hypertension. This diagnosis, therefore remains presumptive until a cure or improvement of hypertension is achieved after anatomical correction of renal artery stenosis with surgery or angioplasty.

Diagnosis is facilitated by the presence of a bruit in the upper quadrant or flank particularly if it remains present during diastole. Many tests have been useful in diagnosis including intravenous pyelography (IVP), simple and captopril isotope renography using ^{131}I-iodohippurate (hippuran), ^{99m}Tc-diethylenetriaminepentacetic acid (DTPA) or 99mTc-mercaptoacetyltriglycine (Mag$_3$), duplex ultrasonography, plasma and renal vein renin, angiography and recently spiral computed tomography (CT) and magnetic resonant angiography (MRA). Of these tests angiography remains the gold standard with approximately 90% sensitivity and specificity supplemented when necessary with isotope renography and renal vein renin. The use of duplex ultrasound, spiral CT and MRA has mostly been restricted to screening purposes.

The low prevalence[21] and lack of certainty in diagnosis of this condition[25] make the decision for interventional treatment quite difficult. The currently accepted indications for treatment of renovascular hypertension are resistance to medical therapy,[25] accelerated or malignant hypertension,[26,27] deterioration of renal function with antihypertensive treatment in general and angiotensin converting enzyme inhibition in particular.[28,29] Further important indications include unexplained or recurrent flash pulmonary oedema in hypertensive patients with good left ventricular function[30] and the development of hypertension following renal vessel trauma.

Assessment of ischaemic nephropathy

The increasing awareness of the detrimental effect of renovascular disease on renal function[31] and the improved success rates of both interventional and surgical revascularization have led to a more liberal attitude towards early treatment. Intervention is generally reserved for patients considered fit for percutaneous transluminal renal angioplasty (PTRA) or reconstructive surgery in whom there is hypertension and unexplained renal insufficiency or a significant size disparity between the two kidneys. The reduction in renal size is the inevitable end result of severe and sustained reduction in renal blood flow and glomerular filtration rate leading to tubular atrophy and nephrosclerosis.

Tests, therefore, should include renal ultrasound examination to measure renal size, assessment of renal function with creatinine clearance or captopril renography with Mag_3 and imaging of the renal arteries similar to that performed for renovascular hypertension. It is worth noting here, that the diagnostic accuracy of functional tests used for renovascular hypertension is reduced in the presence of severe renal insufficiency.[32]

Unlike renovascular hypertension, interventional treatment is probably best reserved for when there is clear evidence of high-grade (> 75%) stenosis affecting the entire renal mass, namely bilateral renal artery stenosis or renal artery stenosis in a solitary kidney. The aim in this situation is to improve renal function or stop its progression to end stage renal failure. The benefit of revascularization for preservation of renal function in a unilateral renal artery stenosis is not clear if the contralateral kidney is anatomically and functionally normal. Dean *et al.*[33] demonstrated this in a retrospective review of 53 patients who underwent surgical revascularization for ischaemic nephropathy. The postoperative glomerular filtration rate was improved in 41 patients treated for bilateral renal artery stenosis, but was unaltered in 12 patients with unilateral renal artery stenosis. There is an exception to this scenario, when the opposite kidney is functioning but affected by parenchymal disease where revascularization of the ischaemic kidney may benefit some patients.

Severity of renal insufficiency as measured by the level of serum creatinine and the rate of deterioration of renal function can influence the results of revascularization for ischaemic nephropathy. Greatest benefit from relief of renal artery stenosis was recorded in patients who suffered rapid deterioration of renal function in the 6 months preceding revascularization,[33] in patients who developed acute renal failure soon after initiation of medical antihypertensive therapy[28,29] and in patients with serum creatinine less than 350 μmol/l.[34,35] Patients with end stage renal failure[36] or with serum creatinine levels greater than 350 μmol/l[34,37] had much poorer outcome unless renal biopsy was positively identified viable glomeruli and excluded severe changes of nephrosclerosis, glomerular hyalinization and cholesterol embolization.[18,34,37–39]

TREATMENT OF RENOVASCULAR DISEASE

The aim of treatment of renovascular disease is to reverse ischaemia. Since to date medical therapy can only control hypertension without a favourable effect on renal ischaemia, a functionally significant renal artery stenosis should therefore be corrected with either endovascular treatment or surgery. Delaying treatment should be avoided as there is clear evidence that the success of interventional treatment is inversely proportional to the duration of renovascular ischaemia.[40] In the future the advent of ever more powerful lipid-lowering agents may allow treatment of atherosclerosis by medical means alone.

When reviewing the results of treatment of renal artery stenosis, one must take into consideration variations in reporting standards. Accurate reporting of cure, improvement, benefit and technical success depends heavily on establishing comparable patient selection, indications, end-points and follow-up. Adding to this problem is the inherent bias in selecting different interventions – i.e. angioplasty vs surgery which relies heavily on the locally available expertise. Thus it is particularly difficult to assess treatment because the literature is characterized by these deficiencies and biases.

In renovascular hypertension cure is defined as a diastolic blood pressure of less than or equal to 90 mmHg without the need for hypertensive medication. Improvement is defined as either a 15% reduction in diastolic blood pressure or a diastolic blood pressure less than or equal to 90 mmHg with reduction of antihypertensive medication. Benefit is considered either cure or improvement.[41] It is always worth remembering that technical success is not always translated into clinical cure which highlights again the value of accurate diagnosis and the appropriate selection of the interventional procedure.

Assessment of success in ischaemic nephropathy treatment is more challenging. Although success is defined as an improvement or stabilization of renal function following intervention, the problem arises when considering the large number of tests used to assess renal function. Most studies used serum creatinine before and after intervention.[34–36] Others, used creatinine clearance, slope plots of serum creatinine[42] or estimation of glomerular filtration rate using various techniques.[33,43]

ENDOVASCULAR TREATMENT OF RENOVASCULAR DISEASE

Percutaneous transluminal renal angioplasty

Since the introduction of this novel treatment modality in 1978,[44] improvements in guide-wire technology, catheters, balloons and introduction of endovascular stents[45] have led to a huge increase in its use.

Percutaneous transluminal renal angioplasty is currently considered the procedure of choice for renovascular hypertension in general and fibromuscular dysplasia lesions in particular. Fibromuscular dysplasia lesions are usually subosteal/truncal or even peripheral in the branches of the renal artery. These lesions dilate easily and since they are fibrotic rather than elastic in nature, recoil is relatively uncommon and healing establishes the dilated state. In atherosclerotic lesions, the majority of the stenotic lesions are osteal or even in the aortic wall itself with the non-osteal lesions responsible for 30–40% of atherosclerotic renal artery stenosis only. These osteal lesions are more difficult and hazardous to treat. Dilatation is usually achieved by splitting rather than extruding or compressing the atheroma which may explain the less satisfactory results found in arteriosclerosis.

The success rates of PTRA for fibromuscular dysplasia are quite high. Technical success rates close to 90% (86–100%) are matched by clinical improvement or cure of hypertension in 75–100% of patients (Table 1). In a meta-analysis of 16 studies,[46] 370 patients were treated with PTRA for fibromuscular dysplasia. The technical success rate was 94%. Their follow-up showed a cure rate of 49% and an improvement in the control of hypertension in 43%. The overall clinical benefit is therefore 92% making PTRA the treatment of choice for this condition. The factors associated with cure were highlighted by Davidson et al.[47] in a study of 23 consecutive patients undergoing PTRA for fibromuscular dystrophy. Twelve (52.2%) of the patients were cured. Using logistic regression, they found younger patients, milder hypertension and shorter duration were independently associated with cure.

In atherosclerosis the beneficial yield of PTRA is lower than that reported for fibromuscular dystrophy. Jensen et al.[48] assessed the results of 180 PTRA performed over a 10-year period: fibromuscular dystrophy was present in 22% and atherosclerotic renovascular disease in 78%. Successful technical dilatation was achieved in 97% of fibromuscular dystrophy patients and in 82% of atherosclerotic renovascular disease patients. A beneficial effect on the blood pressure and the renal function was registered in both groups. The overall cure and improvement rate for hypertension was 86% in the fibromuscular dystrophy group and 64% in the

Table 1. Results of PTRA for treatment of renovascular hypertension in fibromuscular dysplasia

Author	Year	Patients (No.)	Technical success (%)	Cure (%)	Improvement (%)	Benefit (%)
Sos[81]	1983	31	87	59	33	92
Martin[91]	1985	20	82	25	60	85
Millan[92]	1985	16	86	67	25	92
Greminger[93]	1989	34	–	41	47	88
Klinge[84]	1989	52	90	38	55	93
Baert[94]	1990	19	86	58	21	79
Tegtmeyer[95]	1991	66	100	39	59	98
Rodriguez-Perez[87]	1994	27	92	50	25	75
Karagiannis[88]	1995	16	88	71.4	29	100
Jensen[48]	1995	30	97	–	–	86
Von Knorring[89]	1996	12	100	45	55	100
Mali[90]	1997	47	95	35	51	86
Pooled results		370	91	48	42	90

atherosclerotic renovascular disease group after 1 year follow-up. Table 2 summarizes the results of PTRA for atherosclerotic renovascular disease in 13 studies. Technical success varied between 57% and 95% with a mean of 82% and over all clinical benefit varied between 63% and 94% with a mean of 76%. The reported cure rate in this group of patients was only 10–20%, with the remainder requiring additional medical treatment or reintervention. Taking into account that technical failures (20% of these patients) are not included as treatment failures according to the 'intention to treat' principle, simple calculation reveals that the overall success for PTRA in atherosclerotic renovascular disease is therefore no higher than 50–60%. This low yield in terms of blood pressure control and patency of dilation is due to the diffuse nature of atherosclerotic renovascular disease and the predominance of osteal lesions.[49] In a study by Canzanello et al.,[50] 100 patients treated with PTRA for high grade (>75%) atherosclerotic rental artery stenosis, the technical success rate was 73% (72% for non-osteal, 62% for osteal) and the clinical success rate was 43% (53% for non-osteal, 25% for osteal). The poor results associated with the osteal lesion made the role of PTRA in the treatment of atherosclerotic renal artery stenosis rather limited.

Complications from PTRA are rare and occur in approximately 5% of cases.[51] Most of them are minor haematomas at the puncture sites. More serious complications such as false aneurysms, peripheral embolization, embolization into the treated kidney with subsequent infarction and worsening of renal function are less frequent. Local complications at the site of the angioplasty such as thrombosis, dissection or uncontrollable haemorrhage may necessitate emergency surgery and nephrectomies in approximately 0.5% of cases.[52] It is worth remembering that although PTRA is a benign procedure, death can occur as a consequence of these complications or from other associated morbid cardiovascular conditions.

Contraindications to PTRA are few, the most important are high risk of cholesterol embolization and allergy to contrast medium. In a study by Wilms et al.[53] 50 patients

Table 2. Results of PTRA for treatment of renovascular hypertension in atherosclerosis

Author	Year	Patients (No.)	Technical success (%)	Cure (%)	Improvement (%)	Benefit (%)
Sos[81]	1983	51	57	–	–	84
Tegtmeyer[82]	1984	65	94	23	71	94
Miller[83]	1985	34	87	15	49	64
Klinge[84]	1989	134	77	10	68	78
Martin[85]	1992	94	78	22	46	68
Weibull[76]	1993	29	83	12	71	83
Losinno[86]	1994	153	95	12	51	63
Rodriguez-Perez[87]	1994	37	78	0	81	81
Karagiannis[88]	1995	62	72	19	52	71
Jensen[48]	1995	107	82	–	–	64
Von Knorring[89]	1996	38	92	11	74	85
Mali[90]	1997	115	92	10	70	80
Pooled results		919	82	13	63	76

had normal renal function prior to PTRA. Five of these patients (10%) developed renal dysfunction following PTRA, indeed one of them (2%) required temporary haemodialysis. He attributed the deterioration of renal function to contrast medium toxicity and cholesterol embolization. Thus a severely diseased and tortuous aorta is more likely to result in atheroembolism and represents a relative contraindication to PTRA.

One of the other major problems that hindered the long-term results of PTRA is restenosis. It frequently occurs in the first few months after angioplasty and is due either to elastic recoil of the dilated artery, neointimal hyperplasia, or recurrent atheromatous disease.[54] Many imaging studies have confirmed restenosis as the predominant cause of failure following successful PTRA. Restenosis of atherosclerotic lesions occurs in approximately 30% of non-osteal, 50% of osteal lesions, 20% of non-specific aortoarteritis in children[55] and 10% of fibromuscular dystrophy lesions.[56] It is important to stress that all of these lesions are suitable for redilatation without stenting with considerable success.[57]

Endovascular stenting

The use of stent angioplasty was developed as a response to the poor results of PTRA in osteal stenoses and to prevent elastic recoil of stenosed arteries. The idea of endovascular stenting dates back to 1969 when Charles Dotter used stainless steel coils inside normal canine arteries.[58] Since then three types of stents have been developed: shape memory alloy (nitinol), balloon expandable (Palmaz, Strecker) and self-expanding (Wallstent, Gianturcco) stents. The use of stents in the treatment of endovascular disease started in 1989. The most commonly used is the Palmaz stent due to the precision by which this stent can be deployed.

Stent deployment is a very challenging procedure which requires a high level of expertise from the interventional radiologist. The 90 degree angle between the aortic wall and the renal arteries makes the positioning of the stent for osteal stenosis particularly difficult. Renal artery stents are relatively short and inflexible. Protrusion of the stent into the aortic lumen by 2–3 mm is necessary to prevent the elastic recoil of the aortic wall at the renal ostium. Failure to achieve this would necessitate the insertion of a second stent to overcome the problem adding to the expense and possible complications.

The main indications for stenting are osteal stenoses and restenosis. Due to the poor outcome of PTRA in these lesions, many clinicians have adopted a policy of primary stenting. The remaining indications for stent placement are salvage procedures to rescue unsuccessful balloon angioplasty such as residual stenosis greater than 50%, trans-stenotic pressure gradient ≥ 20 mmHg and the occurrence of complications during PTRA such as acute thrombosis and intimal dissection. The results of renal artery stenting from 10 studies are summarized in Table 3. Technical successes varied between 75% and 100% with a mean success of 96%. The impressive 100% success rates seen in the most recent studies represent the growing experience with this technique and the improvement in guide-wires, catheters and balloon technology, all of which are necessary for the appropriate deployment of stents. In these studies restenosis rates after stenting varied between 12% and 25% with a mean rate of 16% which is much lower than that encountered after PTRA alone of similar

Table 3. Results of endovascular stenting for renal artery stenosis

Author	Year	Stent (No.)	Patients (%)	Technical success (%)	Restenosis (%)	Mean follow-up (%)
Kuhn[96]	1991	Strecker	10	75	18	–
Rees[45]	1991	Palmaz	28	97	25	5
Hennequin[97]	1994	Wallstent	21	90	20	29
Raynaud[98]	1994	Wallstent	18	100	12	11
Dorros[99]	1995	Palmaz	76	100	25	6
Van De Ven[100]	1995	Palmaz	24	100	16	6
Iannone[101]	1996	Palmaz	63	99	14	69
Blum[59]	1997	Palmaz	75	100	11	27
Harden[42]	1997	Palmaz	32	100	12	24
Taylor[102]	1997	Palmaz	29	100	16	25
Pooled results			376	96	17	22

lesions. Although the mean follow-up period for accurate assessment of restenosis was short in most studies, many had mean follow-up of 24 months or greater with consistently low restenosis rates.

Complications after stenting appear to be higher than after PTRA. Harden *et al.*[42] reported six complications in 32 patients (18%) and one of them resulted in fatality from a major haemorrhage. Less dramatic were the three minor haematomas reported by Blum *et al.*[59] in a series of 75 patients (4%). This increase in the complication rate after stenting is probably due to the larger introducing cannulae (sheaths) and to cannulation of a second artery for the introduction of a second angiographic catheter.

Endovascular treatment to preserve renal function

Renovascular disease is one of the very few forms of correctable renal failure. Deterioration of renal function as a result of renovascular disease occurs when there is severe bilateral renal artery stenosis, severe unilateral renal artery stenosis with an occlusion of the contralateral renal artery or severe unilateral renal artery stenosis in a solitary functional kidney where the second kidney is absent or affected by parenchymal disease. Traditionally, PTRA in these patients has been contraindicated for fear of precipitating acute exacerbation leading to end stage renal failure in the setting of already compromised renal function. Most of these patients have therefore received surgical treatment in the past. In recent years there have been increasing reports on the use of endovascular treatment for revascularization of bilateral renal artery stenosis or renal artery stenosis in a solitary functioning kidney.

Bilateral PTRA with or without stenting will certainly increase the risk of complications, and authors who declared their willingness to perform bilateral angioplasties, did so, providing that the revascularization procedure on the first renal artery had gone well.

There have been a number of published reports describing the outcome of endovascular treatment in patients with impaired renal function with serum creatinine values of > 150 µmol/l. Early on, Madias et al.[60] noted stabilization or improvement in renal function of seven of 11 patients with severe hypertension and renal impairment after PTRA. Later, Pickering et al.[61] reported his success in 55 patients with atherosclerotic renal artery stenosis and progressive uraemia. Twenty-six patients (47%) had significant and sustained reduction in serum creatinine concentrations during the 2-year follow-up. Table 4 shows a summary of more recent studies of the effect of PTRA and/or stenting on patients with severe renovascular disease and impaired renal function. Approximately 42% of patients had improvement of renal function over a follow-up period of at least 6 months. In a further 32% renal function was stabilized and in 26% renal function deteriorated. Several patients in these series became dialysis independent having already reached end-stage renal failure prior to endovascular intervention.[42,62]

Although all the eight studies in Table 4 reported improvement of renal function after endovascular intervention, many others failed to demonstrate any significant change in the renal function in their patient after similar procedures.[59,63–65] In a case report of four patients, Mikhail et al.[43] showed that the improvement in renal function after PTRA was only temporary, and in all four patients renal function deteriorated again. Repeat angiograms in these patients excluded restenosis in all but one who required a second angioplasty and insertion of stent. In this patient, renal function improved temporarily before deteriorating again, repeat angiogram at this time excluded restenosis. A possible explanation for this and other failures is likely to be the development of nephrosclerosis in the tubules of the revascularized kidney which were previously protected from the systemic effects of hypertension, invariably present in this group of patients. The occurrence of atheroembolism could also provide another more likely explanation.

Table 4.   Results of endovascular interventions (PTRA ± stenting) for ischaemic nephropathy with main indication being renal failure

Author	Year	Patients (No.)	Improved (%)	Stabilized (%)	Deteriorated (%)	No. of patients who came off dialysis (%)
Wilms[53]	1989	29	48	37	13	–
Pattison[103]	1992	60	40	50	10	–
O'Donovan[62]	1992	17	41	23	36	3
Pattynama[104]	1994	40	60	–	40	–
Iannone[101]	1996	29	36	46	18	–
Harden[42]	1997	23	34	34	28	2
Taylor[102]	1997	29	33	29	38	–
Boisclair[105]	1997	17	41	35	24	–
Pooled results		244	42	32	26	5

Surgical treatment of renal artery stenosis

Surgical treatment has until recently been considered as the most effective and reliable method of revascularization for renal artery stenosis. Due to the high success rate of angioplasty in treating renovascular hypertension, PTRA became the first-line treatment particularly for stenoses caused by fibromuscular dystrophy. The early bias towards surgical treatment of osteal atherosclerotic renal artery stenosis has now been reversed by the technical success of endovascular stenting.

Despite this change in renal revascularization, surgery still has a pivotal role to play particularly where the attempted endovascular procedure fails to correct the stenotic lesion or because of development of complications. This secondary or salvaging role for surgery is strengthened by some important primary indications. Surgical revascularization of renal artery disease should be the method of choice for renal artery aneurysm, renal artery occlusion, severe impassable renal artery stenosis, severe bilateral disease, disease in a solitary functioning kidney, stenosis of multiple renal arteries and in renal artery stenosis associated with occlusive or aneurysmal disease of the abdominal aorta.[66] In the extremes of age renal artery stenosis may benefit from planned and controlled operative revascularization.[67]

Although surgical revascularization is aimed at controlling severe hypertension in few cases, most of the indications for this approach is now for salvaging renal[15] function in otherwise a very high-risk group of patients. Intensive preoperative evaluation, optimizing cardiac, respiratory and renal function and perioperative monitoring are all important if serious complication is to be avoided and mortality rates reduced.

The choice of surgical techniques for renal artery reconstruction depends on the underlying pathology and anatomic distribution of the disease. The predominance of unilateral aortorenal bypass as a conduit in the past has been replaced by a variety of innovative extra-anatomical bypasses such as hepato-right-renal, gastroduodenal-right-renal, spleno-left-renal and ilio-renal bypasses[15,66,68] (Fig. 1). These operations are likely to produce less morbidity and mortality by avoiding dissection around the abdominal aorta and obviating the need to use the frequently diseased aortic wall for proximal anastamosis. Cardiac complications are also less likely to occur as clamping of the aorta, which would otherwise increase the stress on the cardiovascular system, is avoided.

Extra-anatomical bypasses are performed by direct anastamosis or by using an intermediate conduit such as polytetrafluoroethyline (PTFE) synthetic graft or non-reversed/reversed long saphenous vein, both proven to be quite durable and successful. An essential prerequisite for performing these bypasses is the presence of a disease-free coeliac axis. In our experience stenoses of the origin of the coeliac axis and the superior mesenteric artery are found in up to 40–50% of these patients. Although less frequently reported by Valentine *et al.* (27%),[69] it remains very important to perform mesenteric angiography with lateral views to exclude any significant stenosis that may impair donor flow. In this situation the aorta as an inflow may therefore still be necessary particularly if bilateral renal artery revascularization is also required (Fig. 2). In the presence of severely diseased infrarenal aorta, alternatives will be either the iliac arteries or the supracoeliac/lower thoracic aorta which are likely to be less affected by atherosclerosis[70] (Fig. 3). In the

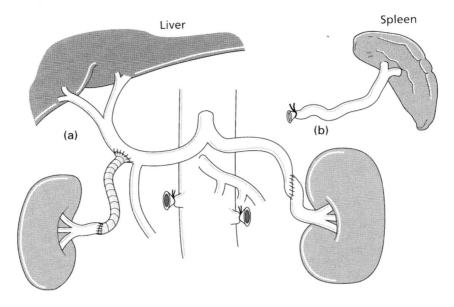

Fig. 1. Extra-anatomical renal bypass; (a) on the right side end-to-end grafting from the hepatic artery using the gastroduodenal artery if big enough (up to 50% of patients) or a saphenous vein or PTFE interposition graft; (b) on the left side an end-to-end anastomosis of the splenic artery into the left renal artery – the spleen does not need to be removed since it will survive on the short gastric arteries and collaterals.

case of simultaneous aortic and renal artery reconstructions, the aortic graft provides an adequate and easy site for the proximal anastomosis.[71]

Another useful operation for renal revascularization is endarterectomy. This operation was the first recorded procedure for renal revascularization when it was performed by Freeman[72] more than 40 years ago. This procedure remains suitable for focal stenosis of the renal ostium (Fig. 4).

Objective assessment of the results of surgical revascularization is extremely difficult. There are as many operations as there are indications for doing them. Most series do not differentiate between the outcome of primary surgical intervention and interventions for salvage of failed endovascular treatment. To further complicate this muddle there is absence of unified reporting standards for morbidity, mortality and early and late failures.

With improvement in antihypertensive therapy and advances in endovascular techniques, surgery is now frequently performed on a much older and sicker cohort of patients. These frequently have more severe forms of renovascular disease with high prevalence of co-morbid conditions such as coronary artery disease and occlusive or aneurysmal disease of the aorta.

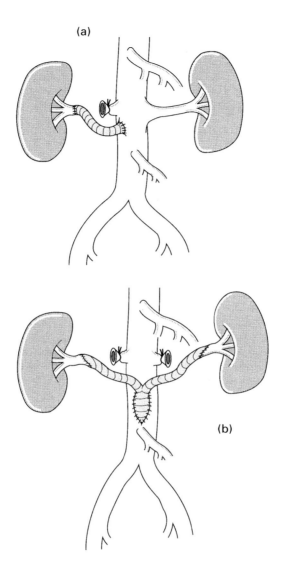

Fig. 2. Aorta-renal bypass grafting; if the infrarenal aorta is sufficiently healthy either a single (a) or bilateral (b) renal revascularization may be performed.

What is clear from the majority of reports is that the patency rate or technical success of surgical procedures is very impressive. Most report primary patency rates between 93%[73] and 97%.[74] Restenosis is also very low, reported in the literature to occur in 3–4%.[75,76] Morbidity rates vary between 6%[74] and 43%[77] with a mean rate of approximately 15%. Mortality rates are 2%[73] to 8%[78] being higher in combined aortic and renal reconstruction than in renal reconstruction alone. Myocardial infarction

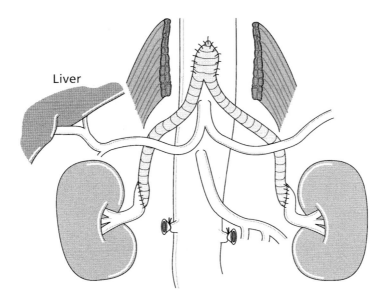

Fig. 3. The use of the supracoeliac aorta as the in-flow site: where the infrarenal aorta is not suitable and does not require resection, division of the crus of the diaphragm via a bilateral subcostal incision allows access to a good length of supracoeliac aorta which is a good site for an in-flow graft – this can be achieved with partial aortic clamping.

and other related cardiac events are the most common cause of postoperative death and morbidity. Cure or improvement of hypertension varied from 63%[79] to 91%[80] with a mean of improvement of 77% in most studies. In renal failure, the successful preservation or restoration of renal function is 33%[79] to 91%[77] with an average success of 72% with many patients being rescued from dialysis.

CONCLUSION

The combination of low complication rate, minimal hospital stay and reasonable technical and clinical success rate, have made PTRA the favoured intervention and treatment of renal artery disease at the present time. The combination of PTRA with use of stents has further improved the primary technical success rate dramatically. As a result there has been a veritable explosion in the use of these interventions. This is based, however, on poor follow-up data over relatively short periods of time.

As always, selection is of vital importance and clearly patients with significant renal artery stenoses only should be considered for intervention. The data are clearly there showing that renal artery stenoses <50% have a very low rate of progression

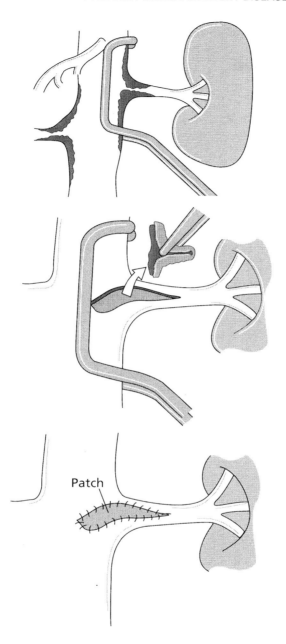

Fig. 4. Renal endarterectomy.

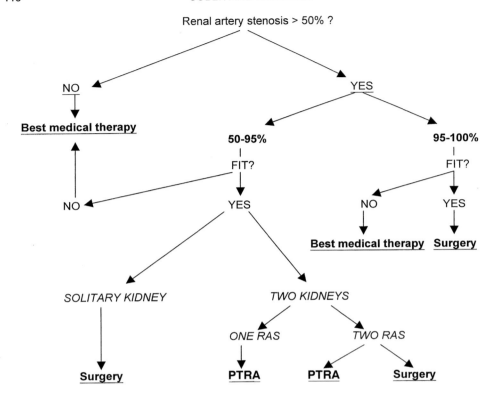

Fig. 5.   Algorithm of management of atherosclerotic renal artery disease (Royal Free
Hospital).

and this group should be treated aggressively by medical intervention in particular,
lipid lowering therapy. In contrast, the reliable follow-up data for angioplasty with or
without stenting that exists shows a disturbingly high restenosis rate for PTRA
overall, being in the region of 40% at 2 years. More worrying still is the high
restenosis rate seen after renal stent angioplasty being approximately 40% at 1
year.[45,106] Restenosis within the stented renal artery is extremely difficult to treat
interventionally and surgical reconstruction is undoubtably made more complex in
the authors' experience and virtually precludes the use of renal endarterectomy.
Longer term analysis of the results of angioplasty including the use of stents suggests
that this treatment modality slows the progression of renal arteriosclerosis and
failure but perhaps only by a period of 1–2 years. The role of aggressive medical
therapy in this situation remains to be defined but may improve the results further.

Individual series generally stress the low morbidity and mortality achieved with
PTRA but a meta-analysis performed in 1993 of published reports of renal
revascularization, showed a similar mortality rate overall for angioplasty at 5% and
surgery at 6%.[107] As in surgery, selection of patients for PTRA is of paramount

importance with obvious contraindications being renal artery occlusion, severely diseased and atheromatous aorta and poor cardiorespiratory status. Perhaps in this small cohort of patients, neither PTRA or surgical revascularization are safe and this group may be better served by renal replacement therapy.

Results of surgical revascularization both from the technical and clinical point of view are good with dramatically lower restenosis rates. The major risk factors in these patients are the underlying cardiac, respiratory and peripheral vascular disease, particularly extracranial disease. Proper selection after exhaustive preoperative assessment for these risk factors will give lower morbidity and mortality. Surgical revascularization avoiding full cross-clamping or replacement of the aorta will also give much better results.

Thus there is a clear case for tailoring the preferred treatment according to the severity of the disease. Patients with good renal function and bilateral renal artery stenoses (>50%) with a good radiological appearance should be treated initially with PTRA. There is a case for performing second- or third-time PTRA without stenting for restenosis rather than using primary stent PTRA.[76] Comparison of repeated PTRA with primary stent PTRA is an important area for future study. Patients with high grade stenoses (>75%), particularly where the aorta is hostile and who are fit for surgery should be considered for a primary surgical intervention, ideally avoiding the aorta. Patients with a solitary functioning kidney, and with renal failure should be considered for surgical intervention rather than angioplasty (Fig. 5 algorithm).

Having expressed our therapeutic bias it is clear that it is now timely to move on to more scientific assessment of these treatment modalities. Agreement on comparable and reliable methods of assessing severity of disease, severity of stenosis and technical and clinical results both in the long- and short-term are required. Finally the most pressing need in the management of renal artery disease is for properly conducted prospective trials assessing the role and importance of aggressive medical therapy, simple and stent PTRA, and surgery.

REFERENCES

1. Greco B, Breyer J: The natural history of renal artery stenosis: Who should be evaluated for suspected ischaemic nephropathy. *Semin Nephrol* **16**: 2–11, 1996
2. Holley KE, Hunt JC, Brown AL *et al.*: Renal artery stenosis: A clinical-pathologic study in normotensive and hypertensive patients. *Am J Med* **37**: 14–22, 1964
3. Olin JW, Melia M, Young JR, *et al.*: Prevalence of atherosclerotic renal artery stenosis in patients with atherosclerosis elsewhere. *Am J Med* **88**: 46–51, 1990
4. Sawiki PT, Kaiser S, Heinmann L, *et al.*: Prevalence of renal artery stenosis in diabetes mellitus-an autopsy study. *J Int Med* **229**: 489–92, 1991
5. Harding MB, Smith LR, Himmelstein SI, *et al.*: Renal artery stenosis: prevalence and associated risk factors in patients undergoing routine cardiac catheterization. *J Am Soc Nephrol* **2**: 1608–16, 1992
6. Jean WJ, Al-Bitar I, Zwicke DL, *et al.*: High incidence of renal artery stenosis in patients with coronary artery disease. *Cathet Cardiovasc Diagn* **32**: 8–10, 1994
7. Vetrovec GW, Landwehr DM, Edwards VL: Incidence of renal artery stenosis in hypertensive patients undergoing coronary angiography. *J Intervent Cardiol* **2**: 69–76, 1989
8. Dustan HP, Meaney TF, Page IH: Comparative treatment of renovascular hypertension. In: Gross F (Ed.) *Antihypertensive Therapy*, pp. 544–56. New York: Springer-Verlag, 1966

9. Wollenweber J, Sheps SG, Davis GD: Clinical course of atherosclerotic renovascular disease. *Am J Cardiol* **21**: 60–71, 1968
10. Zierler RE, Bergelin RO, Davidson RC *et al.*: A prospective study of disease progression in patients with atherosclerotic renal artery stenosis. *Am J Hypertens* **9**: 1055-61, 1996
11. Schreiber MJ, Pohl MA, Novick AC: The natural history of atherosclerotic and fibrous renal artery disease. *Urol Clin N Am* **11**: 383–92, 1984
12. Dean RH, Kieffer RW, Smith BM *et al.*: Renovascular hypertension: Anatomic and renal function changes during drug therapy. *Arch Surg* **116**: 1408–15, 1981
13. Tollefson DFJ, Ernst CB: Natural history of atherosclerotic renal artery stenosis associated with aortic disease. *J Vasc Surg* **14**: 327–31, 1991
14. Hypertension WGOR: Detection, evaluation, and treatment of renovascular hypertension. *Arch Intern Med* **147**: 820–9, 1987
15. Bredenberg CE, Sampson LN, Ray FS *et al.*: Changing patterns in surgery for chronic renal artery occlusive diseases. *J Vasc Surg* **15**: 1018–23, 1992
16. Weaver FA, Kuehne JP, Papanicolaou G: A recent institutional experience with renovascular hypertension. *Am Surg* **62**: 241–5, 1996
17. Novick AC: Options for therapy of ischemic nephropathy: role of angioplasty and surgery. *Semin Nephrol* **16**: 53–60, 1996
18. Vidt DG, Eisele G, Gephardt GN *et al.*: Atheroembolic renal disease: association with renal arterial stenosis. *Cleveland Clin J Med* **56**: 407–13, 1989
19. Robson MG, Scoble JE: Atheroembolic disease. *Br J Hosp Med* **55**: 648–52, 1996
20. Goldblatt H, Lynch J, Hanzal RF *et al.*: Studies on experimental hypertension. 1. The production of persistent elevation of blood pressure by means of renal ischemia. *J Exp Med* **59**: 347–79, 1934
21. Pickering TG: Renovascular hypertension: Medical evaluation and non-surgical treatment. In: Laragh JH, Brenner BM (Eds), *Hypertension*, pp. 1539–60. New York: Raven Press, 1990.
22. Mailloux LU, Napolitano B, Bellucci AG *et al.*: Renal vascular disease causing end-stage renal failure, incidence, clinical corrolates, and outcome: A 20 year clinical experience. *Am J Kidney Dis* **24**: 622–29, 1994
23. Scoble JE, Maher ER, Hamilton G *et al.*: Atherosclerotic renovascular disease causing renal impairment: a case for treatment. *Clin Nephrol* **31**: 119–22, 1989
24. Kellerman PS: Cellular and metabolic consequences of chronic ischaemia on kidney function. *Semin Nephrol* **16**: 33–42, 1996
25. Ram CV, Clagett GP, Radford LR: Renovascular hypertension. *Semin Nephrol* **15**: 152–74, 1995
26. Davis BA, Crook JE, Vestal RE, Oates JA: Prevalence of renovascular hypertension in patients with grade III or IV hypertensive retinopathy. *New Engl J Med* **301**: 1273–76, 1979
27. Ram CV: Diagnosis and management of hypertensive crisis. In: Rippe JM, Irwin RS, Alpert JS, Fink MP (Eds), *Intensive Care Medicine* 2nd edn, pp. 228–38. Boston: Little, Brown and Company, 1991.
28. Hricik DE, Brownin PJ, Kopelman R *et al.*: Captopril-induced functional renal insufficiency in patients with bilateral renal artery stenoses or renal artery stenosis in a solitary kidney. *New Engl J Med* **308**: 373–6, 1983
29. Wenting GJ, Tan-Tjiong HL, Derkx FMH *et al.*: Split renal function after captopril in unilateral renal artery stenosis. *Br Med J* **288**: 886–90, 1984
30. Pickering TG, Herman L, Devereux RB *et al.*: Recurrent pulmonary oedema in hypertension due to bilateral renal artery stenosis: treatment by angioplasty or surgical revascularisation. *Lancet* **2**: 551–2, 1988
31. Jacobson HR: Ischaemic nephropathy: An overlooked clinical entity? *Kidney Int* **34**: 729–43, 1988
32. Wilcox CS: Ischemic nephropathy: Noninvasive testing. *Semin Nephrol* **16**: 43–52, 1996
33. Dean RH, Tribble RW, Hansen KJ *et al.*: Evolution of renal insufficiency in ischemic nephropathy. *Ann Surg* **213**: 446–55, 1991
34. Mercier C, Piquet P, Alimi Y *et al.*: Occlusive disease of the renal arteries and chronic renal failure: the limits of reconstructive surgery. *Ann Vasc Surg* **4**: 166–70, 1990

35. Bedoya L, Ziegelbaum M, Vidt DG *et al.*: Baseline renal function and surgical revascularization in atherosclerotic renal arterial disease in the elderly. *Cleveland Clin J Med* **56**: 415–21, 1989

36. Kaylor WM, Novick AC, Ziegelbaum M, Vidt DG: Reversal of end stage renal failure with surgical revascularization in patients with atherosclerotic renal artery occlusion. *J Urol* **141**: 486–8, 1989

37. Chaikof EL, Smith R3, Salam AA *et al.*. Ischemic nephropathy and concomitant aortic disease: a ten-year experience. *J Vasc Surg* **19**: 135–46, 1994

38. Zinman L, Libertino JA: Revascularization of the chronic totally occluded renal artery with restoration of renal function. *J Urol* **118**: 17–21, 1977

39. Schefft P, Novick AC, Stewart BH *et al.*: Renal revascularization in patients with total occlusion of the renal artery. *J Urol* **124**: 184–6, 1980

40. Barry YM, Davidson RA, Senler S *et al.*: Prediction of cure of hypertension in atherosclerotic renal artery stenosis. *Southern Med J* **89**: 679–83, 1996

41. Kidney DD, Deutsch LS: The indications and results of percutaneous transluminal angioplasty and stenting in renal artery stenosis. *Semin Vasc Surg* **9**: 188–97, 1996

42. Harden PN, MacLeod MJ, Rodger RS *et al.*. Effect of renal artery stenting on progression of renovascular renal failure. *Lancet* **349**: 1133–6, 1997

43. Mikhail A, Cook GJ, Reidy J, Scoble JE:Progressive renal dysfunction despite successful renal artery angioplasty in a single kidney [letter]. *Lancet* **349**, 1997

44. Gruentzig A, Kuhlmann U, Vetter W *et al.*: Treatment of renovascular hypertension with percutaneous transluminal dilatation of a renal artery stenosis. *Lancet* **1**: 801–2, 1978

45. Rees CR, Palmaz JC, Becker GJ *et al.*: Palmaz stent in atherosclerotic stenoses involving the ostia of the renal arteries: preliminary report of a multicenter study. *Radiology* **181**: 507–14, 1991

46. Tegtmeyer CJ, Matsumoto AH, Angle JF: Percutaneous transluminal angioplasty in fibrous dysplasia and children. In: Novick AC, Scoble J, Hamilton G (Eds) *Renal Vascular Disease*, pp. 3636–83. London: WB Saunders Company Ltd., 1996

47. Davidson RA, Barri Y, Wilcox CS: Predictors of cure of hypertension in fibromuscular renovascular disease. *Am J Kid Dis* **28**: 334–8, 1996

48. Jensen G, Zachrisson BF, Delin K *et al.*: Treatment of renovascular hypertension: one year results of renal angioplasty. *Kid Int* **48**: 1936–45, 1995

49. Hayes JM, Risius B, Novick AC *et al.*. Experience with percutaneous transluminal angioplasty for renal artery stenosis at the Cleveland Clinic. *J Urol* **139**: 488–92, 1988

50. Canzanello VJ, Millan VG, Spiegel JE *et al.*: Percutaneous transluminal renal angioplasty in management of atherosclerotic renovascular hypertension: Results in 100 patients. *Hypertension* **13**: 163–72, 1989

51. Rodriguez PJ, Maynar MM, Perez BP *et al.*. [The long-term results on arterial pressure and kidney function after the percutaneous transluminal dilatation of renal artery stenosis]. [Spanish]. *Medicina Clinica* **108**: 366–72, 1997

52. Casarella WJ, Martin LG: Failed percutaneous transluminal renal angioplasty: experience with lesions requiring operative intervention [letter]. *J Vasc Surg* **7**: 821–2, 1988

53. Wilms G, Staessen J, Baert AL *et al.*: Percutaneous transluminal renal angioplasty and renal function. *Radiology* **29**: 195–200, 1989

54. Lenz T, Bussmann WD, Schmidt E, Grutzmacher P: Renal artery dilatation in renovascular hypertension. Acute and long-term outcome in a large patient sample. [German]. *Medizin Klinik* **91**: 442–6, 1996

55. Sharma S, Thatai D, Saxena A *et al.*: Renovascular hypertension resulting from nonspecific aortoarteritis in children: midterm results of percutaneous transluminal renal angioplasty and predictors of restenosis. *Am J Roentgenol* **166**: 157–62, 1996

56. Plouin PF, Darne B, Chatellier G *et al.*: Restenosis after a first percutaneous transluminal renal angioplasty. *Hypertension* **21**: 89–96, 1993

57. Tyagi S, Kaul UA, Satsangi DK, Arora R: Percutaneous transluminal angioplasty for renovascular hypertension in children: initial and long-term results. *Pediatrics* **99**: 44–9, 1997

58. Dotter CT: Transluminally-placed coilspring endarterial tube grafts: Long-term patency in canine popliteal artery. *Invest Radiol* **4**: 329–32, 1969

59. Blum U, Krumme B, Flugel P *et al.*: Treatment of osteal renal-artery stenoses with vascular endoprostheses after unsuccessful balloon angioplasty. *New Engl J Med* **336**: 459–65, 1997

60. Madias NE, Kwon OJ, Millan VG: Percutaneous transluminal renal angioplasty. *Arch Intern Med* **142**: 693–7, 1982

61. Pickering TG, Sos TA, Saddek S *et al.*: Renal angioplasty in patients with azotemia and renovascular hypertension. *J Hypertens* **4**(Suppl 6): 667–9, 1986

62. O'Donovan RM, Gutierrez OH, Izzo JJ: Preservation of renal function by percutaneous renal angioplasty in high-risk elderly patients: short-term outcome. *Nephron* **60**: 187–92, 1992

63. Englund R, Brown MA: Renal angioplasty for renovascular disease: a reappraisal. *J Cardiovasc Surg* **32**: 76–80, 1991

64. Young N, Wong KP: Use of percutaneous transluminal balloon angioplasty to treat renovascular disease. *Australas Radiol* **36**: 289–93, 1992

65. Henry M, Amor M, Henry I *et al.*: Stent placement in the renal artery: three-year experience with the Palmaz stent. *J Vasc Intervent Radiol* **7**: 343–50, 1996

66. Novick AC: Surgical correction of renovascular hypertension. *Surg Clin N Am* **68**: 1007–25, 1988

67. Bendel SM, Najarian JS, Sinaiko AR: Renal artery stenosis in infants: long-term medical treatment before surgery. *Pediatr Nephrol* **10**: 147–51, 1996

68. Stansby GP, Scoble JE, Hamilton G: Use of the hepatic arterial circulation for renal revascularisation. *Ann R Coll Surg Engl* **74**: 260–4, 1992

69. Valentine RJ, Martin JD, Myers SI, *et al.*: Asymptomatic celiac and superior mesenteric artery stenoses are more prevalent among patients with unsuspeted renal artery stenoses. *J Vasc Surg* **14**: 195–9, 1991

70. Novick AC: Use of the thoracic aorta for renal revascularization. *Urol Clin N Am* **21**: 355–60, 1994

71. Allen BT, Rubin BG, Anderson CB *et al.*: Simultaneous surgical management of aortic and renovascular disease. *Am J Surg* **166**: 726–33, 1993

72. Freeman N: Thromboendarterectomy for hypertension due to renal artery occlusion. *J Am Med Assoc* **157**: 1077, 1954

73. Steinbach F, Novick AC, Campbell S, Dykstra D: Long-term survival after surgical revascularization for atherosclerotic renal artery disease. *J Urol* **158**: 38–41, 1997

74. Darling R3, Shah DM, Chang BB, Leather RP: Does concomitant aortic bypass and renal artery revascularization using the retroperitoneal approach increase perioperative risk? *Cardiovasc Surg* **3**: 421–3, 1995

75. Novick AC, Ziegelbaum M, Vidt DG *et al.*: Trends in surgical revascularization for renal artery disease. Ten years' experience. *J Am Med Assoc* **257**: 498–501, 1987

76. Weibull H, Bergqvist D, Bergentz SE *et al.*: Percutaneous transluminal renal angioplasty versus surgical reconstruction of atherosclerotic renal artery stenosis: a prospective randomized study. *J Vasc Surg* **18**: 841–50, 1993

77. Reilly JM, Rubin BG, Thompson RW *et al.*: Revascularization of the solitary kidney: a challenging problem in a high risk population. *Surgery* **120**: 732–6, 1996

78. Cambria RP, Brewster DC, L'Italien GJ *et al.*: Renal artery reconstruction for the preservation of renal function. *J Vasc Surg* **24**: 371–80, 1996

79. Benjamin ME, Hansen KJ, Craven TE *et al.*: Combined aortic and renal artery surgery. A contemporary experience. *Ann Surg* **223**: 555–65, 1996

80. Dean R: Surgical reconstruction of atherosclerotic renal artery disease. In: Branchereau A, Jacobes M (Eds). *Long-term Results of Arterial Interventions*, pp. 205–16. Armonk, NY: Futura Publishing Company, 1997.

81. Sos TA, Pickering TG, Sniderman K *et al.*: percutaneous transluminal renal angioplasty in renovascular hypertensiondue to atheroma or fibromuscular dysplasia. *New Engl J Med* **309**: 274–9, 1983

82. Tegtmeyer CJ, Kellum CD, Ayers C: Percutaneous transluminal angioplasty of the renal artery: Results and long-term follow up. *Radiology* **153**: 77–84, 1984

83. Miller GA, Ford KK, Braun SD *et al.*: Percutaneous transluminal angioplasty vs surgery for renovascular hypertension. *Am J Roentgenol* **144**: 447–50, 1985

84. Klinge J, Mali WP, Puijlaert CB *et al.*: Percutaneous transluminal renal angioplasty: initial and long-term results. *Radiology* **171**: 501–6, 1989

85. Martin LG, Cork RD, Kaufman SL: Long-term results of angioplasty in 110 patients with renal artery stenosis. *J Vasc Intervent Radiol* **3**: 619–26, 1982

86. Losinno F, Zuccala A, Busato F, Zucchelli P: Renal artery angioplasty for renovascular hypertension and preservation of renal function: long-term angiographic and clinical follow-up. *Am J Roentgenol* **162**: 853–7, 1994

87. Rodriguez-Perez J, Plaza C, Reyes R *et al.*: Treatment of renovascular hypertension with percutaneous transluminal angioplasty: experience in Spain. *J Vasc Intervent Radiol* **5**: 101–9, 1994

88. Karagiannis A, Douma S, Voyiatzis K *et al.*: Percutaneous transluminal renal angioplasty in patients with renovascular hypertension: long-term results. *Hypertens Res* **18**: 27–31, 1995

89. Von Knorring J, Edgren J, Lepantalo M: Long-term results of percutaneous transluminal angioplasty in renovascular hypertension. *Acta Radiol* **37**: 36–40, 1996

90. Mali W, Beek E, Kaatee R *et al.*: Endovascular treatment of renovascular disease. In: Branchereau A, Jacobes M (Eds), *Long-term Results of Arterial Interventions*, pp. 235–241. Armonk, NY: Futura Publishing Company, 1997

91. Martin LG, Price RB, Cazarella WJ *et al.*: Percutaneous angioplasty in clinical management of renovascular hypertension: Initial and long-term results. *Radiology* **155**: 629–633, 1985

92. Millan VG, McCauley J, Kopelman RI, Madias NE: Percutaneous transluminal renal angioplasty in nonatherosclerotic renovascular hypertension. Long-term results. *Hypertension* **7**: 668–74, 1985

93. Greminger P, Steiner A, Schneider E *et al.*. Cure and improvement of renovascular hypertension after percutaneous transluminal angioplasty of renal artery stenosis. *Nephron* **51**: 362–6, 1989

94. Baert AL, Wilms G, Amery A *et al.*: Percutaneous transluminal renal angioplasty: initial results and long-term follow-up in 202 patients. *Cardiovasc Intervent Radiol* **13**: 22–8, 1990

95. Tegtmeyer CJ, Selby JB, Hartwell GD *et al.*: Results and complications of angioplasty in fibromuscular disease. *Circulation* **83**: 1155–61, 1991

96. Kuhn FP, Kutkuhn B, Torsello G, Modder U: Renal artery stenosis: preliminary results of treatment with the Strecker stent. *Radiology* **180**: 367–72, 1991

97. Hennequin LM, Joffre FG, Rousseau HP *et al.*: Renal artery stent placement: long-term results with the Wallstent endoprosthesis. *Radiology* **191**: 713–9, 1994

98. Raynaud AC, Beyssen BM, Turmel RL *et al.*: Renal artery stent placement: immediate and midterm technical and clinical results. *J Vasc Intervent Radiol* **5**: 849–58, 1994

99. Dorros G, Jaff M, Jain A *et al.*: Follow-up of primary Palmaz-Schatz stent placement for atherosclerotic renal artery stenosis. *Am J Cardiol* **75**: 1051–5, 1995

100. Van De Ven PJ, Beutler JJ, Kaatee R *et al.*: Transluminal vascular stent for osteal atherosclerotic renal artery stenosis. *Lancet* **346**: 672–4, 1995

101. Iannone LA, Underwood PL, Nath A *et al.*: Effect of primary balloon expandable renal artery stents on long-term patency, renal function, and blood pressure in hypertensive and renal insufficient patients with renal artery stenosis. *Cathet Cardiovasc Diagn* **37**: 243–50, 1996

102. Taylor A, Sheppard D, Macleod MJ *et al.*: Renal artery stent placement in renal artery stenosis: technical and early clinical results. *Clin Radiol* **52**: 451–7, 1997

103. Pattison JM, Reidy JF, Rafferty MJ *et al.*: Percutaneous transluminal renal angioplasty in patients with renal failure. *Quart J Med* **85**: 883–8, 1992

104. Pattynama PM, Becker GJ, Brown J *et al.*: Percutaneous angioplasty for atherosclerotic renal artery disease: effect on renal function in azotemic patients. *Cardiovasc Intervent Radiol* **17**: 143–6, 1994

105. Boisclair C, Therasse E, Oliva VL *et al.*: Treatment of renal angioplasty failure by percutaneous renal artery stenting with Palmaz stents: midterm technical and clinical results. *Am J Roentgenol* **168**: 245–51, 1997

106. Tullis MJ, Zieler RE, Glickerman DJ *et al.*: Results of percutaneous transluminal angioplasty for atherosclerotic renal artery stenosis: A follow up study with duplex ultrasonography. *J Vasc Surg* 25: 46–54, 1997
107. Rimmer JM, Gennari FJ: Atherosclerotic renovascular disease and progressive renal failure. *Ann Intern Med* **118**: 712–19, 1993

Editorial comments by R.M. Greenhalgh

This is a very complete chapter largely reporting results of angioplasty with and without stent for renal artery stenosis and surgical results. The authors are clear that renal artery stenoses of <50% have a very low rate of progression and they do not feel that intervention of any kind is justified. In this sense the thorough review yields one firm conclusion. The algorithm for renal artery stenosis of >50% is stated in Fig. 5 but the justification for choice of treatment is not always absolutely firm. The authors show concern at the high restenosis rate after renal stent angioplasty and note how difficult it is to operate when this problem occurs 40% of the time within a year. Angioplasty is obviously a far less major problem and it has the advantage of seeing if it produces improvement in terms of renal function or hypertension even if the durability of the procedure cannot be guaranteed. In a sense, therefore, it is not an either/or situation and not really either angioplasty or surgery. Nevertheless, having said this, random allocation clinical trials are rather conspicuous by their absence.

What Are the Indications for Intervention in Children with Renal Artery Stenosis?

R.T.A. Chalmers, A Dhadwal, J.E. Deal and J.H.N. Wolfe

INTRODUCTION

Children who are found to have a blood pressure that is above the 95th centile for their age should be considered to suffer from severe hypertension.[1,2] Second only to renal parenchymal disease, renovascular disease has been shown to be the underlying cause of secondary hypertension in up to 20% of children presenting to specialist centres.[3] As it is potentially curable, accurate delineation of the extent and nature of arterial involvement is essential so that appropriate treatment can be given.[4]

In this chapter, we shall describe the place of vascular intervention in the management of children with renal artery stenosis.

AETIOLOGY

Fibromuscular dysplasia of the main renal arteries and/or their branches is the most common cause of renal artery stenosis in children, accounting for up to 70% of cases in published series.[5,6] Often the diagnosis is made on the radiological appearances of the affected vessel alone, without biopsy proof, and so the true incidence of fibromuscular dysplasia may actually be lower. This pathology usually affects the tunica media but has been demonstrated in both the intima and, on occasions, the adventitia. Stanley *et al.* were of the opinion that stenoses thought to be due to fibromuscular dysplasia are actually caused by hypoplasia of the affected arteries and that the lesion represents a failure of normal growth[7] (Fig. 1). Intimal fibromuscular dysplasia of the renal arteries can be found in association with neurofibromatosis and there is also a familial syndrome not associated with neurofibromatosis.[8] Hypertension associated with neurofibromatosis can also be due to either aortic coarctation or the presence of a phaeochromocytoma. The renal arteries can be involved in the so-called mid-aortic syndrome, a condition in which there is severe, diffuse narrowing of the abdominal aorta at visceral vessel level.[9] Histologically, fibrotic changes are seen in the intima and media of the affected arteries. Other eponymous vascular conditions which can include renal artery stenosis are Marfan's syndrome, Klippel-Trenaunay syndrome and Williams syndrome (idiopathic hypercalcaemia), Turner's syndrome and Fuerstein-Mims syndrome.[10] Takayasu's arteritis, more commonly seen in the Asian subcontinent, is another disease that can give rise to stenotic lesions of the aorta and its major branches.[11] Iatrogenic causes of renovascular hypertension include renal artery thrombosis secondary to umbilical artery catheterization in neonates and also the

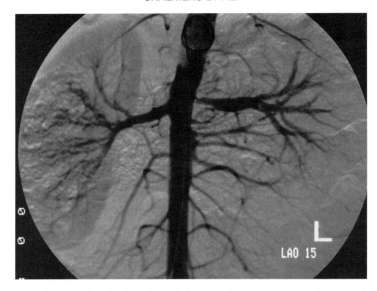

Fig. 1. Arteriogram showing left renal artery stenosis considered unsuitable for balloon angioplasty (patient KB, Table 2). This lesion was treated by aortorenal graft using internal iliac artery (Fig. 5).

development of renal artery stenosis after abdominal radiotherapy. The renal vessels can be compressed by extrinsic pathology, for example, phaeochromocytoma or Wilms' tumour.

DISTRIBUTION OF ARTERIAL LESIONS

In fibromuscular dysplasia, there is a tendency for the lesions to be bilateral and in addition, to affect not only the main renal artery but also branch arteries of the same or contralateral kidney.[5] There are often associated stenotic lesions of the coeliac and superior mesenteric arteries and in reported series, coexisting coarctation of the abdominal aorta or the mid-aortic syndrome is found in a significant proportion of patients. The presence of intracranial arterial disease should be suspected in children with renal artery stenosis who present with neurological symptoms.[10]

PRESENTATION

A proportion of hypertensive children are asymptomatic and are identified at routine physical examination, illustrating the importance of measuring blood pressure in children.[12] Headache is the most frequently described symptom. In accelerated hypertension, irritability, convulsions and even hemiplegia have been reported.[13] A lower motor neuron palsy of the seventh cranial nerve may be present. Other non-specific symptoms include lethargy and failure to thrive in younger children. The presence of associated syndromes should alert the clinician as should other symptoms and signs of arterial disease, for example, a history of claudication or the presence of abdominal and/or carotid artery bruits.[14,15]

INVESTIGATIONS

After a full clinical history and examination, including fundoscopy, blood should be taken for electrolytes and renal function. Routine urinalysis should also be performed. Peripheral plasma renin measurements and plasma and urine catecholamine concentration should be measured as part of the preliminary screening.[16] Electrocardiography and echocardiography identify the presence of cardiac changes secondary to hypertension. Abdominal ultrasound scanning and isotope renography (with 99Tc labelled dimercaptosuccinic acid or DMSA) give information on kidney size and relative function.[17,18] As well as giving baseline

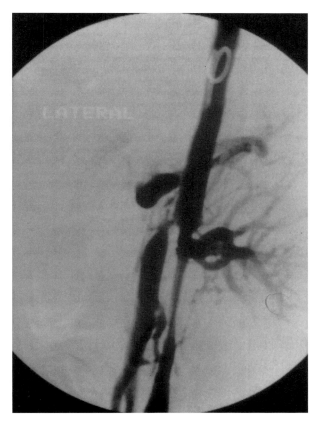

Fig. 2. Lateral aortogram of a child with mid-aortic syndrome showing stenoses of both the coeliac and superior mesenteric artery origins. Bilateral renal artery stenoses also present.

information on renal size and function, serial investigations monitor any deterioration indicating a need to intervene, if this is an option. Isotope studies and duplex scanning also have a role in following patients after vascular intervention. Radionuclide imaging with angiotensin converting enzyme inhibitor drugs administered can help unmask main renal artery or branch artery stenoses. Captopril-primed DMSA scanning had an 80% sensitivity and an 89% specificity in the study by Gordon *et al.*[19] In ordinary circumstances, there is no role for renal biopsy in the investigation of children with renovascular hypertension.

Once renal artery stenosis is suspected as the cause of the child's hypertension, angiography is mandatory.[20] An aortogram and selective anteroposterior and oblique renal artery views should be obtained.[21,22] If a renal artery stenosis is demonstrated, a lateral aortogram should also be performed to show the origins of the coeliac axis and superior mesenteric artery.[23] These vessels are frequently seen to be involved in mid-aortic syndrome (62% involved) (Fig. 2) and in neurofibromatosis (33% involved).[13] It is important to remember to assess the cerebral vasculature if the child has presented with neurological symptoms.[16] In recent years, duplex scanning has been advocated by some authors as giving useful information on the degree of stenosis present.[24] However, this technology is not able to give a full picture when more peripheral branch arteries are involved.[25] Duplex may have an important role in the postoperative monitoring of vascular reconstructions.

Renal vein renin level measurement can include segmental vein sampling and indicate whether there is unilateral or bilateral disease.[10]

MANAGEMENT

The majority of paediatric patients with renovascular hypertension have a pattern of disease that is not amenable to either angioplasty or surgery. In the series by Deal *et al.*, of 54 children studied, only 20 could be treated invasively, the remaining 34 receiving antihypertensive medication only.[16] Regardless of the ultimate treatment plan, be it angioplasty or surgery, it is important to control the patient's blood pressure adequately. Medical therapy consists of beta-blockade combined with either a vasodilator agent or calcium channel blockade. Diuretics are reserved for patients with evidence of fluid or sodium overload and are rarely needed in renal artery disease. The use of angiotensin converting enzyme inhibitors is not recommended as these can compromise renal function by altering glomerular haemodynamics distal to the renal artery stenosis.

Patients treated medically should be monitored regularly. This applies to all children with hypertension, but is especially important in children who have reconstructable disease whose surgical treatment is being delayed, for example, to allow for growth. Frequent blood pressure measurement, urine analysis, annual renal function tests (serum electrolytes and creatinine, isotope renography) regular fundoscopy and annual echocardiography should be performed so that any significant deterioration in renal function or evidence of end-organ damage can be detected early and intervention undertaken.

However, as pointed out by Dean *et al.*, 50% of patients with renovascular hypertension treated with medical therapy alone showed a deterioration in renal function and size over time in spite of adequate blood pressure control.[26] Morris defined 'cure' after definitive therapy as resolution of hypertension without the need for antihypertensives 3 months after intervention and 'improvement' as resolution of hypertension with the need for less antihypertensive medication.[27]

The main invasive treatment modalities are percutaneous transluminal balloon angioplasty (PTBA) and surgery.

THE TIMING OF INTERVENTION

As stated previously, it is only the minority of young patients with renovascular hypertension who have stenoses that are amenable to intervention. When this is the case, the decision to intervene has to take into account some or all of the following factors:

1. Poor blood pressure control on medication.
2. Poor patient compliance with antihypertensive medication.
3. Evidence of deteriorating renal function.
4. Evidence of end-organ effects of hypertension (retinopathy, left ventricular hypertrophy, proteinuria).
5. Treatment of stenosis(es) may preserve renal tissue and/or decrease the requirement for antihypertensive medication.
6. Child's age: surgical reconstruction in the very young may be inadvisable and some allowance for growth should be made, if possible.

PERCUTANEOUS TRANSLUMINAL BALLOON ANGIOPLASTY

The 'ideal' lesion for treatment with PTBA is a short, isolated, non-ostial stenosis due to fibromuscular dysplasia (Fig. 3). This applies to isolated branch artery lesions also. Indeed, PTBA is the treatment of choice for appropriate lesions due to fibromuscular dysplasia. The immediate success rate is quoted in the 80–90% range and such follow-up studies as have been published show that in a reasonable proportion of children, a good outcome is maintained in terms of blood pressure control, freedom from antihypertensive agents and also intact renal function.[28,29] Tegtmeyer *et al.* reviewed the literature and of 25 cases of renal artery stenosis in children due to fibromuscular dysplasia treated with primary PTBA, there was a 92% immediate success rate.[23] Over a median follow-up of 15 months (range: 1–95) 18 patients remained normotensive, two had surgical therapy after recurrence of the stenosis, one required less medication, one had a repeat PTBA, one remained hypertensive and two were lost to follow-up.

Renal artery stenosis as a component of neurofibromatosis does not appear to respond to PTBA so well.[13,30] In a literature review, Tegtmeyer identified 12 patients that had been so treated.[23] Four patients had reverted to normotension, two had a moderate result and still required antihypertensive medication long-term and six

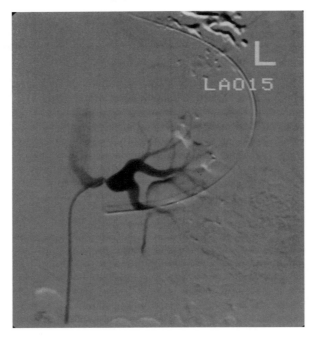

Fig. 3. Pre-angioplasty arteriography demonstrates a tight, focal stenosis of the left renal artery. This was treated successfully by PTBA (patient AA, Table 2).

failed and ultimately underwent surgical treatment. The typical arteriographic appearance of the stenoses in neurofibromatosis are of aortic branch lesions consisting of a stenotic segment continuing into an elongated funnel-shaped channel.

The results of PTBA for renal artery involvement in mid-aortic syndrome and Takayasu's arteritis are discouraging with limited success rates and evidence of early recurrence.[13,31] The exception to this experience is described in a paper by Tyagi *et al.*[32] Reporting the Delhi experience in treating 35 children with renal artery stenosis (89% being due to arteritis, 11% fibromuscular dysplasia) using PTBA as a primary treatment modality they had a 92% immediate success rate and this was sustained in over 90% of the patients over a mean follow-up of 41 months. Deal *et al.*[16] thought that although encouraging, the reported high success rates for PTBA, especially in fibromuscular dysplasic, probably flatter to deceive as the patients reported tend to have 'favourable' lesions and thus represent a super-selected group. The majority of the paediatric renovascular hypertensive population have bilateral, multifocal stenoses and therefore cannot be completely cured. Nevertheless, in such circumstances, PTBA has a role as a temporizing measure allowing for surgical treatment later or at least to palliate a poorly controlled hypertensive child.[10] Indeed, some authors have suggested that in young children, PTBA may act as a reasonable temporary measure for mid-aortic syndrome allowing for growth prior to the definitive surgical procedure.[33]

In general, angioplasty should not be considered as the first-line therapy for patients with renal artery ostial stenoses, long tubular lesions, occlusions, stenoses associated with active arteritis and atherosclerosis (seen as a feature of advanced Takayasu's) or in patients with neurofibromatosis.[23]

There are significant potential complications associated with renal artery PTBA that are specific to the child.[12] Early problems include spasm of the vessel, dissection, thrombosis or embolization. These in turn can lead to renal loss or infarction. For this reason, it is imperative that surgical cover by an experienced vascular surgeon is available whenever the procedure is attempted. Other complications relate to the use of iodine-containing contrast and its potential deleterious effect on renal function.[34] Also, complications due to femoral arterial cannulation have been described.[35]

INDICATIONS FOR SURGICAL TREATMENT

Surgical revascularization is the mainstay of operative treatment. The 'ideal' stenosis in terms of reconstructive vascular surgery is a unilateral, relatively short, ostial or proximal lesion affecting a main renal artery in a patient with unilateral disease (as confirmed by selective renal vein sampling for renin) and no intrarenal disease.[36] However, the majority of patients do not fall into this category and therefore selection for surgery has to take other factors into account. Poorly controlled or completely uncontrolled hypertension in a young patient who manifests high renin output on the affected side and depressed renal function are all important factors in the decision to operate. Even if the disease pattern is complex, vascular reconstruction should still be considered.[37]

Other indications for surgical revascularization are the presence of (short) occlusions and after failed attempts at balloon angioplasty in which renal loss is anticipated.[38,39] Recurrent stenosis after previous angioplasty, especially when repeat angioplasty has been attempted and failed, is best treated by surgery. The lesions associated with neurofibromatosis are best treated by primary surgery where possible.[30] Patients with mid-aortic syndrome and aorto–arteritis tend to have a complex pattern of stenotic (and sometimes coexistent aneurysmal) disease and although PTBA can buy time, when feasible, surgical reconstruction is the treatment of choice.[31]

GENERAL CONSIDERATIONS

A transverse supraumbilical incision is recommended. For lesions other than ostial and proximal stenoses, medial rotation of the viscera allows wide exposure of the renal vessels.[33] Prior to vessel clamping, systemic anticoagulation with heparin is administered and a dopamine infusion initiated together with mannitol. Formerly, especially in patients with complex bilateral disease and coexisting aortic pathology, staged operations were the standard practice, but nowadays, a single-stage procedure is recommended.[7] Anastomoses in smaller or very young children should be performed with interrupted monofilament sutures whereas in teenagers, continuous suture techniques are permissible. Distal graft to renal artery anastomoses are performed end-to-end with a long oblique anastomosis to increase the anastomotic circumference and help prevent the development of late stenoses. It goes without saying that supreme care must be taken in the surgical handling of the grafts and vessels to avoid the subsequent development of traumatic stenoses.

SURGICAL PROCEDURES

Nephrectomy

The place of nephrectomy is a limited. This operation should be reserved for situations where there is complete or virtually complete loss of renal function or where reconstruction is impossible at exploration of the kidney. Partial nephrectomy may be indicated for segmental, distal lesions not amenable to revascularization. Tapper *et al.* stated that infants with severe uncontrolled hypertension and with less than 10% renal function in the affected kidney should have a nephrectomy.[40] They found that severe hypertension caused by renal artery thrombosis due to umbilical catherization in the neonatal period could be cured by nephrectomy.

Intraoperative dilatation

This technique involves the passage of progressively larger rigid dilators through the region of stenosis intraoperatively. This approach has fallen out of favour mostly because it is associated with a high early thrombosis rate and risk of vessel disruption. The unfavourable experience of Stanley *et al.* with operative dilatation led them to abandon the technique and they concluded that their group's poor results with PTBA were mirrored in the outcome of operative dilatation.[7] They postulated that most paediatric renal artery stenoses were due to arterial hypoplasia and that as such PTBA or operative dilatation were not appropriate ways to treat them.

Aortorenal bypass

Over the years, aortorenal bypass grafting has been the most frequently used technique to revascularize the kidney in children.[41] It has been well demonstrated that autologous grafts perform better over time than do prosthetic bypasses (Fig. 4).[42] However, long-term follow-up studies have shown that when vein grafts are placed, up to 20% develop aneurysmal dilatation and this complication is more common in children than in adults.[43,44] In some series, these changes have been described in vein grafts as early as 1 year after placement.[45] Some authors have suggested wrapping the vein graft in prosthetic material at the time of the original bypass procedure to prevent aneurysmal dilatation occurring, but there is not much evidence to suggest that this makes any difference.[46]

    In recent years, the use of the internal iliac artery as the autologous conduit of choice has become popular.[47] There are fewer reported problems with late dilatation,

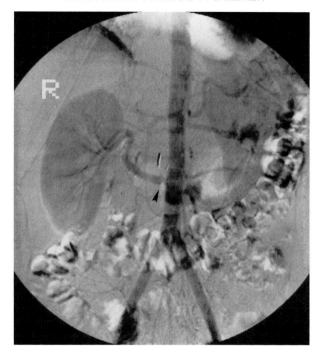

Fig. 4. Follow-up arteriogram of patient BF (Table 2). The apparent stenosis (arrow) at the origin of the right aortorenal Dacron graft (10 years after placement) had no haemodynamic significance by duplex ultrasound and was not treated.

although this may occur if the vessel used is actually abnormal at the time of grafting and this is not appreciated until later.[7] The length available can be a problem for more distal renal artery lesions and in cases requiring bilateral reconstruction.[33] It is recommended that when harvesting the internal iliac artery, the dissection is taken beyond the level of a branch artery so that the two orifices can be conjoined, thereby spatulating the graft and allowing for a wider anastomosis without losing valuable graft length (Fig. 5).

Direct reimplantation of renal arteries

Stenoses involving the ostia or proximal portion of the renal arteries do not respond to PTBA. In recent years, rather than bypass such lesions, Stanley *et al.* have developed the technique of direct reimplantation of the renal artery into the aorta or into an adjacent renal artery or branch artery after transection beyond the stenotic segment.[7] Again, spatulation of the transected artery allows for a safe anastomosis. This approach is clearly dependent upon the aorta being free of disease and therefore is pertinent to the paediatric patient, who, unlike his adult counterpart, has an aorta free of atheroma.

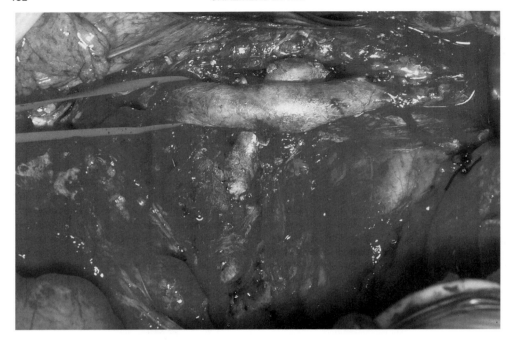

Fig. 5.   Operative photograph (patient KB, Table 2). The completed aortorenal internal
iliac artery autograft is shown.

Splenorenal bypass

This technique involves mobilization of the splenic artery from its origin as far as the
level of the vasa brevia, tunnelling the vessel behind the pancreas (without kinks or
tension) and end-to-end anastomosis to the transected left renal artery. The attraction
of the technique is that an autologous arterial graft of reasonable length is obtained.
However, the reported results in children are not good.[48,49] Early thromboses have
been described. Furthermore, normal-appearing coeliac arteries in young children
can either fail to grow properly or in fact be pathologic such that they develop a
stenosis later in life with recurrence of hypertension. As it is not possible to predict
accurately which patients will develop such problems, splenorenal bypass is not
recommended in children.[41]

Renal autotransplantation

The indications for the use of this approach in paediatric renal artery stenosis include
patients with complex multifocal stenoses particularly when these involve both
extra- and intrarenal vessels simultaneously, renal lesions in association with mid-
aortic syndrome or arteritis, long occlusions of the renal artery with only intrarenal
artery patent, trauma with threat to renal function and in complex reoperation.[50] The

technique involves excision of the kidney (usually with the ureter intact), *ex vivo* cooling, bench-repair of the stenotic lesion(s) if required and anastomosis of the renal vasculature to the iliac vessels with the kidney placed in the iliac fossa.[51] In this way, lengths of saphenous vein can be used to reconstruct multiple stenoses which are not amenable to PTBA or to *in situ* vascular reconstruction.[33]

Mesenteric-renal bypass/iliorenal bypass

Although these methods are utilized in adults with heavily diseased aortas, these operations are performed rarely in children because of problems associated with growth. In his landmark paper, Stanley reported the use of iliorenal vein grafts in only two cases.[7] Reimplantation of a transected renal artery to the superior mesenteric artery did have some place in their practice.

Mid-aortic syndrome

Children who present with this syndrome require revascularization of the kidneys and to a variable extent, the visceral arteries, as well as restoration of adequate circulation to the lower extremities. Some authors have advocated staged operations, but most feel that a single operation is preferable when possible.[52]

The technique adopted for revascularization of the visceral and renal vessels is dictated by the nature of the stenotic disease and may require more than one of the approaches described above in the same patient. The options for aortic reconstruction are either aorto–aortic bypass (Fig. 6) using either Dacron or polytetrafluoroethylene

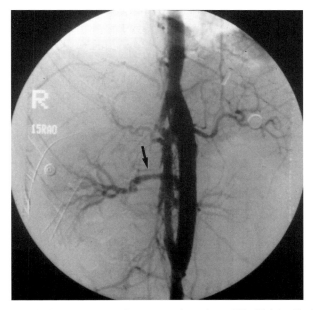

Fig. 6. Follow-up arteriogram of patient ZR (Table 2). The aorto–aortic Dacron graft is seen. There is a saphenous vein graft to the right renal artery (arrow).

(PTFE) or aortic patchplasty.[37] For the former technique, a thoracoabdominal graft is placed and conventionally the renal grafts anastomosed to the prosthesis. However, in order to avoid anastomotic hyperplasia, it is probably better for the renal bypass grafts to originate from the aorta below the level of aortic coarctation.

Stanley *et al.* prefer to perform a patch plasty of the aorta with direct reimplantation of the renal arteries where this is feasible.[7] They use PTFE patch material and try to place a big enough patch to allow for growth. The timing of this operation is important if reoperative intervention is to be avoided, but clearly a balance has to be drawn between delaying too long in a child with poorly controlled hypertension and threat to renal function and the long-term effectiveness of the operation. Reoperation is probably avoided when patchplasty is performed in children aged over 5 years.

Recurrent aortic stenosis can be a problem, however, when this technique is applied to children under 2 years of age. Philosophically, Stanley *et al.* feel that reoperative aortoplasty is technically far easier than reoperation for failed thoracoabdominal bypass.[7] To circumvent this problem, others have suggested autotransplantation of the kidney(s) and PTBA of the aorta to allow for adequate growth, after which decisive patch aortoplasty or aorto–aortic bypass can be performed.[14]

RESULTS OF SURGERY

Bearing in mind that surgical reconstruction can only be applied to a subgroup of paediatric patients with renovascular hypertension and that the results therefore apply to selected patients, the outcome of these operations is good.

In a recent review, Stanley summarized the results of the six largest series in the North American literature (Table 1).[53] The 'cure' rate after surgery ranged from 59% to 84.5% and the majority of the remaining patients with 'improved', such that 'failure' was seen in 0–18.5% of patients.

Table 1.   Results of published series on outcome of surgery for renovascular hypertension in children

		Outcome of surgery (%)		
Institution	*No. patients*	*Cured*	*Improved*	*Failed*
Michigan	57	79	19	2
Cleveland	27	59	18.5	18.5
UCLA	26	84.5	7.5	4
Vanderbilt	21	68	24	8
Pennsylvania	17	76.5	23.5	0
University of California	14	86	7	0
St Mary's	7	86	14	0

(Adapted from ref. 53.)

Over three decades, the Ann Arbor group treated 57 children with renovascular hypertension by surgical intervention;[7] 98% of patients treated benefited from operation. Hypertension was cured completely in 79%, improved with the need for less medication in 19% and unchanged in 2%. There was no operative mortality. Novick *et al.* also have a wide experience in this field.[49] In a series of 27 patients, 16 were cured after surgery, five improved and there were six failures. This outcome was maintained over long-term follow-up. Similar results have also been experienced by Stoney *et al.* who used a variety of surgical approaches, including microvascular bench repair in one patient to achieve excellent long-term control of hypertension in 10 of 14 patients.[54] In the series reported by Welsh *et al.*, 15 children were treated using vascular surgical reconstruction for renal artery stenosis.[55] Five patients had a coexisting coarctation of the abdominal aorta. Over a follow-up period ranging from 1 to 15 years, ten patients had normal blood pressure and only two of these required antihypertensive medicine.

Surgical management of the mid-aortic syndrome also yields good results as far as both hypertension control and preservation of renal function are concerned. In a series of ten patients, Messina *et al.* had excellent outcome over late follow-up in all but one patient.[52] Similarly, of 11 patients aged between 5 months and 15 years treated surgically for mid-aortic syndrome by Lewis and colleagues, nine obtained good late results.[31] It is interesting to note that in this series, PTBA was unsuccessful in three patients. Ellis *et al.* treated six patients with concomitant mid-aortic syndrome and bilateral renal artery stenosis.[14] Their preferred method of surgical reconstruction of the kidneys was autotransplantation which yielded a good outcome in seven kidneys, the remainder being revascularized by PTBA (three) and direct revascularization (two).

At St Mary's Hospital, our recent experience in this field is with ten patients (Table 2). The lesions treated were either isolated renal artery stenoses or more complex multiple stenoses associated with mid-aortic syndrome. Of the eight cases treated surgically, six are normotensive and off all medication, one is normotensive on reduced doses of antihypertensive agents and one patient, originally treated with a splenorenal graft required late reoperation for coeliac stenosis. One child has been successfully treated for an isolated renal artery stenosis with PTBA and a final 8-year-old girl with mid-aortic syndrome is being managed conservatively. Operative intervention is planned for this patient when she has grown.

REOPERATION

Perhaps not surprisingly, reoperation is necessary in a significant percentage (up to 25%) of children who have undergone surgical treatment. The principal reasons for reoperation are perioperative thrombosis, late stenosis and graft dilatation.[42] Early thrombosis is usually secondary to technical problems, poor quality conduit and kinking of the graft. Recurrent hypertension after renal revascularization may be due to parenchymal disease progression but graft stenosis or further renal artery stenosis must be excluded by careful imaging. Stanley *et al.* obtained follow-up arteriograms on their 57 patients, and as a result, 14 underwent a total of 20 secondary procedures.[7] Eleven of 31 vein grafts showed late aneurysmal dilatation, five of which were

Table 2. Vascular intervention for renal artery stenosis in children: St Mary's Hospital experience

Patient	Age	Sex	Diagnosis	Intervention	Pre:post BP	Follow-up	Outcome
DT	22	M	FMD	Renal autotransplantation	180/115:145/75	21 months	Normotensive
KB	19	M	FMD	Aortorenal LSV graft	185/110:120/75	30 months	Normotensive
ZR	21	F	MAS	Aorto–aorto Dacron graft, LSV graft to R renal a	130/90:125/75	43 months	Normotensive
GC	19	M	MAS	Aorto–aorto Dacron graft, LSV graft to R renal artery, reimplantation L renal artery	160/100:130/85	11 months	Normotensive
BF	14	M	FMD	Failed PTBA: Emergency aorto- R renal (Dacron) graft	160/105:125/80	11 years	Normotensive
KB	7	F	NFM	Aorto-L renal (internal iliac artery) graft	150/100:130/90	5 months	Normotensive
RC	19	F	FMD	Splenorenal bypass	130/90	10 years	Coeliac stenosis at 9 years patched
AA	3	F	FMD	PTBA L renal artery stenosis	140/110:110/70	6 months	Normotensive
TW	8	F	MAS	Medical management awaiting surgery			
MM	1	M	MAS	Failed aortic PTBA Thoraco-abdominal Dacron graft	180/110:105/70	3 months	Normotensive

FMD: Fibromuscular dysplasia; MAS: Mid-aortic syndrome; LSV: Long saphenous vein; PTBA: Percutaneous transluminal balloon angioplasty treated by surgical plication. Seven patients required a nephrectomy as further reconstruction was not feasible. Reoperation can be hazardous because of intense scarring in the region of the primary surgery. Also, there is often limited length of remaining artery available and for further revascularization to be achieved *ex vivo* reconstruction and autotransplantation may be the best method employed.[33]

CONCLUSIONS

Renovascular hypertension in children should be investigated thoroughly since, although the majority of patients have complex, multifocal disease, there is a significant number who have disease that is amenable to vascular intervention. The indications for operative intervention are reasonably well defined and are often dictated by the underlying cause of the renal artery stenosis. Surgical revascularization is durable and gives good control of blood pressure and preservation of renal function in the majority of cases. The requirement for antihypertensive medications is often removed altogether.

REFERENCES

1. Report of the Second Task Force on Blood Pressure Control in Children – 1987: *Pediatrics* **79**: 1–25, 1987
2. de Marr SA: Blood pressure in childhood: Pooled findings of six European studies. *J Hypertens* **9**: 109–14, 1991
3. Watson AR, Balfe JW, Hardy BE: Renovascular hypertension in childhood: A changing perspective in management. *J Pediatr* **106**: 366–72, 1985
4. Fry WJ, Ernst CB, Stanley JC, Brinnk B: Renovascular hypertension in the pediatric patient. *Arch Surg* **107**: 692–98, 1973
5. Guzzetta PC, Potter BM, Ruley EJ *et al.*: Renovascular hypertension in children: Current concepts in evaluation and management. *J. Pediatr Surg* **24**: 1236–40, 1989
6. Stanley P, Gyepes MJ, Olson DL *et al.*: Renovascular hypertension in children and adolescents. *Radiology* **129**: 123–31, 1978
7. Stanley JC, Zelenock GB, Messina LM, Wakefield TW: Pediatric renovascular hypertension: A thirty year experience of operative treatment. *J Vasc Surg* **21**: 212–27, 1995
8. Inglefinger JR: Renovascular disease in children. *Kidney Int* **43**: 493–505, 1993
9. Sumboonnanonda A, Robinson BL, Gedoye WMW *et al.*: Middle aortic syndrome: Clinical and radiological findings. *Arch Dis Child* **67**: 501–5, 1992
10. Dillon MJ, Deal JE: Renovascular hypertension in children. In: Novick A, Scobie J, Hamilton G (Eds), *Renal Vascular Disease* pp. 235–44. London: WB Saunders Company, 1992
11. Lagneau P, Michel JB, Virong PN: Surgical treatment of Takayasu's disease. *Ann Surg* **205**: 157–69, 1987
12. Wells TG, Belsha CW: Pediatric renovascular hypertension. *Curr Opin Pediat* **8**: 128–34, 1996
13. Robinson L, Gedoye J, Reidy J, Saxton HM: Renal artery stenosis in children. *Clin Radiol* **44**: 376–82, 1991
14. Ellis D, Shapiro R, Scantlebury VP *et al.*: Evaluation and management of bilateral renal artery stenosis in children: a case series and review. *Pediatr Nephrol* **9**: 259–67, 1995
15. O'Neill JA, Berkowitz H, Fellows KJ, Harmon CM: Midaortic syndrome and hypertension in childhood. *J Pediatr Surg* **30**: 164–72, 1995

16. Deal JE, Snell MF, Barratt TM, Dillon MJ: Renovascular disease in childhood. *J Pediatr* **121**: 378–84, 1992

17. Minty I, Lythgoe M, Gordon I: Hypertension in pediatrics: Can pre- and post-captopril technetium-99m dimercaptosuccinic acid renal scans exclude renovascular disease? *Eur J Nucl Med* **20**: 699–702, 1993

18. de Hollanda R, Giamberardino DD, Bley PCP *et al.*: Renal artery stenosis diagnosed with Tc-99m DMSA scintigraphy. *Clin Nucl Med* **19**: 22–4, 1994

19. Gordon I, Lythgoe M, Minty I, Dillon MJ: Diagnosis of renovascular hypertension: improved specificity of TC99m DMSA using captopril. *Pediatr Nephrol* **7**: C36, 1993

20. Hiner LB, Falkner B: Renovascular hypertension in children. *Pediatr Clin N Amer* **40**: 123–40, 1993

21. Tonkin IL, Stapleton FB, Roy S: Digital subtraction angiography in the evaluation of renal vascular hypertension in children. *Pediatrics* **81**: 150–8, 1988

22. Lanning P, Uhai M: The radiological evaluation of children with hypertension. *Eur J Pediatr* **132**, 147–54, 1979

23. Tegtmeyer CJ, Matsumoto AH, Angle JF: Percutaneous transluminal angioplasty in fibrous dysplasia and children. In: Novick A, Scobie J, Hamilton G (Eds), *Renal Vascular Disease* pp. 363–83. London: WB Saunders Co Ltd, 1992

24. Strauss S, Bistritzer T, Azizi E *et al.*: Renal artery stenosis secondary to neurofibromatosis in children: detection by Doppler ultrasound. *Pediatr Nephrol* **7**: 32–4, 1993

25. Brun P, Kchouk H, Mouchet B *et al.*: Value of Doppler ultrasound for the diagnosis of renal artery stenosis in children. *Pediatr Nephrol* **11**: 27–30, 1997

26. Dean RH, Kieffer RW, Smith BM: Renovascular hypertension. *Arch Surg* **116**: 1408–13, 1981

27. Morris PJ: Renovascular hypertension: The indications for and the results of surgery. In: Bell PRF, Jamieson CW, Ruckley CV (Eds), *Surgical Management of Vascular Disease* pp. 739–50. London: WB Saunders Co Ltd, 1992

28. Casalini E, Sfondrini MS, Fossali E: Two year clinical follow-up of children and adolescents after percutaneous transluminal angioplasty for renovascular hypertension. *Invest Radiol* **30**: 40–3, 1995

29. Simunic S, Winter IF, Radsovinic B *et al.*: Percutaneous transluminal renal angioplasty (PTRA) for renovascular hypertension in children. *Eur J Radiol* **10**: 143–6, 1990

30. Lund G, Swarko A, Castanenda ZW *et al.*: Percutaneous transluminal angioplasty for the treatment of renal artery stenosis in children. *Eur J Radiol* **4**: 254–7, 1984

31. Lewis VD, Merazize SG, McLean GK *et al.*: The midaortic syndrome: diagnosis and treatment. *Radiology* **167**: 111–3, 1988

32. Tyagi S, Kaul UA, Stasangi DK, Arora R: Percutaneous transluminal angioplasty for renovascular hypertension in children: initial and long-term results. *Pediatrics* **99**: 44–9, 1997

33. Jenkins AMcL: Operations for renal ischaemia. In: Bell PRF, Jamieson CW, Ruckley CV (Eds), *Surgical Management of Vascular Disease* pp. 751–66. London: WB Saunders Co Ltd, 1992

34. Norling LL, Chevalier RL, Gomez RA, Tegtmeyer CJ: Use of interventional radiology for hypertension due to renal artery stenosis in children. *Child Nephrol Urol* **12**: 162–6, 1992

35. Mali WPThM, Puijlaert CBAJ, Kouwenberg HJ *et al.*: Percutaneous transluminal renal angioplasty in children and adolescents. *Radiology* **165**: 391–4, 1987

36. Stanley JC: Surgical intervention in pediatric renovascular hypertension. *Child Nephrol Urol* **12**: 167–74, 1992

37. Stanley JC, Fry WJ: Pediatric renal artery occlusive disease and renovascular hypertension. Etiology, diagnosis and operative treatment. *Arch Surg* **116**: 669–76, 1981

38. Guzzetta PC, Potter BM, Kapur S *et al.*: Reconstruction of the renal artery after unsuccessful percutaneous transluminal angioplasty in children. *Am J Surg* **145**: 647–51, 1983

39. Valdes F, Sareh C, Kramer A: Surgical treatment of complete renal artery occlusion in pediatric patients. *Ann Vasc Surg* **4**: 490–3, 1990

40. Tapper D, Brand T, Hickman R: Early diagnosis and management of renovascular hypertension. *Am J Surg* **153**: 495–500, 1987

41. Novick AC: Percutaneous transluminal angioplasty and surgery of the renal artery. *Eur J Vasc Surg* **8**: 1–9, 1994
42. Stanley JC, Whitehouse WMJ, Zelenock GB *et al.*: Reoperation for complications of renal artery reconstructive surgery. *J Vasc Surg* **2**: 133–41, 1985
43. Dean RH, Wilson JP, Burko H, Foster JH: Saphenous vein aorto-renal bypass grafts: serial arteriographic study. *Ann Surg* **180**: 469–76, 1974
44. Stanley JC, Ernst CB, Fry WJ: Fate of 100 aortorenal vein grafts: Characteristics of late graft expansion, aneurysmal dilatation and stenosis. *Surgery* **74**: 931–9, 1973
45. Novick AC, Straffon RA, Stewart BH, Benjamin S: Surgical treatment of renovascular hypertension in the pediatric patient. *J Urol* **119**: 794–801, 1978
46. Berkowitz HD, O'Neill JA Jr: Renovascular hypertension in children: Surgical repair with special reference to the use of reinforced vein grafts. *J Vasc Surg* **9**: 46–55, 1989
47. Stoney RJ, DeLuccia N, Ehrenfeld WK, Wylie EJ: Aorto-renal arterial autografts. Long-term assessment. *Arch Surg* **116**: 1416–21, 1981
48. Novick AC, Burowsky LH, Stewart BH, Straffon RA: Splenorenal bypass in the treatment of renal artery stenosis. *Trans Am Soc Genitourin Surg* **69**: 139–45, 1977
49. Novick AC, Benjamin S, Straffon RA: Stenosing renal artery disease in children: clinicopathologic correlation and results of treatment. *Nephron* **22**: 182–95, 1978
50. Sicard GA, Valentin LI, Freeman MB *et al.*: Renal autotransplantation: an alternative to standard renal revascularization procedures. *Surgery* **104**: 624–30, 1988
51. Jordan ML, Novick AC, Cunningham RL: The role of autotransplantation in pediatric and young adult patients with renal artery disease. *J Vasc Surg* **2**: 385–91, 1985
52. Messina LM, Reilly LM, Goldstone J *et al.*: Middle aortic syndrome: Effectiveness and durability of complex arterial revascularization techniques. *Ann Surg* **204**: 331–9, 1986
53. Stanley JC: Surgical treatment of renovascular hypertension. *Am J Surg* **174**: 102–10, 1997
54. Stoney RJ, Cooke PA, String ST: Surgical treatment of renovascular hypertension in children. *J Pediatr Surg* **10**: 631–9, 1975
55. Welsh P, Repetto R: Renovascular hypertension in pediatric patients. *J Cardiovasc Surg (Torino)* **28**: 505–9, 1987

Editorial comments by P.R.F. Bell

This chapter sets out all details of renal artery stenosis and hypertension in children. It makes the usual points that intervention is required if there is poor blood pressure control, poor patient compliance, deterioration in renal function etc. Balloon angioplasty as is the case in most centres, is mentioned as the best form of treatment for this condition which turns out to be as expected. There then follows a description of a number of procedures which can be done for the disease in children and the summary of the results available. Experiences with nine patients are covered, five of whom had operations. The chapter concentrates on the results of balloon angioplasty and surgery in the few patients mentioned.

AORTIC QUESTIONS AND INDICATIONS

When Should We Operate and When Should We Not?

W. Bruce Campbell and David Hewin

INTRODUCTION

Mortality after operation for ruptured abdominal aortic aneurysm (RAAA) remains very high, with most recent series reporting death rates around 50%.[1-12] It could be argued that since this condition is fatal without surgery, all patients should be offered operation. However, many surgeons try to practice some preoperative case selection – on clinical, compassionate, and perhaps financial grounds.

From a clinical point of view, very major surgery on a patient with minimal chance of survival is hard to justify. From a compassionate and humanitarian standpoint operation and often prolonged intensive care is questionable management if the chance of survival is low, and especially if quality of life is then likely to be poor. Finally, there are financial arguments for directing the expensive treatment required for RAAA towards those with greatest chance of benefit.[4] Unfortunately only the occasional series[13] includes information about the numbers of patients who do not have operations, and the reasons for these decisions.

This chapter considers the problems in deciding when to operate and when not to operate, and presents the published data on factors which may influence this decision. The current views and practices of vascular surgeons in the UK and Ireland are also described, based on a recent questionnaire study undertaken by the authors.

HOW MANY PATIENTS DO NOT HAVE OPERATIONS?

Many patients never reach surgeons for assessment either because they die very rapidly or because the diagnosis is missed,[14-17] or perhaps because primary care doctors may decide not to refer some who are elderly or frail. Those making long journeys to tertiary referral centres may die in transit.

Two separate epidemiological studies in the UK,[18,19] covering the early 1980s, showed almost identical figures, with about one-third of all RAAA patients dying in the community, and one-quarter reaching hospital but having no operation. A longer term review by Ingoldby et al.,[20] and a similar study from Scandinavia[2] both reported similar results. All these figures relate to fairly well defined populations of patients, and it is clear that pre-hospital selection for some tertiary referral centres is even more intense. For example, Lawrie et al.[21] dealt with only 61 cases of rupture (4.4%) in a cohort of 1363 aneurysm operations: by contrast, large British hospitals receive about 40% of their aortic aneurysm patients after rupture.[18,22,23] These variations are seldom taken into account in series describing the results of surgery for RAAA of patients, but Callam *et al.*[24] have pointed out how seriously they may skew results. The proportion of patients who die in the community may also influence the degree of case selection after reaching hospital.

WHAT CRITERIA MIGHT BE USED IN CASE SELECTION?

Numerous series have been reported of patients having operations for RAAA, in which various factors have been analysed for an association with postoperative death (Table 1). Other studies have concentrated on intraoperative[5,9,16,21,25-28] and postoperative[4,5,7,8,10,27] factors which may predict a reduced chance of survival: these may help with decisions about whether to persevere with intensive care after operation, but they are no help in preoperative case selection.

Table 1.   Preoperative factors associated with increased mortality in patients with ruptured abdominal aortic aneurysm.

Increasing age[3,8.11,21,23,26,33,35]
Hypotension[1,3,5,7,9,23,25,27,29,31,36]
Myocardial ischaemia[8,16,23,25-27,31,33,36]
Renal dysfunction[1,5,8,23,25,33]
Cardiac arrest[7,8,25,33]
Anaemia[25,26,33,35]
Coagulation abnormalities[6,8,37]
Loss of consciousness[8,31,33]
Respiratory disease[1]
Cerebrovascular disease[32]
Acidosis[31]

WHAT ARE THE PROBLEMS IN USING SINGLE CRITERIA FOR CASE SELECTION?

Certain factors – such as age, hypotension, and myocardial disease – have been quite consistently shown to increase the risk of death after operation for RAAA. However, the problem of using any single criterion in preoperative case selection is that none offers reliable prediction of mortality. Age is the simplest and perhaps the most powerful predictor of survival,[11] and provides a good example of the difficulties. McCready *et al.*[3] showed that those over 70 fared significantly worse (mortality 63%) than those under 70 (mortality 34%): but conversely 37% of those over 70 survived, and in any event, using 70 years as a threshold would exclude the majority of all RAAA patients having operations in the United Kingdom from surgical treatment! Few publications give a clear description of the age range of survivors, but a proportion of even very elderly patients can survive surgery,[7,29] making it impossible to use age as a criterion for case selection with absolute confidence. Similar arguments apply to hypotension – another consistent predictor of increased mortality – a proportion of seriously hypotensive patients survive.[5]

Many of the other factors associated with high mortality are often difficult to elucidate and to quantify: there may be a history of cardiac or renal problems, but just how severe are they? Obtaining any information about the patient may be difficult in the emergency setting. Time is short, particularly when the patient is shocked, and the least delay in controlling the aorta gives the best chance of survival. The patient himself may be able to give some medical history, but is often in great pain, confused, or unconscious, so information about his premorbid condition, quality of life, and risk factors may be absent or unreliable. Medical notes may not be available, and there may be no relative present to provide information. Pressure of time also creates difficulties in getting the results of blood tests: this is an important reason why laboratory tests which may aid prediction of survival are not widely used.

Finally, it is worth noting that even some patients who have been advised against elective surgery after full assessment may then survive operation for RAAA despite their recognized risk factors.[30]

CAN WE USE COMBINATIONS OF CRITERIA FOR CASE SELECTION?

The fact that no single factor can predict outcome reliably has led to investigation of combinations of criteria with a view to case selection.

In 1985, Donaldson et al.[26] published a series of 81 patients whose risk factors had been analysed, and for whom computerized discriminant function analysis using age, haematocrit and blood pressure had then been applied to predict survival: this retrospective attempt at prediction was only correct in 70%.

Another retrospective study, published in 1987 by Shackleton et al.[31] used multivariate analysis to determine risk factors, and then stratified patients for risk of postoperative death using coefficients generated from a model based on their data. The factors they used were unmeasured anion gap, a history of congestive cardiac failure, and level of consciousness before operation (unmeasured anion gap is the difference between serum sodium, and the sum of chloride and total carbon dioxide content – it is a measure of acidosis). Their four subgroups had mortalities of 100%, 75%, 28%, and 12%. The fact that all five of their patients in the highest risk category died suggests a possibly useful system, but the figures and calculations required to use a system like this are unattractive (and impractical) in the ordinary emergency setting, and the authors even pointed out that 'the prediction rules often perform best in the data set that generated them'.

More recently, Samy et al. have proposed[32] and evaluated[23] the Glasgow Aneurysm Score to predict mortality risk, based on simple clinical criteria. This score was calculated as: (age in years) + (17 points for shock) + (7 points for myocardial disease) + (10 points for cerebrovascular disease) + (14 points for renal disease). In a prospective study of 320 patients[23] having operations for ruptured and non-ruptured aneurysms, they defined four levels of risk, with patients scoring over 85 having a mortality of 35%. They justified combining all ruptured and non-ruptured cases on the basis that shock was a better predictor of poor outcome than rupture, but unfortunately they did not at any stage describe patients with RAAA separately, so it is difficult to draw any conclusions about how well this system works for those patients. Based on the available data, it would seem that this system cannot select out with any certainty those patients in whom operation is not justified – it can simply identify a group at higher risk. The authors nevertheless deserve credit for their attempt to test a simple system prospectively.

Two separate studies were published in 1996 which produced similar conclusions about factors which might be used in mortality prediction. Based on logistic regression analysis in a series of 157 RAAA patients, Chen et al.[8] proposed a model for predicting mortality based on age, level of consciousness, and cardiac arrest. Although no group could be predicted to have 100% mortality, the model predicted mortality rates for unconscious patients who had sustained a cardiac arrest at age 60, 70, 80, and 90 years as 88%, 93%, 96%, and 99% respectively. A model which can predict such high chances of death would appear to offer practical possibilities, althought the sceptic might argue that such patients are ones who would be excluded from operation on simple clinical grounds, without the need to apply mathematical modelling.

The second recent study was by Hardman et al.[33] who again used logistic regression analysis on a retrospective series (154 patients) to define risk factors, and then to stratify patients into risk groups. This study has attracted particular interest, because it identified a group (albeit only eight patients) with 100% mortality. Two of the criteria used in prediction were clinical – age over 76 years and loss of consciousness – and three required special tests – creatinine >0.19mmol/l, haemoglobin <9g/dl, and electrocardiographic ischaemia. The authors reported mortalities of 37%, 72%, and 100% for patients with one, two, and three or more risk factors respectively. Two studies have tested these criteria by case note review, and the results are shown in Table 2. Prance et al.[12] concurred with Hardman's observations that all patients with three or more risk factors died, while Irvine et al.[34] had 40% (two of five) such patients survive: however, all five of their patients with loss of consciousness after admission died, supporting this as a powerful risk factor. These numbers are all small, but Hardman's set of criteria represent one of the most promising approaches to date for case selection.

Table 2. Mortality (%) in three case series using the criteria described by Hardman et al.[33] (age>76, loss of consciousness, creatinine >0.19mmol/l, haemoglobin<9g/dl, and electrocardiographic ischaemia)

No. of factors	Hardman et al.[33] n=154	Prance et al.[12] n=46	Irvine et al.[34] n=30
0	16%	25%	11%
1	37%	45%	22%
2	72%	65%	57%
3 or more	100%	100%	60%

WHAT UNPUBLISHED FACTORS MAY INFLUENCE CASE SELECTION?

Factors relating to quality of life often play an important part in decisions not to operate. Patients severely disabled by Parkinson's disease or stroke, the demented, those in long-term care, and the very elderly without any close relatives, are all people for whom some surgeons would decide against operation on compassionate grounds. Decisions of this kind may be very difficult, and the potential to make them may be very different in different countries. For example, there is generally much greater pressure to operate regardless of future quality of life in the USA than in the UK: this is driven by medicolegal pressures.

Almost nothing is documented about the current practices and views of vascular surgeons in general regarding the factors which influence their decisions against operation for RAAA, and it was for this reason that we investigated the issue in a questionnaire based study.

WHAT ARE THE CURRENT VIEWS AND PRACTICES OF VASCULAR SURGEONS?

Questionnaires were sent to all 404 members of the Vascular Surgical Society of Great Britain and Ireland at the end of 1996. The questionnaire was entitled *Ruptured aortic aneurysm: the decision not to operate* and asked about provision of services for RAAA, followed by detailed questions about criteria which might influence the decision not to operate, about preoperative assessment and about attitudes towards medicolegal considerations. Surgeons were asked to indicate how specified criteria would influence their decision not to operate – no influence; may influence; would seldom operate; would never operate.

The response rate to the questionnaire was 81% (323 completed, and four returned by surgeons who had retired). Eleven (3%) surgeons operated on all cases of RAAA, but 308 (97%) decided not to operate on some patients. The influences of specified factors on these decisions are shown in detail in Table 3. Factors which influenced the majority of surgeons strongly against operation ('operate seldom or never') were age over 85 years (54%), severe neurological disease (75%), and a combination of two or more comorbidities (including cardiac, pulmonary, renal, and neurological disease) (74%). Prolonged hypotension had some influence on the decision for 73% surgeons, and 17% surgeons said they would seldom or never operate on patients who had been hypotensive for a long time.

It is interesting to look at the influence of the other criteria recently documented by Hardman *et al.*[33] and by Chen *et al.*,[8] which have been discussed above, and which seem to be powerful predictors when used in combination. Cardiac arrest influenced 85% surgeons, and 36% would seldom or never operate on these patients: for loss of consciousness the proportions were 74% and 26% respectively. However, haemoglobin <9g/dl had no influence at all on decisions for 70% surgeons: this may reflect the fact that many surgeons make their decisions about operation on clinical grounds alone.

Some insight into the extent of preoperative assessment and use of laboratory tests

Table 3. The way in which specific criteria influenced vascular surgeons in their decision not to operate on RAAA (all figures are %)

	No influence	May influence	Seldom operate	Never operate
Over 75 years	67	33	0	0
Over 80 years	23	55	22	0
Over 85 years	11	35	36	18
Severe neurological disease	1	24	57	18
Limiting cardiac disease	7	71	21	1
Severe pulmonary disease	8	63	27	2
Renal dysfunction	12	68	18	2
Two or more of the above	1	25	51	23
Cardiac arrest	15	49	28	8
Loss of consciousness	26	48	19	7
Prolonged hypotension	27	56	14	3
Haemoglobin <9g/dl	70	28	2	0
Long-term care (e.g. nursing home)	13	53	30	4
Absence of close caring relative	67	31	2	0

was provided by the single question about surgeons' usual policies in preoperative management. This question offered alternatives of 'Selected cases' or 'Always' to two possible management policies – (a) immediate transfer to theatre for emergency operation without any investigations, or (b) a period of assessment (+ resuscitation) to obtain more medical details/do blood tests/consider wisdom of operation. A selective approach was used by 55%, while 37% practised immediate transfer to theatre (although this immediate transfer was combined with a period of assessment by 14%).

Social factors swayed few surgeons strongly against operation (Table 3). Long-term care (e.g. nursing home) influenced 87% to some extent, but only 34% would seldom on never operate on these grounds; while absence of a close caring relative had no influence at all for 67%.

Surgeons were asked 'Do possible medicolegal consequences of not operating influence your decision?' Seventy eight percent said that they never did so; 20% were influenced 'occasionally'; 2% 'often'; and no surgeon was 'always' influenced by medicolegal considerations.

These results provide some insight into current practices in the UK, although the need to keep any questionnaire simple prohibited exploring each issue in greater depth. In particular, it was difficult to pose questions about different combinations of criteria and the reasons for surgeons' practices. However, the study showed that almost all surgeons do practice case selection, and that every one of the criteria which has been documented as influencing postoperative survival adversely (apart from haemoglobin level) has some influence on the decisions of more than 70% vascular surgeons.

CONCLUSION AND A PERSONAL VIEW

If only to provoke criticism, I (BC) will state some of my own current practices in case selection for RAAA. I never operate on patients aged 90 or over, and consider patients much over 80 very carefully, tending to advise against operation if they have serious disease in more than one system. I am very strongly influenced by quality of life and social factors. I seldom operate on the demented or those who are very seriously disabled (e.g. advanced Parkinson's disease); or on those with known incurable cancer (with the possible exception of prostatic malignancy). Existence in long-term care or absence of a close caring relative influence me strongly against operation in the very elderly, unless the patient is known to have an active and happy independent existence. Conversely, the presence of a spouse sways me towards operation even in some very high risk patients. The younger patients are, the more difficult it is to deny them surgery, but I take the grossly obese 64-year-old with a bad cardiac history to the operating theatre with a sense of pessimism.

These are personal views and are presented to demonstrate my own bias. Each surgeon's policy will be dictated their own experience and their personal concepts of compassion, kind management, and use of resources. No regimented set of criteria is ever likely to be applicable to all patients – each presents a unique set of considerations. However, open discussion about policies, and more rigorous presentation of data on patients who are excluded from operation, will help vascular surgeons to make decisions about case selection with greater confidence.

REFERENCES

1. Ouriel K, Geary G, Green RM *et al.*: Factors determining survival after ruptured aortic aneurysm: the hospital, the surgeon, and the patient. *J Vasc Surg* **11**: 493–96, 1990
2. Bengtsson H, Bergqvist D: Ruptured abdominal aortic aneurysm: a population-based study. *J Vasc Surg* **18**: 74–80, 1993
3. McCready RA, Siderys H, Pittman JN *et al.*: Ruptured abdominal aortic aneurysms in a private hospital: a decade's experience (1980–1989). *Ann Vasc Surg* **7**: 225–28, 1993
4. Tromp Meesters RC, van der Graaf Y, Eikelboom BC: Ruptured aortic aneurysm: early postoperative prediction of mortality using an organ system failure score. *Br J Surg* **81**: 512–16, 1994
5. Johnston KW: The Canadian Society for Vascular Surgery Aneurysm Study Group: Ruptured abdominal aortic aneurysm: six-year follow-up results of a multicenter prospective study. *J Vasc Surg* **19**: 888–900, 1994
6. Bradbury AW, Bachoo P, Milne AA, Duncan JL: Platelet count and the outcome of operation for ruptured abdominal aortic aneurysm. *J Vasc Surg* **21**: 484–91, 1995
7. Panneton JM, Lassonde J, Laurendeau F: Ruptured abdominal aortic aneurysm: impact of comorbidity and postoperative complications on outcome. *Ann Vasc Surg* **9**: 535–41, 1995
8. Chen JC, Hildebrand HD, Salvian AJ: Predictors of death in nonruptured and ruptured abdominal aortic aneurysms. *J Vasc Surg* **24**: 614–23: 1996
9. Farooq MM, Freischlag JA, Seabrook GR: Effect of the duration of symptoms, transport time, and length of emergency room stay on morbidity and mortality in patients with ruptured abdominal aortic aneurysms. *Surgery* **119**: 9–14, 1996
10. Kazmers A, Jacobs L, Perkins A *et al.*: Abdominal aortic aneurysm repair in Veterans Affairs medical centers. *J Vasc Surg* **23**: 191–200, 1996
11. Rutledge R, Oller DW, Meyer AA *et al.*: A statewide, population-based, time-series

analysis of the outcome of ruptured abdominal aortic aneurysm. *Ann Surg* **223**: 492–505, 1996

12. Prance S, Wilson YG, Cosgrove C *et al.*: Ruptured abdominal aortic aneurysm: preoperative selection of patients for surgery. *Br J Surg* **84**: 567, 1997

13. Campbell WB, Collin J, Morris PJ: The mortality of abdominal aortic aneurysms. *Ann R Coll Surg Engl* **68**: 275–78, 1986

14. Armour RH: Survivors of ruptured abdominal aortic aneurysm: the iceberg's tip. *Br Med J* **2**: 1055–77, 1977

15. Gaylis H, Kessler E: Ruptured aortic aneurysm: *Surgery* **87**: 300–04, 1980

16. Hoffann M, Avellone JC, Plecha FR *et al.*: Operation for ruptured abdominal aortic aneurysms: a community-wide experience. *Surgery* **91**: 577–602, 1982

17. Marston WA, Ahlquist R, Johnson G, Meyer AA: Misdiagnosis of ruptured abdominal aortic aneurysms. *J Vasc Surg* **16**: 17–22, 1992

18. Thomas PRS, Stewart RD: Abdominal aortic aneurysm. *Br J Surg* **75**: 733–36, 1988

19. Budd JS, Finch DRA, Carter PG: A study of the mortality from ruptured abdominal aortic aneurysms in a district community. *Eur J Vasc Surg* **3**: 351–54, 1989

20. Ingoldby CJ, Wujanto R, Mitchell JE: Impact of vascular surgery on community mortality from ruptured aortic aneurysms. *Br J Surg* **73**: 551–53, 1986

21. Lawrie GM, Morris GC, Crawford ES *et al.*: Improved results of operation for ruptured abdominal aortic aneurysms. *Surgery* **85**: 483–88, 1979

22. Fielding JWL, Black J, Ashton F *et al.*: Diagnosis and management of 528 abdominal aortic aneurysms. *Br Med J* **283**: 355–59, 1981

23. Samy AK, Murray G, MacBain G: Prospective evaluation of the Glasgow Aneurysm Score. *J R Coll Surg Edinb* **41**: 105–07, 1996

24. Callam MJ, Haiart D, Murie JA: Ruptured aortic aneurysm: a proposed classification. *Br J Surg* **78**: 1126–129, 1991

25. Wakefield TW, Whitehouse WM, Wu S-C *et al.*: Abdominal aortic aneurysm rupture: statistical analysis of factors affecting outcome of surgical treatment. *Surgery* **91**: 586–96, 1982

26. Donaldson MC, Rosenberg JM, Bucknam CA: Factors affecting survival after ruptured abdominal aortic aneurysm. *J Vasc Surg* **2**: 564–70, 1985

27. Bauer EP, Redaelli C, von Segesser LK, Turina MI: Ruptured abdominal aortic aneurysms: predictors for early complications and death. *Surgery* **114**: 31–35, 1993

28. Marty-Ane CH, Alric P, Picot E *et al.*: Ruptured abdominal aortic aneurysm: influence of intraoperative management on surgical outcome. *J Vasc Surg* **22**: 780–86, 1995

29. Butler MJ, Cnant ADB, Webster JHH: Ruptured abdominal aortic aneurysms. *Br J Surg* **65**: 839–841, 1978

30. Burke PM, Sannella NA: Ruptured abdominal aortic aneurysm: a community experience. *Cardiovasc Surg* **1**: 239–42, 1993

31. Shackleton CR, Schechter MT, Bianco R, Hildebrand HD: Preoperative predictors of mortality risk in ruptured abdominal aortic aneurysm. *J Vasc Surg* **6**: 583–89, 1987

32. Samy AK, Murray G, MacBain G: Glasgow aneyrysm score. *Cardiovasc Surg* **2**: 41–44, 1994

33. Hardman DTA, Fisher CM, Patel MI *et al.*: Ruptured abdominal aortic aneurysms: who should be offered surgery? *J Vasc Surg* **23**: 123–29, 1996

34. Irvine C, Ruddle A, Mitchell D, Lear P: Risk stratification for ruptured aneurysm: is it reliable? *Proc S West Vasc Surg* 1997

35. Katz SG, Kohl RD: Ruptured abdominal aortic aneurysms: a community experience. *Arch Surg* **129**: 285–90, 1994

36. Browning NG, Long MA, Barry R *et al.*: Ruptured abdominal aortic aneurysms – prognostic indicators and complications affecting mortality. *S Afr J Surg* **33**: 21–25, 1995

37. Davies MJ, Murphy WG, Murie JA *et al.*: Preoperative coagulopathy in ruptured abdominal aortic aneurysm predicts poor outcome. *Br J Surg* **80**: 974–76, 1993

Editorial comments by P.R.F Bell

This is a well organized chapter which looks at the criteria for selection for aneurysm surgery. It reports on data obtained after a written questionnaire was sent to members of the Vascular Society of Great Britain and Ireland. The case is made for not treating certain groups of patients who have aneurysms and who are over the age of 80. The author has analysed the results of a postal survey which clearly show that there is much variation in practice but patients over the age of 80 and also those who are not leading an independent life are probably best not operated upon. This seems a perfectly reasonable point of view with the proviso that age is not everything, some patients of 85 are very young and some of 60 very old.

Is It Feasible to Treat Contained Aortic Aneurysm Rupture by Stent–Graft Combination?

S.W. Yusuf and B.R. Hopkinson

INTRODUCTION

Despite improvements in the perioperative care and intensive care support, the operative mortality rate for ruptured aortic aneurysm has remained unchanged over the last two decades and on an average nearly 50% of patients treated with open surgery die during the perioperative period.[1,2] There is therefore a significant potential for improvement in the results of surgery for ruptured aneurysms. Physiological studies show that elective endovascular repair is associated with fewer haemodynamic changes,[3] fall in colonic intramucosal pH[4] and subclinical renal injury[5] and improved postoperative respiratory function[6] compared with open surgery. Endovascular surgery could therefore be expected to reduce the operative mortality rate. Nearly 50% of aneurysm surgery is performed for ruptured aneurysms[7] and this could become an important indication for the use of endovascular method of repair. Although endovascular repair of a ruptured aneurysm was first reported in 1994,[8] limited data are so far available on the use of endovascular surgery for ruptured aneurysms and it is not possible to discuss this indication with the support of scientific evidence. This chapter will therefore focus on the technical aspects and feasibility of endovascular repair of contained rupture of an aortic aneurysm.

CHOICE OF PROCEDURE

Despite being the most simple in design and requiring shortest deployment time, aorto–aortic graft is now rarely used for endovascular repair. Few patients are found to have a distal aortic neck[9] and the results of those patients who have been treated with an aorto–aortic graft have been disappointing with a high rate of distal endoleak.[10] Bifurcated grafts have a relatively higher suitability rate but the currently available devices are suitable for less than one-third of aneurysms[9] and the insertion or deployment of the contralateral iliac limb may be time consuming in a modular or unitary prosthesis. However, recently a commercially available modular device has been successfully used for endovascular repair of a contained rupture (personal communication, M. Wyatt). In selected patients where the anatomy is suitable and a bifurcated graft readily available such a repair should be possible. Aorto–uni–iliac device is not only suitable for the majority of aneurysms,[9] but it can also be deployed in a relatively short time. Based on the information obtained from previous studies on aneurysm morphology in our unit we have been able to keep a stock of sterile tapered endoprosthesis for an aorto–uni–iliac repair suitable for majority of aneurysms. For these reasons and because we have found this type of repair to be effective in elective cases,[11] we use the aorto–uni–iliac device in the management of ruptured aneurysm. The aorto–uni–iliac endoprosthesis consists of a thin-walled uncrimped graft (Vascutek, Renfrewshire Scotland) which is supported by Gianturco stents (William Cook Europe, Denmark) throughout its length (Fig. 1, p. 222, this volume). In addition the emergency graft has an uncovered stent at the top for deployment above the renal arteries.

Preoperative assessment

A contrast enhanced computerized tomography (CT) scan is required to assess the anatomical suitability for endovascular repair, estimation of the graft size, and finally to confirm the diagnosis of a ruptured aneurysm. This investigation adds a delay of up to one hour in surgery and only those patients who are stable at presentation are considered for endovascular repair. As patients with a ruptured aneurysm can rapidly deteriorate from a stable state, careful monitoring by a team of vascular surgeon and anaesthetist is maintained throughout this period. An intra-aortic balloon catheter has been developed in our unit in collaboration with William Cook Europe, to provide rapid temporary control of haemorrhage by occluding the aorta (Fig. 1). This is a dual purpose balloon catheter designed to act as an aortic occlusion balloon catheter and a marker angiographic catheter. Once this catheter has been placed, intra-aortic injection of contrast through this catheter can provide better contrast enhancement during CT scan, particularly in a compromised circulatory state, and should the patient become unstable, inflation of the balloon can provide immediate control.

Multiplanar reconstruction of CT images does allow a more detailed analysis and perhaps provide a more accurate measurement of aortic neck and particularly the iliac diameter and time permitting this should be undertaken, while other preparations are being made in the operating theatre. On the other hand if the time and or expertise for multiplanar reconstruction is not available then estimates from the axial slices have to be used and the graft is oversized at the top end by 10–15%.

In elective cases it is desirable to obtain detailed information about the aorto–iliac anatomy preoperatively. However, in an emergency it may not be possible or appropriate to obtain a CT or magnetic resonance scan. A study was therefore undertaken to assess whether an on-table calibrated angiogram could provide the necessary information to allow selection of an appropriate endoprosthesis. A blind review of on-table calibrated angiogram performed by two observers showed that the measurements of neck length, diameter and iliac diameter obtained from the calibrated angiogram did not agree closely with the measurements obtained from spiral CT reconstruction. However, with graft oversizing of 10–15% at the proximal end and about 10% at the iliac end, it was possible to select an appropriate endoprosthesis for 60% of the cases (unpublished data) from a calibrated angiogram alone. The reliability of using measurements from on-table calibrated angiogram alone for ruptured aneurysms needs further prospective evaluation.

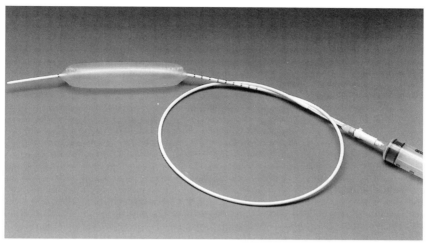

Fig. 1a. Aortic occlusion balloon catheter. This is a catheter witha 40-mm diameter balloon and 1-cm radiopaque markers to allow calibrated angiography.

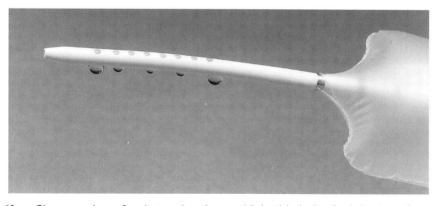

Fig. 1b. Close-up view of catheter showing multiple side-holes for injection of contrast.

Method of graft deployment

The procedure can be started with exposure of the femoral arteries under local anaesthesia. Once the delivery system is ready to be introduced general anaesthesia is administered. Elective endovascular repair entirely under local anaesthesia has recently been reported[12] and it may have advantages in patients with ruptured aneurysm. For an aorto–uni–iliac repair, a preliminary angiogram is performed to obtain measurement of the aorto–iliac length, determine the position of the renal arteries and choose the favourable iliac artery for the introduction of the delivery system and implantation of the stent-graft. As it may not be possible to assess the anatomy carefully in an emergency, routine use of a suprarenal uncovered stent provides additional security in case the aneurysm neck is short. Once the graft is deployed, the contralateral iliac is occluded with an occluding device and a femorofemoral bypass performed. Completion angiogram is performed in two planes and a contrast enhanced CT scan is obtained to make sure that the aneurysm is effectively excluded from the circulation.

EVIDENCE OF FEASIBILITY

Infrarenal aortic aneurysms

In our unit endovascular repair of contained aneurysm rupture has been attempted on nine patients. On two occasions the patients became unstable during transfer to theatre and died before the stent–graft could be deployed. The remainder of seven cases remained haemodynamically stable with a systolic blood pressure ≥ 90 mmHg. In these seven cases it was possible to implant a device and achieve effective exclusion of aneurysm. All seven patients survived the procedure but one 84-year-old patient with an excluded aneurysm died 2 weeks postoperatively from renal failure, without any evidence of renal artery occlusion. On an intention-to-treat basis successful repair was achieved in 7/9 (77.7%) with an overall perioperative mortality rate of 3/9 (33.3%). The anatomy was particularly complex and challenging in 5/7 patients, and significant co-morbid conditions were present in 6/7 patients. One patient had been deemed unsuitable for elective endovascular repair on the basis of unfavourable anatomy and poor cardiovascular status (Fig. 2). However, when he presented with a ruptured aneurysm, an endovascular repair was successfully achieved. This patient is alive more than 1 year after repair and the aneurysm has shown a remarkable reduction in size. Similar reduction in aneurysm size has been observed in the other two patients who had their aneurysm repaired more than 1 year ago (Fig. 3).

Thoracic aneurysms

Endovascular repair of contained rupture of thoracic aneurysm has been reported from Stanford University Medical Center, USA. This group has acquired substantial experience with the elective endovascular repair of thoracic aneurysms since 1992 and has recently reported endovascular repair in six patients with rupture of thoracic aneurysm contained within the mediastinum.[13] The Endoprosthesis was assembled using an ironed woven polyester graft (Cooley Veri-Soft Dacron, Meadox/Boston Scientific, Watertown, MA) and Gianturco Z-stent (Cook, Bloomington, IN) endoskeleton. Rupture had occurred within the preceding 7 days and was confirmed with preoperative imaging in all cases. All six patients survived the procedure and there was one death at 28 days which was considered to be unrelated to the procedure. No patient developed postoperative spinal cord or renal complications. In our unit successful endovascular exclusion of a ruptured thoracic aneurysm has recently been performed and the patient is still recovering in hospital. These results are very encouraging as open surgery for ruptured thoracic aneurysm is associated with a high morbidity and mortality rate even in the most experienced centres.[14,15]

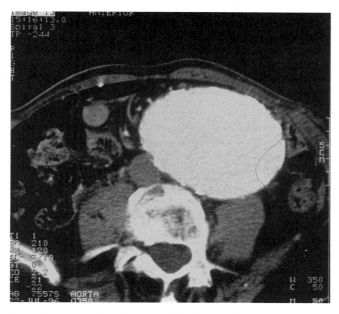

Fig. 2a. Preoperative CT scan showing a 9.6-cm diameter aortic aneurysm with no thrombus inside.

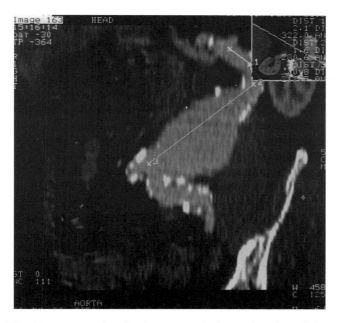

Fig. 2b. Reconstruction in the coronal plane showing right angle bends at the aorto–iliac junction and between the neck and the aneurysm with calcification of the iliac.

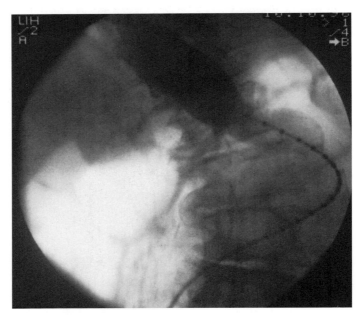

Fig. 3a. On-table angiogram showing marked tortuosity of the aneurysm. Tortuosity combined with a large empty sac makes estimation of the graft length difficult in this case.

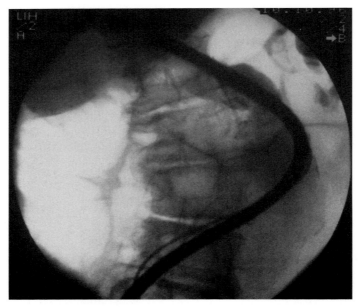

Fig. 3b. Delivery sheath showed following the curved lumen making introduction of graft difficult.

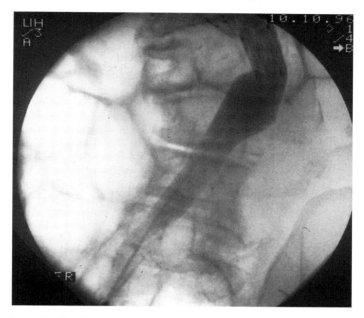

Fig. 3c.   Graft takes a shorter course, and a satisfactory exclusion is achieved.

FUTURE TRIALS

The technical feasibility of treating contained rupture of both abdominal and thoracic aneurysms has now been demonstrated in a few cases. However, there are many issues that need to be resolved through controlled trials before endovascular repair could make an impact on the outcome of ruptured aneurysms.

One of the concerns about the use of endovascular repair is that a preoperative CT scan may cause a delay which may adversely influence the outcome in some patients. However, there is some evidence that transfer of stable patients for open surgery may be safe.[16–18] The vascular surgical community in the UK is now supporting the move towards centralization of vascular services that will require such transfers between hospitals.[19] It could therefore be argued that a short delay caused by CT scan may not result in an increase in avoidable deaths.

While there is some data regarding the anatomical suitability of intact aneurysms, there is little information about the suitability of ruptured aneurysms, which may represent a different subpopulation. It seems from our relatively small experience that patients presenting with ruptured aneurysms usually have adverse anatomical features and it is therefore possible that a higher proportion of ruptured aneurysms may be anatomically unsuitable for endovascular repair using the commercially available devices than that estimated from the study on elective cases.[9]

Endoleaks following elective repair have been observed with all devices. The primary endoleak rate following elective repair is between 5 and 44%[20–23] depending

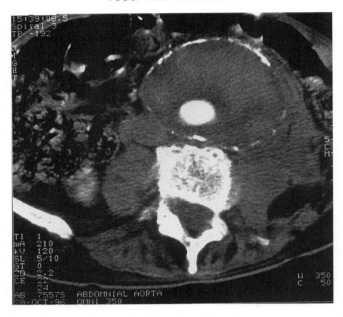

Fig. 4a.   Same patient as in Fig. 2a with a haematoma around the
aneurysm and an endovascular graft with no endoleak.

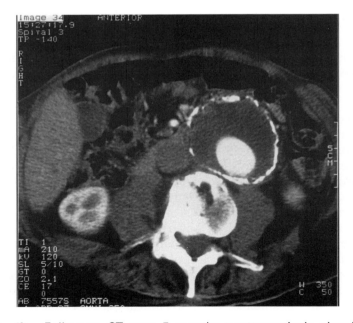

Fig. 4b.   Follow-up CT scan 5 months postoperatively showing
resolution of retroperitoneal haematoma, no endoleak and a
significant reduction in the size of the aneurysm.

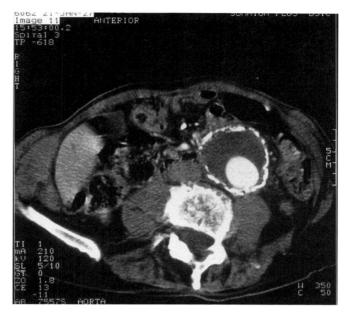

Fig. 4c. Further reduction in the size seen on a CT scan performed at 1 year.

to some extent on the type of endoprosthesis used. Many of these endoleaks can be treated expectantly or by additional procedures at the time of elective surgery but persistent endoleak following endovascular repair of a ruptured aneurysm could have more serious consequences.

Conversion of a failed elective endovascular procedure to an open procedure is known to make the open procedure more difficult than a primary open procedure.[23] Endovascular repair of ruptured aneurysm should not be undertaken by centres during their learning curve as the outcome in patients with conversions is likely to be worse than those undergoing primary open repair.[24]

Timely efforts are being made to organize a multicentre randomized trial of open vs endovascular surgery to define the role of endovascular repair. Data from the European (EUROSTAR) registry[25] and the UK (RETA) registry[26] indicate that the randomized trials could fail to show significant advantage with endovascular repair in elective cases, in terms of perioperative mortality rates.

Although the data from these registries include the learning curve with endovascular repair and also inclusion of high risk patients, many of whom may not be suitable for open surgery, it is possible that the randomized trials show no benefit with endovascular repair and if the cost of endovascular repair is found to be significantly greater than open repair than it may have to be abandoned for elective cases. In which case the expertise for performing endovascular repair in emergencies (where there may be an advantage) will no longer be available. It is therefore imperative that concurrent randomized trial of endovascular vs open surgery for ruptured aneurysm is undertaken by those centres that have sufficient expertise and resources. Such a trial will no doubt require considerable enthusiasm, energy and

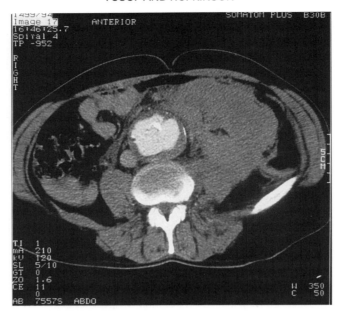

Fig. 5a. Extensive retroperitoneal haematoma on the preoperative CT scan.

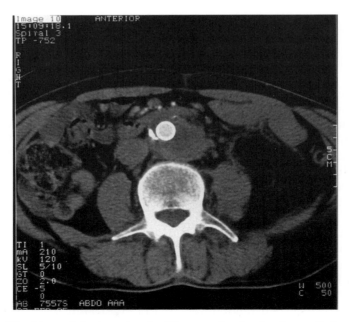

Fig. 5b. No endoleak and a significant reduction in size on follow-up
CT scan done 5 months postoperatively.

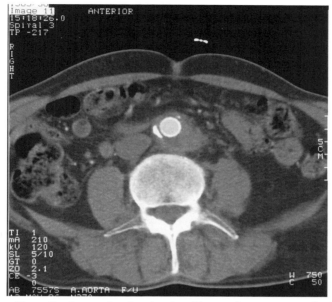

Fig. 5c. Further reduction in size 17 months postoperatively.

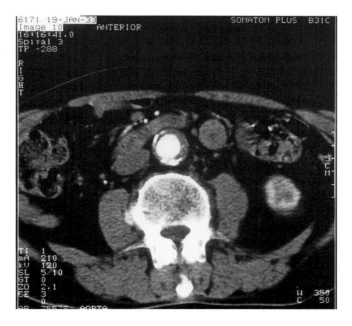

Fig. 5d. A very small aneurysm left at 36 months postoperatively.

resources but the results of such a trial could have a major impact on the outcome of patients with ruptured aneurysm.

REFERENCES

1. Ernst CB: Abdominal aortic aneurysms. *New Engl J Med* **328**; 1167–72, 1993
2. Callam MJ, Haiart D, Murie JA *et al.*: Ruptured aortic aneurysm: a proposed classification. *Br J Surg* **78**; 1126–9, 1991
3. Baxendale BR, Baker DM, Hutchinson A *et al.*: Haemodynamic and metabolic response to endovascular repair of infra-renal aortic aneurysm. *Br J Anaesthes* **77**; 581–5, 1996
4. ElMarasy N, Yusuf SW, Lonsdale RJ *et al.*: Study on the effect of Endovascular repair on colonic perfusion. *J Endovasc Surg* **3**; 95, 1996
5. Baker DM, Wenham PW: Renal damage. In: Hopkinson BR, Yusuf SW, Whitaker SC, Veith FJ (Eds), *Endovascular Surgery for Aortic Aneurysms*. London: WB Saunders Co, Ltd, 1997
6. Boyle JR, Thompson JP, Thompson MM *et al.*: Improved respiratory function and analgesia control after endovascular AAA repair. *J Endovasc Surg* **4**; 62–5, 1997
7. Bradbury AW, Makhdoomi KR, Adam DJ: Ruptured abdominal aortic aneurysm (AAA): A 12 year experience. 30th Annual Conference of the Vascular Surgical Society of Great Britain and Ireland. Bournemouth 20–22 November 1996
8. Yusuf SW, Whitaker SC, Chuter TAM *et al.*: Emergency endovascular abdominal aortic aneurysm repair. *Lancet* **344**; 1645, 1994
9. Armon MP, Yusuf SW, Lateif K *et al.*: The anatomical suitability of abdominal aortic aneurysms for endovascular repair. *Br J Surg* **84**; 178–80, 1997
10. Armon MP, Yusuf SW, Whitaker SC *et al.*: The anatomy of abdominal aortic aneurysms: Implications for sizing of endovascular grafts. *Eur J Vasc Endovasc Surg* **13**; 398–402, 1997
11. Yusuf SW, Whitaker SC, Chuter TAM *et al.*: Early results of endovascular abdominal aortic aneurysm repair with aorto–uni–iliac graft and femoro-femoral bypass. *J Vasc Surg* **25**; 165–72, 1997
12. Papasoglu K, Christu T, Iordanidis K *et al.*: Endovascular AAA repair with percutaneous transfemoral prosthesis deployment under local anesthesia. Initial experience with a new, simple to use, tubular and bifurcated device, in the first 27 cases. Presented to the XI Annual Meeting of the European Society for Vascular Surgery, Lisbon 1997
13. Semba CP, Kato N, Kee ST *et al.*: Acute rupture of the descending thoracic aorta: repair with the use of endovascular stent-grafts. *JVIR* **8**; 337–42, 1997
14. Moreno-Carbal CE, Miller DC, Mitchell RS *et al.*: Degenerative and atherosclerotic aneurysms of the thoracic aorta. *J Cardiovascular Surg* **88**; 1020–32, 1984
15. Crawford ES, Hess KR, Cohen ES *et al.*: Ruptured aneurysms of the descending thoracic and thoraco-abdominal aorta: analysis according to size and treatment. *Ann Surg* **213**; 417–26, 1991
16. Adam DJ, Mohan IV, Stuart WP *et al.*: Transferring patients with ruptured abdominal aortic aneurysm to a regional vascular surgery unit does not prejudice outcome. Presented to the 31st Annual Conference of the Vascular Surgical Society of Great Britain & Ireland, London, 1997
17. Barros D'Sa AAB: Optimal travel distance before ruptured aortic aneurysm repair. In: Greenhalgh RM, Mannick JA, Powell J (Eds), *The Causes and Management of Aneurysms*. London: WB Saunders, 1990
18. Farooq MM, Freischlag JA, Seabrook GR *et al.*: Effect of duration of symptoms, transport time, and length of emergency room stay on morbidity and mortality in patients with ruptured abdominal aortic aneurysms. *Surgery* **119**; 9–14, 1996
19. The provision of Vascular Services: A document prepared for the Vascular Surgical Society of Great Britain and Ireland by the Vascular Advisory Committee, 1997
20. White GH, Yu W, May J *et al.*: Three year experience with the White–Yu endovascular GAD graft for transluminal repair of aortic and iliac aneurysms. *J Endovasc Surg* **4**; 124–35, 1997

21. Blum U, Voshage G, Beyersdorf F *et al.*: Two-center German experience with aortic endografting. *J Endovasc Surg* **4**; 137–46, 1997
22. Malina M, Ivancev K, Chuter TAM *et al.*: Changing aneurysmal morphology after endovascular grafting: relation to leakage or persistent perfusion. *J Endovasc Surg* **4**; 23–30, 1997
23. Moore WS, Rutherford R: Transfemoral endovascular repair of abdominal aortic aneurysm: Results of the North American EVT phase I trial. *J Vasc Surg* **23**; 543–53, 1996
24. May J, White GH, Yu W *et al.*: Conversion from endoluminal to open repair of abdominal aortic aneurysms: A hazardous procedure. *J Endovasc Surg* **4**(Suppl 1); I27–I28, 1997
25. Gilling-Smith GL, Cuypers P, Buth J, Harris PL for Eurostar Collaborators: Endovascular repair of abdominal aortic aneurysms: Results of a European multicentre study. Presented to the XI Annual meeting of the European Society for Vascular Surgery, Lisbon, 17–20 September 1997
26. Beard J on behalf of the VSS & SIR Registry of Endovascular treatment of aneurysms (RETA): Preliminary results. Presented to the XI Annual meeting of the European Society for Vascular Society, Lisbon, 17–20 September 1997

Editorial comments by P.R.F. Bell

This paper discusses an interesting extension of the use of endovascular stenting for enclosed ruptures of aneurysms. Nine cases are discussed and the point about a non-customized graft is well made. Maintaining the patient's condition with intra-aortic ballon while CT scanning is done has been advocated here but this seems unacceptable. The authors have also looked at calibrated angiography on the table to examine the measurements and find, not suprisingly, that this is not sufficient. However, by oversizing the upper end of the stent and using aorto–uni–iliac grafts they were able to deal with six cases. It might be worthwhile, rather than making this statement, to give some data about that particular situation as the only practical way of dealing with these patients is going to be using non-customized grafts and assessing the neck on the table by use of angiography and an intra-aortic balloon. The paper does, however, show that it is feasible and makes the point that this may be the best use of endovascular repair in the sense that it would be cost-effective if used in an emergency situation. I think more details from the authors of how they manage patients and the difficulties encountered would be appropriate.

When Should We Intervene for Aortic and Arterial Dissections?

Barbara Theresia Müller, Klaus Grabitz, Bernd Luther and
Wilhelm Sandmann

AORTIC DISSECTIONS

Acute aortic dissection probably occurs at a rate of 5 to 10 per million inhabitants per year.[1-3] The life-threatening disease starts with an intimal tear (entry) in the ascending aorta (type A) or distally to the left subclavian artery (type B). The dissecting haematoma in the outer half of the media may extend antegrade or retrograde and re-enter into the tube arterial channel, resulting in a spontaneous cure (re-entry), or rupture to the outside, leading in general to death. The dissections are 'acute' when onset is less than 2 weeks before and become 'chronic' when more than 2 weeks have elapsed.[4]

Predisposing factors are cystic medial necrosis, which was first described by Erdheim[5] and congenital diseases of the connective tissue such as Marfan's syndrome and Ehlers–Danlos syndrome type IV.[6-9] Congenital bicuspid aortic valves may be a risk for development of type A dissections while aortic atherosclerosis and hypertension often accompany type B dissections.[10] It is our impression, that the incidence of aortic dissection is increasing and only a few patients appear to have the above-mentioned risk factors.

Without treatment the prognosis of acute aortic dissection is very poor. In 1958 Hirst reviewed 505 cases and found out that 21% of his patients died within 24 hours of onset and only 9% survived 6 months.[11] Causes of death in untreated type A patients include intrapericardial and free intrapleural rupture, acute aortic valve insufficiency and to a minor extent cerebral and coronary malperfusion. In patients with type B dissections, free rupture of the aorta is less frequent. They usually die of peripheral vascular complications resulting in organ failure.[12-14]

To improve the natural course of the disease, de Bakey *et al*. developed a new surgical treatment of the dissected aorta by excision of the intimal tear, obliteration of the false lumen and insertion of a prosthetic graft. The results were outstanding with an overall mortality of 21% and a mortality of 23% in the acute stage.[15,16] However, the experiences of other workgroups[17] were not as successful as those reported by de Bakey *et al*., who developed a new medical treatment to influence the hydrodynamic forces of the bloodstream based on the theory that blood pressure and the steepness of the pulse wave are propagating the dissecting hematoma. The first drugs used were ganglionic blockers, later replaced by propanolol, a beta-adrenergic blocker and sodium nitroprusside, which selectively relaxes vascular smooth muscle.[1,17] A summary of 219 patients, treated either surgically or medically in six separate centres, revealed a bad outcome of patients with type A dissections, treated with drugs only. They had a mortality rate of 74% compared with only 30% when surgical intervension was performed. On the other hand, in patients with acute type B dissection, drug therapy alone yielded a survival rate of 80% compared with 50%, when surgical intervention was added.[1] Several other groups confirmed these results with high mortality rates of patients with type A dissections when treated with pharmacological agents only, compared with high survival rates of patients with type B dissections.[2,17-22]

Current therapy of type A aortic dissections consists of early surgical treatment by replacement of the involved ascending aorta and if necessary the aortic valve or reconstruction of these structures.[23-24]

Nowadays, the management of acute uncomplicated Stanford B dissections in most centres of the world is medical.[12-14,16,18-22,25-27] The appropriate diagnostic method is a contrast computed tomography to evaluate the extension of the dissection and its relation to major branches of the aorta. The patients should be admitted to an intensive care unit to allow careful monitoring while antihypertensive and negative inotropic drugs as well as analgesics are administered. The intention is for the medical treatment to stabilize the aortic dissected wall and to prevent further dissection and perforation.

Immediate surgical intervention becomes necessary if there is an expansion or rupture of the false lumen or if there is evidence for obstruction of a major aortic branch or lower extremity ischaemia.[12-14,18-22,25-27] In cases of peripheral vascular complications, angiography should be carried out first to see the exact cause of ischaemia. There are different mechanisms for aortic branch obstruction in acute dissection. Organ arteries may be perfused by the true or the false lumen. Therefore bulging or thrombosis of the false lumen may produce obstruction of the orificium. On the other hand, aortic dissection may proceed into the branch itself and lead to stenosis or thrombosis.[12]

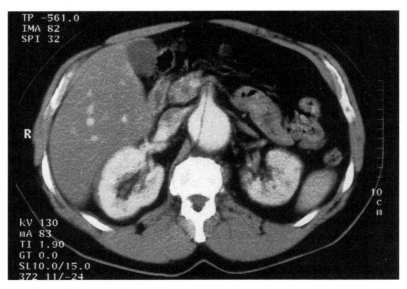

Fig. 1.   Chronic aortic dissection, the superior mesenteric artery is perfused by the true and false lumen.

Peripheral vascular complications occur in about one-third of the type B patients. Most frequent are lower extremity ischaemia and renal ischaemia, while perfusion of visceral arteries appears in about 10–20%. Paraplegia due to spinal cord ischaemia is rare.[12-14]

The therapeutic approach to these complications of acute aortic dissection remains controversial. Some centres prefer a resection of the dissecting membrane and replacement of the diseased aortic segment by a graft.[14,25,26] Others, like ourselves, tend to local reconstructions such as fenestration and extra-anatomic bypass grafting and performed these procedures in 15 cases.[12,13,27-29] Our only indication for total aortic replacement in the acute stage of dissection is aortic perforation or penetration. Aortic surgery in this early stage of dissection is a dangerous procedure. The aortic tissue is extremely friable and does not hold sutures and prosthesis well.[13,16] As intimal re-entry and the end of the false channel are either in the aorta itself or in one of the iliac arteries, one or both iliac arteries are always free of dissection and can be used as a donor vessel for extra-anatomic bypass surgery. If only one aortic branch

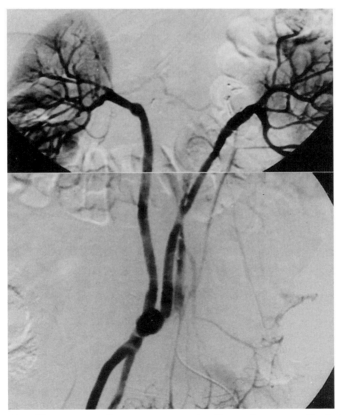

Fig. 2. Treatment of an acute aortic dissection complicated by kidney failure due to dissection of both renal arteries. Iliacobirenal bypass performed by an upside down 14/8 mm Dacron bifurcation graft.

needs revascularization, we use saphenous vein for bypass grafting. Otherwise an upside down Dacron bifurcation graft is used and revascularization is performed between the two graft branches and the renal or visceral arteries.

Limb ischaemia is treated by local removal of the iliac dissecting membrane often combined with thrombectomy or by femorofemoral bypass grafting. Abdominal aortic fenestration, first performed in 1935,[30] is carried out, if several organ arteries are occluded by the false lumen, or if paraplegia due to intercostal artery occlusion develops.

Endovascular catheter techniques are rather newer approaches to solve peripheral vascular complications. The Stanford group treated 11 patients with complicated aortic dissections by aortic stent and/or by balloon fenestration of the intimal flap. They were successful with relief of clinical symptoms in nine patients and had a 30-day mortality rate of 9%.[31,32] Other reports also show the possible effectiveness of endovascular treatment.[25,33,34]

Efficient medical treatment with antihypertensive and negative inotropic drugs, even in normotensive patients, is essential to prevent redissection and further dilatation of the aorta.[4,25] In particular, beta-adrenergic blockers reduce the progression of aortic dilatation.[35]

Table 1. Results of treatment of non-dissected thoracoabdominal aortic aneurysm (Crawford's classification used[78])

		No. of patients all groups	Paraparesis/ paraplegia all groups (%)	No. of patients group II	Paraparesis/ paraplegia group II (%)
Crawford[36]	1986	503	11	102	21
Sandmann[37]	1995	179	13.5	66	27.2

Table 2. Results of treatment of dissected thoracoabdominal aortic aneurysm (Crawford's classification used[78])

		No. of patients all groups	Paraparesis/ paraplegia all groups (%)	No. of patients group II	Paraparesis/ paraplegia group II (%)
Crawford[36]	1986	102	30.4	57	41
Sandmann[37]	1995	43	25.5	29	31

Table 3. Rate of postoperative complications in thoracoabdominal aortic replacement (Sandman[37])

	No. of patients	Postoperative dialysis (%)	Mortality (%)
Without dissection	179	13 (7.5)	19 (10.5)
Dissection	43	8 (18.5)	8 (18.5)

About 20% of the patients with type B dissections develop aneurysmal dilatation in later follow-up.[1,13,27] Indications for surgical intervention in chronic aortic dissection are expanding aneurysms which exceed 6 cm in diameter, painful symptomatic aneurysms and local vascular complications.[25]

The decision for operation should be reflected thoroughly because thoracoabdominal aortic replacement in aortic dissection has the highest risk of paraplegia and a high risk of postoperative kidney failure[25,36,37] (Tables 1, 2, 3).

ARTERIAL DISSECTIONS

Spontaneous dissections of visceral and renal arteries are rare, whereas dissections of the internal carotid artery are diagnosed more often.[38–41] They are produced by intramural bleeding of the vasa vasorum or by an intimal tear.[38] The intramural medial haematoma may expand toward the adventitia and cause aneurysmal dilatation or may extend more subintimally and cause stenosis.[42,43]

The pathogenesis is unclear. Frequently fibromuscular dysplasia can be found together with dissections of the internal carotid artery and renal artery dissections.[38,43–50,66] Some patients developed dissections of renal and carotid arteries at the same time, due to fibromuscular dysplasia.[41,46] Spontaneous bilateral internal carotid artery dissections are not rare. Even dissections of several organ arteries at the same time can be seen, as we treated a female patient with dissection of one renal and the coeliac artery. Internal carotid artery dissections are often attributed to mild or severe head and neck trauma.[43,51–57,66] Although renal artery dissections can be traumatic, they are more often seen after endovascular procedures.[41]

Dissection of the internal carotid artery

Due to recent advances in neurodiagnostic techniques, cervical artery dissection is an increasingly recognized cause of stroke, especially in young adults.[38,58–60,66] Most common signs are headache, bruit, oculosympathetic paresis and infrequent, homolateral disturbances of basal cranial nerves.[38,44,61–63,66] Mokri found focal cerebral symptoms in two-thirds of his patients, one-third presented with stroke.[44] Others observed stroke as initial symptom in nearly half of their cases.[63,65]

Different from atherosclerotic lesions, internal carotid artery dissection usually starts distally to the carotid bulb, where the elastic type of vessel changes to the muscular type,[81] and terminates at the entrance of the artery into the petrous bone.[38]

Radiological findings represent different stages of the disease,[63] including tapered pseudoocclusion of the internal carotid artery, and long irregular luminal stenosis with sudden reconstitution of the lumen, often at the carotid foramen and aneurysmal dilatation mostly near to the skull base.[44,63] Sensitive, non-invasive diagnostic methods are Doppler ultrasound and duplex scanning.[63,64]

Nearly all reports show the benign course of the disease with marked improvement or complete resolution of the dissected carotid artery and good clinical recovery of most patients with spontaneous dissections,[44,51,63] whereas residual dissecting aneurysms and occlusions seem to occur more frequently with traumatic dissections of the extracranial internal carotid artery.[79]

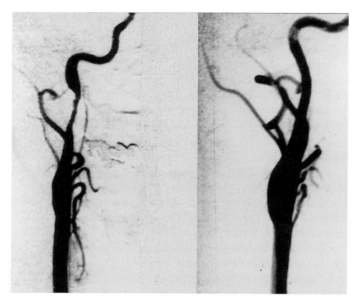

Fig. 3. Restitution of a spontaneous internal carotid artery dissection 6 months after onset treated by anticoagulation only.

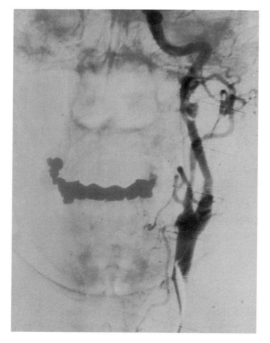

Fig. 4. Chronic dissection of the internal carotid artery complicated by an aneurysm near the skull base.

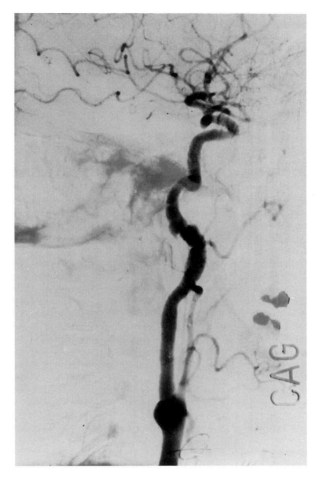

Fig. 5.   Resection of the dissected internal carotid artery and
the aneurysm, replacement by a vein interposition graft.

Steinke *et al.* used Doppler ultrasound investigation in 33 patients with dissection of the internal carotid artery. Initially nearly 29.8% presented as pseudoocclusion, 11.8% had a subtotal stenosis, the others had mild stenosis. Follow-up of these patients revealed a recanalization in 73.6%. In 8.8% the internal carotid artery remained occluded. Of these cases, 5.8% of the patients underwent reconstructive surgery at our institution because of a persisting aneurysm.[63]

In consideration of the high rate of spontaneous recanalization in internal carotid artery dissections, management is primarily non-surgical. Most surgeons recommend anticoagulation in symptomatic dissections to prevent further thromboembolic complications.[44,62,66,68] In patients without focal neurological signs and without severe stenosis or aneurysms, antiplatelet agents may be reasonable.[44] Frequent investigations with Doppler ultrasound, duplex scanning and in case of aneurysm, angiography are important to control the dissected lesions.

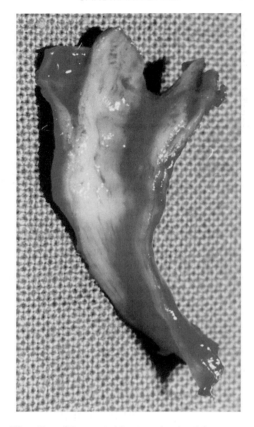

Fig. 6. Dissected internal carotid artery.

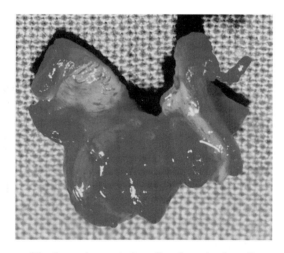

Fig. 7. Aneurysm with thrombus at the distal end of a dissected internal carotid artery.

Indications for surgical intervention are persisting or newly developed aneurysms and persisting severe internal carotid artery stenosis.[65,67–70,80]

From 1982 until now a total of 44 surgical procedures in 43 patients with internal carotid artery dissections was performed at our institution. Indications were persisting aneurysm, stenosis and floating thrombus.

As all aneurysms were located above the Blaisdell line, an imaginary anatomic line between the tip of the mastoid and the angle of the jaw,[71] resection of the diseased internal carotid artery and vein graft replacement had to be carried out in 32 cases. In five cases dissection ended more proximally and thromboendarterectomy with patch angioplasty could be done. In five cases aneurysmal dilatation reached into the skull. Reconstruction was impossible. Dilatation of the stenotic internal carotid artery and patch angioplasty was performed twice.

One patient died of intracranial bleeding, which appeared at the end of surgery; five (11%) patients suffered a minor stroke (none with persisting neurological deficits); 20 (45%) patients developed perioperative loss of function of one or more cranial nerves. After a follow-up of 6 months a deficiency remained in eight patients (18%), mostly of the glossopharyngeal nerve. Only three patients had severe dysphagia. During follow-up of 2–156 months (average 60 months), no one developed focal neurological signs, such as transitoric ischaemic attack or stroke.

Table 4. Indications for operative intervention

Cause	No. (%)
Aneurysm	25 (57)
Stenosis	7 (16)
Stenosis and aneurysm	10 (23)
Floating thrombus	2 (5)

Table 5. Aetiology of dissection

Cause	No. (%)
Trauma	21 (48)
Fibromuscular dysplasia	7 (16)
Atherosclerosis	7 (16)
Spontaneous	9 (20)

Table 6. Operative technique

Technique	No. (%)
Resection, vein interposition graft	32 (73)
Ligation	5 (11)
Thromboendarterectomy + patch angioplasty	5 (11)
Dilatation + patch angioplasty	2 (5)

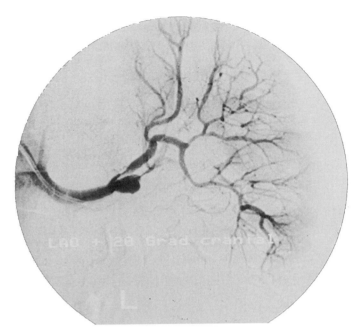

Fig. 8.   Traumatic dissection of the main renal artery and one primary branch.

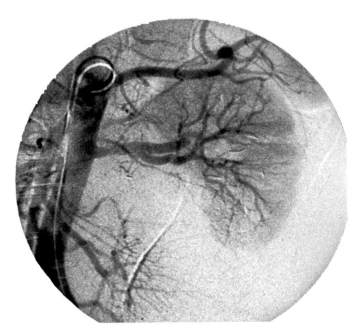

Fig. 9.   Resection of the dissected renal artery and a primary branch. Replacement by
two vein interposition grafts. Revascularization *in situ*.

Renal artery dissection

Acute spontaneous or traumatic dissections of the renal arteries are rare. Flank pain, haematuria, sudden onset of hypertension and headache may lead to diagnosis.[47,72-77] The radiological findings are often very impressive: dissection often involves main, primary and secondary branches. Renal infarction is frequent, but does not always occur.[4,72-77] Acute symptomatic dissection of the renal artery requires immediate intervention for kidney salvage. In the case of unilateral disease the decision to attempt revascularization in patients whose angiographies show total occlusion, may be difficult. In these cases local thrombolysis could be an alternative.[77]

Chronic dissections are usually discovered during evaluation for hypertension.[75] Aneurysmal enlargement is a common finding. In the case of renovascular hypertension caused by stenosis of the dissected renal artery, resection and vein graft interposition become necessary.[73-75] Asymptomatic aneurysms without hypertension should be resected when they exceed 1.5 cm in diameter.[74]

Within the last 15 years 20 patients with chronic dissection and two patients with acute dissection of the renal artery underwent operation at our institution. Nearly all (17 of 20) patients with chronic renal artery dissection had hypertension and 11 of them presented with aneurysmal dilatation. Two patients suffered from recurrent renal embolism. The acute renal artery dissections were caused by trauma.

REFERENCES

1. Wheat MW, Wheat MD: Acute dissecting aneurysms of the aorta: diagnosis and treatment-1979. *Am Heart J* **99**: 373–87, 1980
2. Jamieson WRE, Munro AI, Miyagishima RT *et al.*: Aortic dissection: Early diagnosis and surgical management are the keys to survival. *Can J Surg* **25**: 145–9, 1982
3. Fradet G, Jamieson WRE, Janusz M *et al.*: Aortic dissection. A six years experience with 117 patients. *Am J Surg* **155**: 697–700, 1988
4. de Bakey ME: Dissections of the thoracic aorta. In: Greenhalgh RM (Ed.), *Indications in Vascular Surgery*. London: WB Saunders Co Ltd, 1988
5. Erdheim J: Medionecrosis aortae idiopathica cystica. *Virchows Arch* **276**: 187–229, 1930
6. Ragunath M, Nienaber C, Kodolitsch Y: 100 Jahre Marfan-Syndrom- eine Bestandsauf-nahme. *Dt Ärztebl* **94**: A-772–9, 1997
7. Pyeritz RE, McKusick VA: The Marfan syndrom: diagnosis and management. *New Engl J Med* **300**: 772–9, 1979
8. Coselli JS, Le Maire SA, Büket S: Marfan syndrome: The variability and outcome of operative management. *J Vasc Surg* **21**: 432–43, 1995
9. Serry C, Agomuhoh O, Goldin M: Review of Ehlers Danlos syndrome Type IV. *J Cardiovasc Surg* **29**: 530–43, 1988
10. Larson EW, Edwards W: Risk factors for aortic dissection: A necropsy study of 161 cases. *Am J Cardiol* **53**: 849–55, 1984
11. Hirst AE, Johns VJ, Kime SW: Dissecting aneurysma of the aorta: a review of 505 cases. *Medicine* **37**: 217–79, 1958

12. Cambria RP, Brewster DC, Gertler J *et al.*: Vascular complications associated with spontaneous aortic dissection. *J Vasc Surg* 7: 199–207, 1988
13. Da Gama AD: The surgical management of aortic dissection: from university to diversity, a contineous challenge. *J Cardiovasc Surg* 32: 141–53, 1991
14. Fann JI, Sarris GE, Mitchell RS *et al.*: Treatment of patients with aortic dissection presenting with peripheral vascular complications. *Ann Surg* 212: 705–13, 1990
15. de Bakey ME, Cooley DA, Creech O: Surgical considerations of dissecting aneurysm of the aorta. *Ann Surg* 142: 586–610, 1955
16. de Bakey ME, Henly WS, Cooley DA *et al.*: Surgical management of dissecting aneurysm of the aorta. *J Thorac Cardiovasc Surg* 49: 130–47, 1965
17. Wheat MW, Palmer RF, Bartley TD, Seelman RC: Treatment of dissecting aneurysm of the aorta without surgery. *J Thorac Cardiovasc Surg* 58: 364–71, 1965
18. Vecht RJ, Bestermann EMM, Bromley LL, Eastcott HHG: Acute dissection of the aorta: long term review and management. *Lancet* **i**: 109–10, 1980
19. Vecht RJ, Bestermann EMM, Bromley LL, Eastcott HHG: Acute aortic dissection: Historical perspective and current management. *Am Heart J* 102: 1087–9, 1981
20. Fradet G, Jamieson WRE, Janusz MT *et al.*: Aortic dissection: A six year experience with 17 patients. *Am J Surg* 155: 697–700, 1988
21. Glower DD, Speier RH, White WD: Management and long term outcome of aortic dissection. *Ann Surg* 214: 31–41, 1990
22. Hashimoto A, Kimata S, Hosoda S: Acute aortic dissection: A comparison between the result of medical and surgical treatments. *Jap Circ J* 55: 821–3, 1991
23. Borst HG, Laas J, Frank G, Haverich A: Surgical decision making in acute aortic dissection type A. *Thorac Cardiovasc Surg* 35: 134–5, 1987
24. Heinemann M, Borst HG: Kardiovaskuläre Erkrankungen des Marfan Syndroms. *Dt Ärztebl* **93**B: 934–8, 1996
25. Coselli JS: Thoracoabdominal aortic aneurysm. In: Rutherford RB (Ed.), *Vascular Surgery*. London: WB Saunders Co Ltd, 1995
26. Carrel T, Jenni R, Segesser LK, Turina M: Behandlungsstrategie von vaskulären Komplikationen der akuten Aorten-dissektion. *Helv Chir Acta* 59: 575–81, 1991
27. Kogel H: Die Behandlung des disseziierenden Aortenaneurysmas Typ B-Standortbestimmung und Kontroversen. *Angio* 14: 189–97, 1992
28. Shah PM, Clauss RH: Dissecting hematoma presents as acute lower limb ischemia: diagnostic patient profile and management. *J Cardiovasc Surg* 24: 649–53, 1983
29. Elefteriades JA, Hammond GL, Gusberg RJ, Kopf GS, Baldwin JC: Fenestrastion revisited. A safe and effective procedure for descending aortic dissection. *Arch Surg* 125: 786–91, 1990
30. Gurin D, Bulmer JW, Derby R: Dissecting aneurysm of the aorta: diagnosis of operative relief of acute arterial obstruction due to this cause. *N Y State J Med* 35: 1200–2, 1935
31. Slonim SM, Nyman UR, Semba CP *et al.*: True lumen obliteration in complicated aortic dissection: Endovascular treatment. *Radiology* 201: 161–6, 1996
32. Walker PJ, Dake MD, Mitchell RS, Miller DC: The use of endovascular techniques for the treatment of complications of aortic dissection. *J Vasc Surg* 18: 1042–51, 1992
33. Farber A, Gmelin E, Heinemann M: Transfemorale Fensterung und Stentimplantation bei aorto-iliacaler Dissektion. *Vasa* 24: 389–91, 1995
34. Marty-Anè CH, Alric P, Prudhomme M *et al.*: Intravascular stenting of traumatic abdominal aortic dissection. *J Vasc Surg* 23: 156–61, 1996
35. Shores J, Berger KR, Murphy EA, Pyeritz R: Progression of aortic dilatation and the benefit of long-term beta-adrenergic blockade in Marfan's syndrome. *New Engl J Med* 330: 1335–41, 1994
36. Crawford ES, Crawford JL, Safi HJ *et al.*: Thoracoabdominal aortic aneurysms: preoperative and intraoperative factors determining immediate and long-term results of operations in 605 patients. *J Vasc Surg* 3: 389–404, 1986
37. Sandmann W, Grabitz K, Torsello G *et al.*: Chirurgische Behandlung des thorakoabdominalen Aortenaneurysmas. Indikationen und Ergebnisse. *Chirurg* 66: 845–56, 1995
38. Hart RG, Miller VT: Dissections. *Stroke* **14**: 925–6, 1985

39. Hagemann JH, Smith RF, Szilagy DE, Elliott JP: Aneurysms of the renal artery: Problems of prognosis and surgical management. *Surgery* **84**: 563–78, 1978

40. Tham G, Ekelund L, Herrlin K *et al.*: Renal artery aneurysms. *Ann Surg* **197**: 348–52, 1984

41. Mokri B, Stanson AW, Houser OW: Spontaneous dissections of renal arteries in a patient with previous spontaneous dissections of the internal carotid arteries. *Stroke* **16**: 959–63, 1985

42. Luken MG, Asherl GF, Corell J, Hilal SK: Spontaneous dissecting aneurysm of the extracranial internal carotid artery. *Clin Neurosurg* **26**: 353, 1979

43. Mokri B: Traumatic and spontaneous extracranial internal carotid artery dissections. *J Neurol* **237**: 356–61, 1990

44. Mokri B, Sundt TM, House OW, Piepgras D: Spontaneous dissection of the cervical internal carotid artery. *Ann Neurol* **19**: 126–138, 1986

45. Mokri B, Piepgras DG, Wiebers DO, Houser OW: Familial occurrence of spontaneous dissection of the internal carotid artery. *Stroke* **18**: 246–51, 1987

46. Amarenco P, Seux-Levieil ML, Cohen A: Carotid artery dissection with renal infarcts. Two cases. *Stroke* **25**: 2488–91, 1994

47. Edwards BS, Stanson AW, Holley KE, Sheps SG: Isolated renal artery dissection. *Mayo Clin Proc* **57**: 564–71, 1982

48. Reilly LM, Cunningham CG, Maggisano R *et al.*: The role of arterial reconstruction in spontaneous renal artery reconstruction. *J Vasc Surg* **14**: 468–77, 1991

49. Perry MO: Spontaneous renal artery dissection. *Cardiovasc Surg* **32**: 54–9, 1982

50. Meyers DS, Grim CE, Keitzer WF: Fibromuscular dysplasia of the renal artery with medial dissection. *Am J Med* **56**: 412–6, 1974

51. Dannemaier B, Eppinger B, von Reutern GM, Schumacher M: Spontane Rückbildung von hochgradigen Stenosen und Verschlüssen der Arteria carotis interna. *Nervenarzt* **63**: 363–70, 1992

52. Kaech D, Maeder P, Uske A *et al.*: Traumatische Dissektiionen der Arteria carotis interna. *Unfallchirurg* **93**: 6–10, 1990

53. Bewermeyer H, Neveling M, Dreesbach HA, Wiedemann G: Traumatisch bedingte Dissektion und Pseudokklusion der Arteria carotis interna mit spontaner Rekanalisierung. *Fortschr Röntgenstr* **140**: 728–9, 1984

54. Bauer KF, Hoffmann W, Garaguly G: Traumatisch bedingter Verschluß mit spontaner Rekanalisierung der Arteria carotis interna. *Chirurg* **68**: 187–9, 1997

55. Gee W, Kaupp HA, McDonald KM *et al.*: Spontaneous dissection of internal carotid arteries. *Arch Surg* **115**: 944–9, 1980

56. Maxeiner H, Finck GA: Traumatischer Hirninfarkt bei mehrzeitig verlaufender Dissektion der extrakraniellen Arteria carotis interna. *Unfallchirurg* **92**: 321–7, 1989

57. Hoffmeister AW, Neumann MFC: Spontane Dissektion der Arteria carotis interna. *Fortschr Med* **29**: 25–29, 1992

58. Bogousslavsky J, Regli F: Ischemic stroke in adult younger than 30 years of age. *Arch Neurol* **44**: 479–82, 1987

59. Hart RG, Miller VT: Cerebral infarction in young adults: a practical approach. *Stroke* **14**: 110–4, 1983

60. Adams HP, Kapelle LJ, Biller J *et al.*: Ischemic stroke in young adults. *Arch Neurol* **52**: 491–4, 1995

61. Budmiger H, Bollinger A: Die Dissektion der Arteria carotis interna – ein oft verkanntes Krankheitsbild. *Vasa* **17**: 219–24, 1988

62. Treimann GS, Treimann RL, Foran RF *et al.*: Spontaneous dissection of the internal carotid artery: A nineteen-year clinical experience. *J Vasc Surg* **24**: 597–605, 1996

63. Steinke W, Aulich A, Hennerici M: Diagnose und Verlauf von Carotisdissektionen. *Dtsch Med Wochenschr* **114**: 1869–75, 1989

64. Early TF, Gregory RT, Wheeler JR *et al.*: Spontaneous carotid dissection: Duplex scanning in diagnosis and management. *J Vasc Surg* **14**: 391–7, 1991

65. Ehrenfeld WK, Wylie EJ: Spontaneous dissection of the internal carotid artery. *Arch Surg* **11**: 1294–300, 1976

66. Stillhard G, Waespe W, Germann D: Die Karotisdissektion. *Schweiz Med Wschr* **188**: 1933–40, 1988

67. Sundt TM, Pearson BW, Piepgras DG, Houser OW, Mokri B: Surgical management of aneurysms of the distal extracranial internal carotid artery. *J Neurosurg* **64**: 169–82, 1986

68. Zelenock GB, Kazmers A, Whitehouse WM *et al.*: Extracranial internal carotid artery dissections. *Arch Surg* **117**: 425–32, 1982

69. Schievink WI, Piepgras DG, McCaffrey TV, Mokri B: Surgical treatment of extracranial internal carotid artery dissecting aneurysms. *Neurosurgery* **35**: 809–15, 1994

70. Sandmann W, Kniemeyer HW, Jaeschock R *et al.*: Techniques to facilitate the surgical approach to high artery lesions. In: Veith FJ (Ed.), *Current Critical Problems in Vascular Surgery*. St Louis: Quality Medical Publishing Inc, 1992

71. Blaisdell FW, Clauss RH, Galbraith JG *et al.*: Joint study of extracranial arterial occlusion. IV. A review of surgical considerations. *J Am Med Assoc* **209**: 1889, 1969

72. Salvis SA, Hodge EE, Novick AC, Maatman T: Surgical treatment for isolated dissection of the renal artery. *J Urol* **144**: 233–7, 1990

73. Veeckman PH, Voss EU: Die spontane Nierenarteriendissektion (AND). *Vasa* **21**: 310–5, 1992

74. Hageman JH, Smith RF, Szilagyi DE, Elliott MD: Aneurysms of the renal artery: Problems of prognosis and surgical management. *Surgery* **84**: 563–71, 1978

75. Smith Bruce M, Holcomb GW, Richie RE, Dean RH: Renal artery dissection. *Ann Surg* **200**: 134–44, 1984

76. Vogt J, Kutkuhn B, Sandmann W *et al.*: Spontane Nierenarteriendissektion. *Z Kardiol* **81**: 512–4, 1992

77. Klein RM, Niehus R, Hollenbeck M *et al.*: Lokale Lyse-Therapie bei spontaner Nierenarteriendissektion mit arterieller Thrombose. *Dtsch Med Wsch* **117**: 1185–90, 1990

78. Crawford ES, Snyder DM, Cho GC, Rochin JOF: Progress in treatment of thoracoabdominal and abdominal aortic aneurysms involving celiac, superior mesenteric and renal arteries. *Ann Surg* **188**: 404, 1978

79. Mokri B, Piepgras DG, Houser OW: Traumatic dissections of the extracranial internal carotid artery. *J Neurosurg* **68**: 189–97, 1988

80. Sandmann W, Hennerici M, Aulich A *et al.*: Progress in carotid artery surgery at the base of the skill. *J Vasc Surg* **1**: 734–43, 1984

81. Heine H, Dalith F: Stammes- und entwicklungsgeschichtliche Ursachen lokalisierter Wandveränderungen im Bereich des Aortenbogens und der brachiocephalen Gefäßstämme des Menschen und Huhnes. *Z Anat Entwickl-Gesch* **140**: 231–44, 1973

Editorial comments by C.V. Ruckley

Lying as it does in the no man's land between cardiac and vascular surgery, aortic dissection tends not to be well managed and to carry a high mortality and morbidity. Being uncommon and presenting with symptoms which may be non-specific it is a diagnosis frequently arrived at late. The authors provide a clear, pragmatic and well reasoned approach to management.

Dissection of peripheral arteries is even more uncommon, although as the authors indicate, there is a predilection for the carotid system. In reporting 43 patients treated surgically for the complications of carotid dissection the authors may have a unique series, with excellent outcomes.

Management of arterial dissection requires the full resources of advanced radiology, cardiology, cardiac surgery, peripheral vascular surgery and intensive care. Furthermore it is noted that 21 of the carotid and two renal dissections were caused by trauma. There is currently national debate in the UK, and no doubt elsewhere, on the merits of centralizing vascular services and the extent to which they should be networked to other services. The variety of surgical procedures adopted in the series of aortic and peripheral aneurysms reported in this chapter, the concentration of surgical experience, the high levels of expertise implicit, together with the range of supporting services required, constitute a salutary reminder of the benefits to be gained from linking centralized vascular units to regional trauma centres and to the full range of acute services.

Is Intensive Care Support Essential for Open Abdominal Aortic Aneurysm Surgery?

Anthony E.B. Giddings and Nial Quiney

THE AUTHORS' CHOICE

It is important to define the most appropriate system of care for patients undergoing abdominal aortic surgery whether by open operation or endovascular technique as endovascular procedures carry a significant risk of conversion to an open operation.

In Guildford, the Royal Surrey County Hospital serves a population of 240 000 and has 504 beds but only three or four of these are in use as intensive care unit (ICU) beds, a minimum number and far fewer than the 1–2% recommended in the UK.[1,2] In the USA, ICU beds may constitute up to 10% of acute hospital beds, currently numbering 7400 and accounting for 22% of all hospital costs.[3,4] Between 1972 and 1992, ICU beds in the USA increased from 2.5% to 8.6% of total hospital beds. In the UK, they remain at 2.6%.[5]

There are no high dependency unit beds (HDU)[6] beds in Guildford, despite a vigorous 5-year campaign and therefore, the authors have only the choice of ICU, or ward management for patients undergoing aortic surgery. However, it must be stated at the outset that no firm evidence for the benefit of ICU in improving the outcome of abdominal aortic aneurysm surgery exists, despite reasonable suggestions,[7] although many vascular surgeons and anaesthetists believe that organization of care in ICU confers advantages and their support for HDU is based on similar perceptions.

Open abdominal aortic aneurysm surgery is a procedure of potentially high risk, undertaken for two quite different indications. Elective operation is advised to prevent the risk of rupture and to restore the life expectancy of the patient to almost normal.[8] Ruptured aneurysm carries a mortality of 78%[9] and is the cause of death in 1.2% of men and 0.6% of women over the age of 65 years in the USA.[10] Two-thirds of abdominal aortic aneurysm patients, however, will die of another cause. Elective operation can, therefore, only be justified when perioperative mortality is near zero, requiring expertise and vigilance in preoperative preparation, intraoperative care and postoperative support. The lowest perioperative mortality from elective abdominal aortic aneurysm surgery is about 2.4%[11] in individual series, while hospital figures in the USA vary from 3.5% in some to 10.5% in community-wide surveys.[9] A 5-year regional survey in England suggested much higher figures with a surgeon-specific mortality sometimes exceeding 20% and up to 100% for emergencies.[12] Mortality following operation for ruptured abdominal aortic aneurysm is less in patients with confined rupture (Fig. 1) but is over 90% in those with a free intraperitoneal rupture (Fig. 2).

Intra- and postoperative cardiac problems are unpredictable. Campbell[13] reported 45 consecutive abdominal aortic aneurysm operations, 41 of which were initially

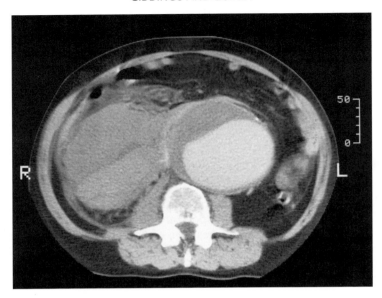

Fig. 1. Computer-assisted tomography with contrast enhancement demonstrating an abdominal aortic aneurysm which has ruptured. The rupture is confined to the retroperitoneal tissues.

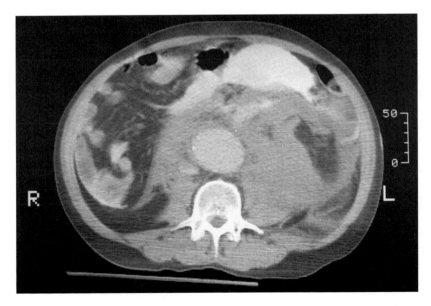

Fig. 2. Computer-assisted tomography demonstrating an abdominal aortic aneurysm with free intraperitoneal rupture, demonstrated by extravasation of contrast.

managed in the ICU. Of these patients 80% had adverse medical events within 48 hours, most of which could be managed in the HDU, and 59% of their patients had more than one episode which could not be predicted from preoperative assessment. It could be argued that hospitals without HDU will manage critically ill patients who need HDU care expensively in ICU or inefficiently and dangerously in the wards. Access to intensive monitoring and effective critical care are mandatory. In hospitals without HDU facilities, ICU is likely to be the best place and some authors[13] think ICU support is essential.

Few would deny that ICU was essential for patients with a free rupture of an abdominal aortic aneurysm.[14] Such patients often arrive in theatre, unprepared and shocked, to suffer the additional trauma of haemorrhagic surgery. The need for effective critical care is self-evident and probably incapable of clinical trial. Intensive care facilities must be to hand when needed until the patient is stable enough to be moved to a lower level of care. Although for patients with ruptured abdominal aortic aneurysm, the authors always use the ICU, it is interesting to reflect that mortality from ruptured abdominal aortic aneurysm has remained stubbornly at 50% for the last three decades despite improvements in elective mortality[15] and the enhancement of ICU support.

OPTIONS AVAILABLE

At present, three levels of surgical care can be identified in the UK, provided by ICU, HDU and surgical wards, and the Department of Health has issued guidelines on admission and discharge criteria (Table 1). The intensity of nursing and medical care

Table 1. Guidelines on admission to and discharge from intensive care and high dependency units (Department of Health, March 1996)

Intensive care is appropriate for	High dependency care is appropriate for
Patients requiring or likely to require advanced respiratory support alone (e.g. IPPV)	Patients requiring support for a single failing organ system but excluding those needing advanced respiratory support
Patients requiring support of two or more organ systems	Patients who can benefit from more detailed observation or monitoring than can be safely provided on a general ward
Patients with chronic impairment of one or more systems sufficient to restrict daily activities (co-morbidity) and who require support for an acute reversible failure of another organ system	Patients no longer needing intensive care but who are not yet well enough to return to a general ward
	Postoperative patients who need close observation or monitoring for longer than a few hours

IPPV: Intermittent positive pressure ventilation.

varies from high to low across this spectrum. The concept of progressive patient care implies transfer between facilities as requirements change.[6] ICU and HDU are compared in Table 2.

In the UK, however, neither the skills nor the manpower of surgical wards are seen to be ideally suitable for the immediate postoperative care of aortic patients, particularly 'out of hours'.[16] In fact less than 7% of surgeons questioned in one series were not routinely using either HDU or ICU facilities[17] but 77% of vascular surgeons are thought to use ICU routinely. There is, however, good evidence that HDU reduces inappropriate use of ICU by patients requiring a lower intensity of monitoring or therapy.[18] A recent survey suggests that not all anaesthetists would insist on postponing elective aortic surgery if no ICU bed were available, although many would be concerned if there were no HDU.[19]

Table 2. A comparison between intensive care and high dependency units

Intensive care unit	High dependency unit
History Established nationally in the 1950s and 1960s – an essential component of all acute general hospitals	Slow and sporadic evolution from traditional ward practice
Definitions A service for patients with potentially recoverable diseases who can benefit from more detailed observation than is generally available in standard wards and departments	A standard of care intermediate between that available on the general ward and that in the ICU, providing monitoring and support for patients at risk of developing organ failure, including facilities for short term ventilatory support and immediate resuscitation
Monitoring Pulmonary artery catheters, transoesophageal ultrasound, invasive cardiac output and systemic vascular resistance measurements	Arterial oxygenation, blood pressure (invasive/non-invasive), CVP, urine output
Therapy Mechanical ventilation, haemofiltration and inotropic support	Oxygen therapy, epidural infusion, vasodilators and low dose inotropes
Nursing One nurse to each patient	One nurse to two patients
Medical cover Resident doctor immediately available and experienced in critical care. Medical staff generally intensivists or anaesthetists	Experienced staff on call within the hospital
Distribution Percentage of acute hospitals with ICU facility – 90%.	Percentage of acute hospitals with HDU facility – 20%.

CVP: Central venous pressure

THE PHYSIOLOGICAL CHALLENGE OF AORTIC SURGERY

Elective patients will usually be over the age of 60 and coexisting disease is common, 48% having clinically important coronary artery disease.[20] Additional hazards include pulmonary disease and smoking, diabetes mellitus and renal impairment, all of which adversely affect outcome.

Several algorithms for stratification of risk have been suggested for example by Goldman in 1977[21] and Detsky in 1986.[22] In 1987 Goldman[23] also highlighted the difficulties of predictive scores. Reliability requires definition of risk factors and outcome criteria as well as clinical relevance proved by prospective trials. This has not been achieved and the level of postoperative support required for an individual cannot be predicted from these algorythms.

In a prospective study of abdominal aortic aneurysm patients by Jeffery et al.,[24] the Goldman Cardiac Risk Index using the criteria shown in Table 3, predicted a better outcome than that which was observed in Class I aortic surgery patients, that is, those thought to be at low risk. Several methods have been suggested to improve patients' chances, including admission of higher risk patients to ICU preoperatively for 'invasive haemodynamic monitoring and optimization' or 'tune-up'[25] but there is no evidence that optimization of cardiac performance and oxygen delivery preoperatively confer any benefit. It is essential, however, to achieve these goals from the commencement of surgery and to maintain them throughout the operation.

D'Angelo et al.[26] in a retrospective review of 113 consecutive abdominal aortic aneurysm patients showed there to be no significant difference in cardiac events, complications and mortality between those having electrocardiograms (ECG) only and those having more extensive cardiac investigations. They concluded that their policy of intensive intraoperative monitoring and management was the most important factor in determining the outcome and that intensive preoperative investigations had little benefit.

Preoperative tests can be difficult to perform. For example, the use of exercise ECG is limited in patients with leg ischaemia and angina. Mason et al.[27] examined the role of coronary angiography and revascularization before non-cardiovascular surgery, showing better outcome in the group which did not undergo preoperative coronary angiography and cardiac interventions. Echocardiography and angioscintigraphy may be useful to demonstrate reduced cardiac reserve and left ventricular dimensions which may accurately reflect the presence of coronary artery disease and

Table 3. Criteria used in calculating Goldman Cardiac Risk Index

1. Myocardial infarction in the last 6 months
2. Age >70
3. Aortic stenosis
4. Third heart sound or jugular venous distention
5. ECG non-sinus rhythm
6. More than five premature ventricular beats per minute
7. Poor general medical condition
8. Abdominal or thoracic aortic surgery
9. Emergency procedures

a degree of decompensation[28] but benefit is unproven. Ramsay[29] highlighted the belief that most cardiac events take place in the first 72 hours after surgery and intensive monitoring for this period using continuous ECG, pulmonary artery catheter or transoesophageal ultrasound is generally believed to be useful, but they showed no incontrovertable evidence.

Whatever method of preoperative assessment is chosen, treatment of coexisting pathology and optimization of the patient's medication are the goals of the preoperative period. Much of this can be carried out on an outpatient basis and most patients are admitted to the general ward rather than ICU or HDU during the 24 hours before surgery.

Assuming that patients are fit enough to be nursed on the general ward immediately before operation, it must, therefore, be the success of the surgical technique and anaesthetic management which will dictate the level of care required in the immediate postoperative period. Whatever the approach to the aorta,[30-32] pathophysiological changes are of a similar nature and these dictate the patient's need for critical care.

PATHOPHYSIOLOGICAL CHANGES WITH AORTIC SURGERY (Table 4)

Cardiovascular system: reduced perfusion

Aortic cross-clamping causes an increased afterload, increased systemic vascular resistance with a risk of myocardial ischaemia and/or decrease in cardiac output. Monitoring of cardiac output, oxygen delivery and myocardial ischaemia will identify those patients who are at greatest risk of myocardial ischaemia or infarction. Appropriate use of fluids, vasodilators and inotropes will reduce postoperative complications.[25] This, in effect, requires intensive care in theatre (Fig. 3).

Respiratory system: cellular hypoxia

This may be affected by cardiac performance, reperfusion injury and pain. Intraoperative intubation and ventilation should not preclude early extubation. Effective postoperative analgesia by a thoracic epidural will allow most patients to be extubated immediately after operation but careful monitoring will need to be continued (Figs. 4, 5).

Table 4.   Pathophysiological changes with aortic surgery

1.	Cardiovascular system, reduced perfusion
2.	Respiratory system, cellular hypoxia
3.	Hypothermia
4.	Renal and visceral ischaemia
6.	Blood loss and coagulation disorders
5.	Reperfusion injury

Hypothermia

Cooling during open aortic surgery is due to two causes, first to heat loss from the immobile and exposed patient, in particular from the uninsulated abdomen by radiation and evaporation, and, second, by the infusion of cool or refrigerated intravenous fluids. Mild hypothermia (33°C to 36°C) had been accepted as unavoidable until the significant effects on the patient were appreciated. Below a core temperature of 34°C, intense vasoconstriction gives rise to generalized hypoperfusion, increasing mortality from 1.5% to 12.1% in the 262 abdominal aortic aneurysm patients (all of whom were cared for in the ICU) reported by Bush in 1995.[33] Blood loss and the need for postoperative transfusion is increased[34] and there is a higher incidence of myocardial ischaemia.[35] Good haemostasis and short operation time are ideal but insulation, aggressive warming of the patient by convective air blowers, heating blankets, heat and moisture exchangers in the patient's breathing system and the warming of intravenous fluids will all help maintain patient temperature (Fig. 3).

Renal and visceral ischaemia

Infrarenal cross-clamping may cause a profound reduction in renal and splanchnic blood flow.[36] Maintenance of intravascular volume, cardiac output and perfusion pressure will reduce renal damage. Although mannitol, frusemide and dopamine may increase urine volume, they may not protect renal function.[37]

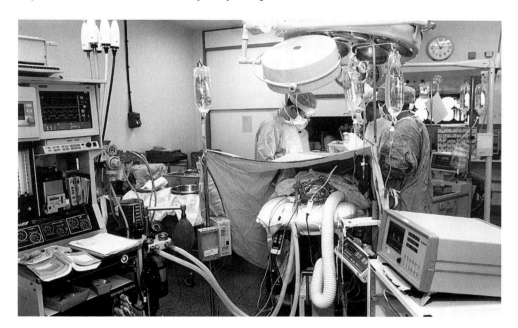

Fig. 3. An example of intensive care in the operating theatre, showing a system for intravenous fluid warming and a convective air warming apparatus. Syringe drivers for vasodilators and intropes are also available, together with transoesophageal Doppler ultrasound cardiac output measurement.

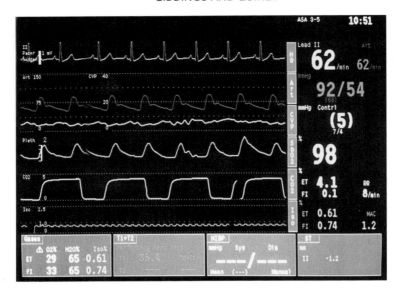

Fig. 4. Example of monitoring in theatre, showing pulse rate and invasive blood pressure measurement, central venous pressure measurement, pulse oxymetry, end tidal CO$_2$, a volatile agent, and, at the bottom right-hand corner, ST segment analysis of the ECG. Nasopharyngeal temperature is also recorded.

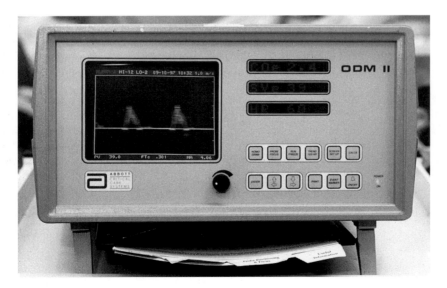

Fig. 5. An example of the display on a cardiac output monitor with estimated cardiac output and estimated stroke volume.

Blood loss and coagulation

Blood loss and homologous blood transfusion can be kept to a minimum by careful surgical technique, predonation, blood salvage and maintenance of normothermia.

Reperfusion injury

The flow of oxygenated blood to ischaemic tissues is associated with the release of highly reactive oxygen species. These cause both local damage and widespread systemic effects, including impaired oxygen exchange in the pulmonary bed and a reduction in cardiac contractility. Mannitol may reduce the pulmonary injury associated with reperfusion and may also reduce renal reperfusion injury.[38]

INDICATORS OF THE NEED FOR CRITICAL CARE

Increased operation time, volume deficit, multiorgan failure and female gender are all known to be adverse influences. Whalley *et al.*[36] showed in 20 patients that increased systemic vascular resistance on aortic cross-clamping was also associated with an increase in the base deficit after clamp removal, indicating visceral ischaemia. Lactate started to rise as soon as the cross-clamp was placed with a shift to anaerobic metabolism, a depletion of antioxidants which normally protect from free radicals and capillary membrane damage, disorders of permeability, pulmonary oedema and renal failure which may be heralded by microalbuminuria. Khaira[39] studied ischaemia and reperfusion in abdominal aortic aneurysms, correlating antioxidant levels with a reduction in central venous pressure and inferior mesenteric blood flow. Hypovolaemia is known to reduce splanchnic blood flow disproportionately and this has been used as an indicator of adequacy of systemic perfusion and tissue oxygenation. Boyd[40] studied variations in gastric pH with blood pressure and found a good correlation between gastric intramucosal pH and arterial base deficit in critically ill patients, reflecting the systemic nature of the problem which was not a selective splanchnic effect. Gastric intramucosal pH was also studied in the first 24 hours postoperatively by Maynard,[41] showing that, in patients with ruptured abdominal aortic aneurysms, the pH was higher in survivors. Studies in Guildford have similarly demonstrated that arterial base deficit may be used as an indicator of outcome in postoperative patients following abdominal aortic aneurysm surgery.[42] A strongly negative base deficit is an indicator of severe metabolic disturbance, the need for intensive care and the likelihood of mortality. The role of surgical and anaesthetic management should be to avoid this situation.

THE GOALS OF MANAGEMENT

The aim is to produce a situation in which a patient wakes rapidly after operation, warm, free of pain and haemodynamically stable (Figs 6,7). Postoperative management should include the use of supplementary oxygen, maintenance of

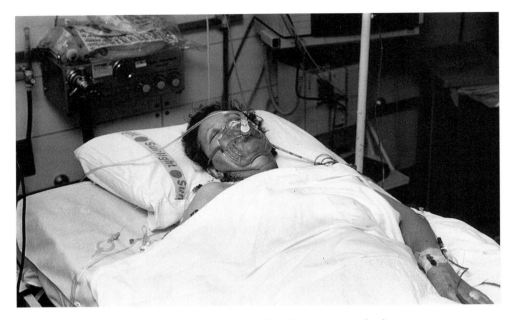

Fig. 6.   A patient immediately postoperatively.

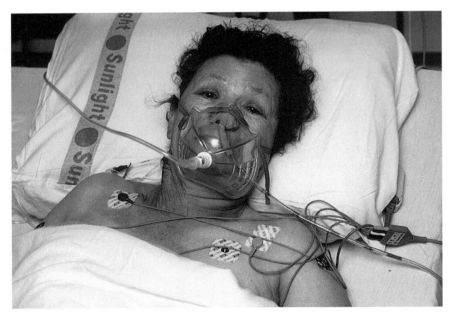

Fig. 7.   The same patient 1 hour later, awake and free of pain. (Reproduced with
permission from the patient.)

analgesia and haemodynamic stability. Such patients may be adequately managed in an HDU. If the above goals are not identified and achieved, the patient may be cold, in pain, haemodynamically unstable and require large volumes of blood and other intravenous fluids to support blood pressure. The patient may be ventilated due to poor oxygenation and inadequate pain relief and ICU facilities may be considered essential.

EVIDENCE

Evidence from the literature is confined to reports of costs and current practice. The overall costs of nursing treatment and diagnostic services, excluding the overheads, in the Royal Surrey County Hospital have been approximately £55 per patient per day on the ward and £566 per patient per day in the ICU but figures including overheads raise these costs to at least £250 for the ward and £1000 for the ICU. Comparable figures are found in other UK centres.[43,44] In the USA, ICU beds are more extensively used and one day in the ICU can increase patient costs by 12.5%,[45] while the costs of one organ failure have been estimated at $125 000.

There is strong evidence that many patients are admitted to the ICU inappropriately. In the UK, 33% of ICU admissions could have been managed in the HDU.[46] In the USA 32% of admissions were inappropriate in a 10-year retrospective review[47] and, in another study in the USA, 49% of patients were admitted to an ICU for observation rather than for treatment.[48] There can be little doubt that the availability of approximately 7% of acute beds for HDU use would relieve ICUs from a significant number of inappropriate admissions but, in the UK, only about 20% of acute general hospitals have an HDU and, in recent years, some of those few have been closed.[18] There is good evidence that less than 5% of HDU patients need to be transferred to ICU.[49,50]

Edbrooke in 1996 speculated on the cost implications and benefits of HDU. It would be expected that the fuller use of HDU rather than ICU might result in considerable cost savings but the expectations were not met in reality.[50] There is no direct evidence that such an arrangement may improve the quality of care, although it has been postulated that effective HDU care may have a role in reducing overall hospital stay after major operations by reducing morbidity. Gamil and Fanning[7] reported a 5% incidence of serious complications in the first 24 hours postoperatively in 2153 general patients. They also suggested that 17% of the recorded deaths might have been avoided if HDU facilities had been available.

The lack of clear evidence of benefit from one system or another in the care of abdominal aortic aneurysm patients gives an opportunity to reappraise the essentials of care, focusing on the task rather than on the environment in which it is to be performed. The ICU/HDU debate may be seen as a distraction when fundamental questions about the intra- and postoperative management of patients need to be answered. For example, is the goal-directed therapy as advocated by Shoemaker[51] which could be suitable for the management of a young trauma victim an appropriate model for the postoperative care of a patient after aortic surgery? There is some evidence to suggest that patients having surgery for non-elective abdominal aortic aneurysm do less well with vigorous fluid and inotrope support than those managed less aggressively.[52] It seems likely that an elderly cardiopathic patient will have different requirements from that of a young and resilient patient without significant co-morbidity. As always, the aim of the surgeon and anaesthetist should be to reduce the need for intensive or high dependency care by good surgical technique and appropriate intraoperative care.

TRIALS

Good clinical management would be facilitated if it were possible to predict risk in an individual patient and if the goals of management could be matched to that risk. In some disciplines, for example cardiac surgery, reliable indicators of the operative risk have been established. This allows better assessment of the performance of individual surgeons and trials of intervention but no such evidence-based system is available for aortic surgery. Further clinical trials of management strategies are required to identify appropriate physiological targets in cardiac output, fluid volume and oxygen delivery to optimize the patient's condition during and after aortic operation. It will be difficult to interpret trials of management strategy for aortic surgery until a reliable method for the assessment of individual patient risk is established.

CONCLUSIONS

In our present state of knowledge, it would seem adventurous to argue that patients suffering ruptured aneurysm should go anywhere other than to an ICU in the immediate postoperative period. It is hoped that those who do well will need to stay a relatively short time and might then be moved to an HDU for the management of fluid balance and analgesia. For elective aortic surgery, the position is less clear. A minority of patients may benefit from a preoperative admission to the ICU for a 'tune up' but there is no evidence to suggest that this preoperative preparation is superior to appropriate intraoperative management. There is at present no evidence to permit stratification of risk in such a way as to direct elective aortic patients to ICU or to HDU facilities with the certainty that the decision is correct. It is likely that there will continue to be some patients who, having declared no special risk factors, will present with difficulties which will require postoperative ventilation and, therefore, the services of an ICU. Similarly, the onset of renal failure may be unpredictable and require ICU support. For the majority of patients, however, in whom elective operation is undertaken because they are expected to fall within the low risk criteria mandated by the requirements of prophylactic surgery, management by HDU facilities should be sufficient to monitor blood volume, temperature and give effective pain relief. The goals of management should be to provide effective pre- and intraoperative cardiac support and efficient surgical technique so that demand for the expensive facilities of ICU can be minimized. There is certainly no proof that the huge expense and inconvenience of prolonged intensive care is effective in avoiding a fatal outcome if surgical or anaesthetic management allow the development of severe haemodynamic and metabolic shock.

REFERENCES

1. *Intensive Care Services – Provision for the Future*. London: Association of Anaesthetists of Great Britain and Ireland, 1988
2. Oh TE: *Intensive Care Manual* 3rd edn. Sydney: Butterworth, 1990
3. Halpern NA *et al.*: Federal and nationwide intensive care units and healthcare costs: 1986–1992. *Crit Care Med* **22**: 2001–7, 1994
4. Halpern NA *et al.*: Critical care medicine: Observations from the Department of Veterans Affairs intensive care units. *Crit Care Med* **22**: 2008–12, 1994
5. Brydon CW: Organization and function of intensive care and high dependency units. *Surgery* 493–5, 1993
6. *The High Dependency Unit – Acute Care in the Future*. London: Association of Anaesthetists of Great Britain and Ireland, 1991
7. Gamil M, Fanning A: The first 24 hours after surgery: a study of complications after 2153 consecutive operations. *Anaesthesiology* **46**: 712–5, 1991
8. Stonebridge PA *et al.*: Comparison of long-term survival after successful repair of ruptured and non-ruptured abdominal aortic aneurysm. *Br J Surg* **80**: 585–6, 1993
9. Taylor LM, Porter JM: Basic data related to clinical decision-making in abdominal aortic aneurysms. *Ann Vasc Surg* **1**: 502–4, 1986
10. US Department of Health and Human Services: *Vital Statistics of the United States* Vol II: *Mortality*, Part A. Hyattsville: National Center for Health Statistics, 1988
11. Lloyd WE *et al.*: Results of 1000 consecutive elective abdominal aortic aneurysm repairs. *Cardiovasc Surg* **4**: 724–6, 1996
12. Giddings AEB: What are the true morbidity and mortality rates of abdominal aortic aneurysm surgery in the UK? *Br J Surg* **84**: 568, 1997
13. Campbell WB *et al.*: Intensive care after abdominal aortic surgery. *Eur J Vasc Surg* **5**: 665–8, 1991
14. Brimacombe J, Berry A: A review of anaesthesia for ruptured abdominal aortic aneurysm with special emphasis on preclamping fluid resuscitation. *Anaesthesia Intens Care* **21**: 311–23, 1993
15. Katz DJ *et al.*: Operative mortality rates for intact and ruptured abdominal aortic aneurysms in Michigan: an eleven year statewide experience. *J Vasc Surg* **19**: 804–17, 1994
16. Crosby DL *et al.*: The role of the high dependency unit in post-operative care: an update. *Ann R Coll Surg Engl* **72**: 3090–12, 1990
17. Michaels JA *et al.*: A survey of methods used for cardiac risk assessment prior to major vascular surgery. *Eur J Vasc Endovasc Surg* **11**: 221–4, 1996
18. Coggins R, de Cossart L: Improving post-operative care: the role of the surgeon in the high dependency unit. *Ann R Coll Surg Engl* **78**: 163–7, 1996
19. Woods AW, Wylie P: Cancellation of elective AAA due to lack of ICU beds. *Anaesthesia* **52**: 1115–6, 1997
20. Wolf YG, Bernstein EF: A current perspective on the natural history of abdominal aortic aneurysms. *Cardiovasc Surg* **2**: 16–22, 1994
21. Goldman L *et al.*: Multifactorial index of cardiac risk in noncardiac surgical procedures. *New Engl J Med* **297**: 845–50, 1977
22. Detsky AS: Predicting cardiac complications in patients undergoing non-cardiac surgery. *J Int Med* **1**: 211–9, 1986
23. Goldman L: Multifactorial index of cardiac risk in noncardiac surgery: ten year status report. *J Cardiothorac Anaesth* **1**: 237–44, 1987
24. Jeffery CC *et al.*: A prospective evaluation of cardiac risk index. *Anesthesiology* **58**: 462–4, 1983

25. Varon AJ *et al.*: Pre-operative intensive care unit consultations: accurate and effective. *Crit Care Med* **21**: 234–9, 1993

26. D'Angelo *et al.*: Is preoperative cardiac evaluation for abdominal aortic aneurysm repair necessary? *J Vasc Surg* **25**: 152–6, 1997

27. Mason JJ *et al.*: The role of coronary angiography and coronary revascularization before noncardiac vascular surgery. *J Am Med Assoc* **273**: 1919–25, 1995

28. Coriat P, Kieffer E: Pre-operative risk stratification in vascular surgical patients. *Acta Anaesth Scand* **109** (Suppl): 127–30, 1996

29. Ramsay J, Thomas B: Pre-operative cardiac evaluation and peri-operative monitoring for noncardiac surgery. *J Am Med Assoc* **274**: 1671–2, 1995

30. Darling III RC *et al.*: Advances in the surgical repair of ruptured abdominal aortic aneurysms. *Cardiovasc Surg* **4**: 720–2, 1996

31. Todd GJ, DeRose JJ: Retroperitoneal approach for repair of inflammatory aortic aneurysms. *Ann Vasc Surg* **9**: 525–34, 1995

32. Chen MHM *et al.*: Laparoscopically assisted abdominal aortic aneurysm repair: a report of 10 cases. *Surg Endosc* **10**: 1136–9, 1996

33. Bush HL *et al.*: Hypothermia during elective abdominal aneurysm repair: the high price of avoidable morbidity. *J Vasc Surg* **21**: 392–402, 1995

34. Schmied H *et al.*: Mild hypothermia increases blood loss and transfusion requirements during total hip arthroplasty. *Lancet* **347**: 289–92, 1996

35. Frank MS *et al.*: Perioperative maintenance of normothermia reduces the incidence of morbid cardiac events: a randomised clinical trial. *J Am Med Assoc* **277**: 1127–34, 1997

36. Whalley DG *et al.*: Haemodynamic and metabolic consequences of aortic occlusion during abdominal aortic surgery. *Br J Anaesth* **70**: 96–8, 1993

37. Badwin L *et al.*: Effect of postoperative low-dose dopamine on renal function after elective major vascular surgery. *Ann Int Med* **120**: 744–7, 1994

38. Paterson IS *et al.*: Pulmonary edema after aneurysm surgery is modified by mannitol. *Ann Surg* **219**: 796–801, 1989

39. Khaira HS *et al.*: Antioxidant depletion during aortic aneurysm repair. *Br J Surg* **83**: 401–3, 1996

40. Boyd O *et al.*: Comparison of clinical information gained from routine blood-gas analysis and from gastric tonometry for intramural pH. *Lancet* **341**: 142–6, 1993

41. Maynard ND *et al.*: Gastric intramucosal pH predicts outcome after surgery for ruptured abdominal aortic aneurysm. *Eur J Vasc Endovasc Surg* **11**: 201–6, 1996

42. Jeddy T *et al.*: Use of base deficit as a predictor of outcome following abdominal aortic surgery. *Br J Surg* **83** (Suppl): 4, 1996

43. Crosby DL *et al.*: The role of the high dependency unit in post-operative care: an update. *Ann R Coll Surg Engl* **72**: 309–12, 1990

44. Coggins R *et al.*: Use of a general surgical HDU in a district general hospital. (in prep) 1998

45. Collier PE: Do clinical pathways for major vascular surgery improve outcomes and reduce costs? *J Vasc Surg* **26**: 179–85, 1997

46. Bodenham AR, Klein H: High dependency units: role and need. *Br J Hosp Med* **56**: 192–3, 1996

47. Nelson JB Jr: The role of an ITU in a community hospital: a ten year review with observations on utilisation past, present and future. *Ann Surg* **120**: 123–6, 1985

48. Knaus WA *et al.*: The range of intensive care services today. *J Am Med Assoc* **246**: 2711–16, 1981

49. Zimmerman JE *et al.*: Planning patient services for intermediate care units: insights based on care for intensive care unit low-risk monitor admissions. *Crit Care Med* **24**: 1626–32, 1996

50. Edbrooke DL: The high dependency unit: where to now? *Ann R Coll Surg Engl* **78**: 161–2, 1996

51. Shoemaker WC *et al.*: Prospective trial of supranormal values of survivors as therapeutic goals in high-risk surgical patients. *Chest* **94**: 1176–86, 1988

52. Sandison AJP *et al.*: ICU protocol affects the outcome of non-elective abdominal aortic aneurysm. *Eur J Vasc Endovasc Surg* (in press) 1998

Editorial comments by B.R. Hopkinson

This is a very important chapter in light of the current excess of demand over supply for intensive care unit (ICU) beds which is affecting all of the UK. There is no doubt that ICU beds have their place and that they are very expensive but it is also equally clear that they are not always necessary. Certainly in the 1960s before they commonly existed we used to manage patients after abdominal aortic surgery quite happily on the surgical wards but at that time we had extremely good, experienced nursing staff who would 'special' the patient and give them very intensive care. As ICUs became more popular so more critically ill patients went to them. The skills of looking after ill patients on the ward were lost. Currently in most hospitals, especially at night time, there is not the senior and experienced staff available to look after particularly ill patients on the ward. That is why high dependency units (HDUs) and ICUs have become more necessary. Giddings argues well that patients with ruptured aneurysms who need ventilating postoperatively are best looked after in ICUs. Once the ventilator is no longer necessary they would probably be just as well looked after in an HDU.

On the other hand the perfectly fit patient who has a straightforward elective aortic aneurysm repair and does not need to go to an ICU or an HDU can be just as well looked after on an ordinary surgical ward. The greatest problem is stratifying risk. Goldman, Detsky and other risk-stratification with their predictive score have not achieved the level of helpfulness that might have been hoped for. We definitely need much better risk-stratification to predict better or worse outcomes.

There is one further option available which is for the patients to be held in recovery after surgery for a longer time than usual until they are clearly fit to return to the ward. They would not need to go to the HDU or ICU.

This chapter gives many pros, cons and difficulties but comes to no firm conclusion other than that more work is required to stratify the risks of patients, the effectiveness of the surgery and need of the ICU.

Authors' reply

We do not agree with this comment. We clearly state that for the majority of elective abdominal aortic aneurysms, HDUs are appropriate, and that the goal of management should be to avoid the need for an ICU. These are our firm conclusions.

Should Size of Aneurysm Determine Procedure Type for Endovascular Stent-Grafting for Aortic Aneurysm?

J.C. Parodi

INTRODUCTION

In 1990 we began implanting a stent–graft combination to exclude aneurysms.[1] This procedure was very soon extended to treat dissections, vascular trauma and occlusive diseases of the arteries. In all these procedures the basic mechanism of the proposed treatment was to line the lumen of the artery creating a new conduit inside the vascular segment; in this way aneurysms could be excluded, intimal tears of dissections sealed, as well as orifices created by trauma. Suffice it to say that until now, all we have proven is that those procedures were feasible but we have not demonstrated that they were safe and effective for every patient.[2] There is no question that this method has very special characteristics that we still have to learn mostly in relation to the long-term effects after implantation of the stent–graft combination in a diseased artery. We have, however, learned important lessons during these last 7 years and technology has moved us a step forward providing new and more reliable devices.[3]

In the present chapter we will describe our experience and thoughts about the application of the endoluminal method to treat aneurysms, the type of procedure applicable, depending on the morphology of the aneurysm, and the differences encountered in the outcome of aneurysms of diverse sizes.

In order to organize the present chapter we will develop the following topics:

1. Description of devices used.
2. Technical aspects of stent–graft application in small and large aneurysms.
3. Changes elicited in the artery in which the stent–graft was implanted in relation to the size of the aneurysm.
4. The fate of backflow from the inferior mesenteric and lumbar arteries in small and large aneurysms.
5. Long-term results. Concerns and new ways to cope with problems.

DESCRIPTION OF DEVICES USED

Initial cases

The combination of an 'Extralarge' Palmaz stent and a thin polyester graft attached at the mid-portion of the stent was used in the first eight cases.

Second system

In spite of the excellent results obtained in the experimental work with animals,[4] we very soon learned that we needed a second stent to seal the distal end of the graft. Only two of the initially successful cases had good long-term outcome. One patient survived 37 months after having sealed an infrarenal dissection which created a large and rapidly growing infrarenal aneurysm. The second patient still lives free of aneurysmal growth after 6 years of exclusion of a small aortic aneurysm which caused spontaneous embolization. The rest of the patients treated using only the proximal stent, developed endoleaks and had to be treated by placing a second distal stent. This last method was used in 38 patients.

Third system

Most large aneurysms do not have a distal neck or cuff. Thus in 1992, we started to use an aorto–uni–iliac device and 46 patients were treated with it.

Fourth system

The Bifurcated Mihale-Mintec and later the Vanguard device were applied in 32 patients. The Vanguard system described in several publications consists of a modular system constructed of a totally supported thin polyester woven graft and a skeleton of Nitinol (Cragg stent).

TECHNICAL ASPECTS OF STENT–GRAFT APPLICATION IN SMALL AND LARGE ANEURYSMS

The morphology of aneurysms varies according to several factors, and size is the main one. For the purpose of this chapter we define large aneurysms as those in which the maximum diameter exceeds 7 cm. Small or medium size are those smaller than 6.9 cm. This division is for the most part arbitrary and used simply to define characteristics of aneurysms which significantly change as the aneurysm grows larger.

In the first stage of aneurysm development (3.5–4.5 cm), both proximal and distal necks are long, the proximal always being longer than the distal (>2 cm proximal and >1.5 cm distal) during this initial stage. Iliac arteries are generally not affected by dilatation and their axes are straight. As the aneurysm grows (4.5–5.5 cm), the distal end becomes shorter and finally vanishes. The proximal neck remains unchanged in most of the cases. Iliac arteries are still straight. When the aneurysm becomes larger than 7.0 cm, only rarely can a distal neck be visualized and the proximal neck measurements often indicate that the neck is wider and shorter than smaller aneurysms. The axes of the neck, the aneurysm and the iliac arteries are no longer straight and frequently an angle exceeding 60 degrees is found between the proximal neck and the aneurysm. Iliac arteries in this stage are more tortuous and in a significant proportion aneurysmatic.

The above description accounts for most cases with few exceptions. The morphology of the aneurysm predicts in general the problems that will be encountered during the endoluminal deployment of the device.

Access was the first problem that we faced when dealing with large aneurysms with tortuous iliac arteries. Our three initial devices needed a 25 F sheath (outer diameter) at the beginning. This fact plus the addition to the rigidity of these systems explained the extreme difficulties we found at that time. We dealt with this problem by miniaturizing the device to reach 21 F which was a great accomplishment. Using a through-and-through rigid (Superstiff) guide-wire passed from the brachial artery down to the femoral artery and applying tension to it, helped to overcome many problems of access. The rigid guide-wire was inside a catheter in order to protect the subclavian artery when tension was applied to both ends.

The Vanguard system is significantly more flexible than the initial systems and this accounts for the greater ease we experienced in accessing the aortic aneurysm using this system.

The adaptability of the two different systems (balloon-expandable and self-expandable) to the variable geometry of the proximal necks deserves a short comment. The more plastic and malleable balloon-expandable stent acquired the shape of the neck; when this latter was heavily calcified and not cylindrical, a partially compliant balloon (Balt, Paris, France) was utilized. Angles exceeding 60 degrees caused problems of initial endoleaks when the Vanguard system was applied. Several studies demonstrated that not all necks are cylindrical. Some of them have an ovoid section, others a conical shape and a few have rings in the middle of the neck (hourglass). The morphology of every single case should be studied thoroughly if excellent results are to be achieved using this technology. Measurement of diameters, lengths and angles are crucial not only for the selection of patients but also for the selection of the device and for determining the size needed for a specific patient. Initially we relied upon measurements performed using a pigtail catheter with radioopaque marks placed every 5 mm and using quantitative angiography. Early in our experience, however, we learned that very often this method failed. Mostly, measurement of length underestimated the actual length. The reason for miscalculation was the presence of curves created by the elongation of the artery. The length of the centre line of the flow is much more accurate than the measurement using marked catheters to define the length of device needed. In order to obtain the centre of the flow length we used pure geometrical calculations using the Pythagoreas theorem and lately we produced a three-dimensional reconstruction in our workstation of the spiral CT scan. The company Medical Media Systems developed a very reliable software to be used for this purpose. Their results were validated using phantom models of known dimensions. With this software even volumes can be easily calculated.

As this chapter deals with differences found in aneurysms of different sizes it should be said that accuracy in calculating sizes and angles is much more demanding in cases of large aneurysms. Intravascular ultrasound seems to be an alternative for obtaining measurements. In our experience, this method was accurate in measuring diameters but only when the transducer was precisely located at the centre of the lumen. Calculation of lengths was not reliable with intravascular ultrasound. This method is by all means the best for assessing completeness of the device deployment and presence of kinks, folds or external compressions.

Initial endoleaks were the second problem encountered during the procedures. Leaks resulted from incomplete sealing of the graft at the ends of the device. Endoleaks using the initial system resulted from applying the system in the presence of short proximal or distal ends. The segment of the stent covered with graft was left inside the aneurysm without providing a watertight sealing of the end of the graft. Endoleaks caused catastrophic consequences later on if left untreated. No initial endoleaks from the ends or connections were detected in our experience using the Vanguard device.

Initial and later endoleaks were found with higher frequency in large aneurysms compared with small and medium size aneurysms. The cause of this difference in our cases was not the dilatation of the aorta but rather the incorrect implantation of devices in contact with thrombus at either end. Because large aneurysms had a shorter or even non-existent neck, (distal) leaks developed more frequently in those aneurysms.

Embolization accounted for the first fatal complications we had in the present series. Four massive microembolizations resulted from complicated procedures in which excessive instrumentation inside the aneurysmal sac was needed. All four cases of massive embolization resulted in large aneurysms. Large aneurysms are more tortuous and longer; these characteristics probably accounted for the disruption of mural thrombus that precipitated embolization. This is one of the differences we found between small and large aneurysms. Furthermore, we had three cases of small aneurysms treated endoluminally after causing spontaneous embolization and by using careful techniques no one embolized during the procedure. We had no cases of embolization in straightforward procedures even in the presence of large aneurysms. Special care has to be taken to deal with large and tortuous aneurysms. The site of access has to be chosen in relation to the presence of thrombus and its location in relation to the axes of the iliac arteries. A rigid guide-wire usually prevents disruption of mural thrombus when the sheath is introduced inside the aneurysm. The through-and-through technique described previously helps a great deal in preventing thrombus disruption.

In summary, procedure success varies significantly according to the size of the aneurysm. The larger the aneurysm the more problems in access and incomplete sealing we encountered; in addition, risk of embolization in our series was directly related to the size of the aneurysm.

CHANGES ELICITED IN THE AORTA AFTER ENDOLUMINAL EXCLUSION OF AN ANEURYSM

From September 1990 until October 1997 we treated 133 patients with aortic aneurysms. The initial success rate for aorto–aortic procedures with one stent was 87.5%; for the aorto–aortic procedures with two stents it was 72.7%. Aorto–uni-iliac system resulted successfully in 71%; for bifurcation systems (Mintec, Vanguard) it was 88.8%. Late success was obtained in 12.5% of the patients who had only the proximal stent placed, in 68% of the aorto–aortic cases with two stents; 85% of the aorto–uni–iliac cases resulted successfully in the long term and in 88% of those who had a bifurcated system implanted. These results indicate clearly that the aorto–uni–iliac and the bifurcation systems had by far the best long-term results.

In order to investigate further the causes of failures, we reviewed the changes in diameters that occurred in those patients treated with endoluminal grafts. Twenty-three patients had at least three CT scans performed in a period exceeding 3 years after treatment and had only the primary treatment performed. Analysis of these data indicate that the diameter of the aneurysm increases when a leak is present. There were no significant increases in diameters of the aorta at three levels measured, at the level of the superior mesenteric artery, renal arteries and neck of the aneurysm (see Tables 1, 2, 3 and 4).

In summary, these studies demonstrated that aneurysmal growth after exclusion indicated the presence of endoleaks. No significant changes were found in the diameter of the proximal neck, at the level of the renal and superior mesenteric

Table 1.

Proximal neck diameters
Before treatment: 23.31 mm (SD: 3.57)
After treatment: 24.23 mm (SD: 3.83)
    NS (p > 0.30)

Diameters at the level of the renal arteries
Before treatment: 24.15 mm (SD: 3.48)
After treatment: 24.23 mm (SD: 3.42)
    NS (p > 0.25)

Table 2.

Diameters at the level of the superior mesenteric artery
Before treatment: 25.69 mm (SD: 3.35)
After treatment: 26.08 mm (SD: 3.77)
    NS (p > 0.30)

Table 3.

Diameters of abdominal aortic aneurysm (total)
Before treatment: 51.92 mm (SD: 13.82)
After treatment: 57.62 mm (SD: 18.07)
    S (p < 0.05)

Table 4.

Diameters of abdominal aortic aneurysm with leak treatment
Before treatment: 52.87 mm (SD: 12.92)
After treatment: 62.63 mm (SD: 17.50)
    S (p < 0.05)

Diameters of abdominal aortic aneurysm leak treatment
Before treatment: 50.4 mm (SD: 15.01)
After treatment: 49.6 mm (SD: 17.63)
    NS

arteries during a mean follow-up of 5 years and 2 months. Only one case of 23 examined showed a significant increase in the diameter of the proximal neck. These findings are in disagreement with the results of Illig et al.[5] who encountered significant dilatation of the neck of the aneurysm after open surgical graft replacement. The reason for these quite different results is not clear, but we can speculate that perhaps the presence of the metal stent which generates a layer of myointimal hyperplasia covering the stent and the reinforcement of the wall of the

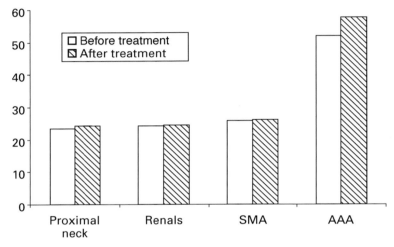

Fig. 1. Variation in diameter after endovascular treatment of abdominal aortic aneurysms (AAA). SMA: Superior mesenteric artery.

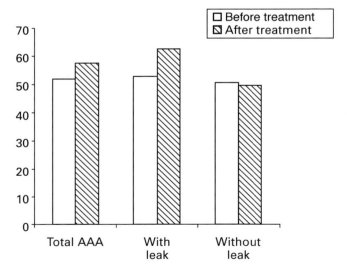

Fig. 2. Variation in diameter after endovascular treatment of abdominal aortic aneurysms (AAA), showing results with and without leaks.

artery which had incorporated the stent as part of its architecture could create more resistance to dilatation of the arterial segment.

THE FATE OF BACKFLOW FROM THE INFERIOR MESENTERIC OR LUMBAR ARTERIES

In our initial experience, we had no opportunity to see any endoleak caused by backflow from the inferior mesenteric or lumbar arteries. The reason for this was clear, our patients had very large aneurysms or small ones which had embolized spontaneously. All these patients had mural thrombus covering the entire circumference of the aneurysm. In a study we helped to start, performed by Eton *et al.*[6] it was proven experimentally that branches thrombose after aneurysmal exclusion. In the experience of the group of Shah *et al.*[7] using the surgical exclusion technique only very few patients needed to be treated because of the persistence of backflow from branches. Lately as we have started to treat smaller aneurysms, we have seen on several occasions perigraft flow caused by backbleeding from branches. This backflow has not caused any aneurysmal growth as yet and we are following these patients closely. What has become evident is that backflow is far more frequent in small aneurysms and it is an issue that will have to be addressed when treatment of small aneurysms is undertaken.

Several investigators[8,9] have reported cases of persistent perigraft flow caused by backflow from branches and some have undertaken an endoluminal treatment of this condition. Eikelboom *et al.*[10] presented recently a study demonstrating that the incidence of persistent backflow from branches depended upon the number of lumbar arteries open before the endoluminal treatment as well as the presence of thrombus and its localization (presence of posterior wall thrombus had less incidence of backflow).

If in the future these branches can be coil-embolized before they persist, or treated laparoscopically when they do, is not yet clear. Their optimal treatment is not yet certain.

LONG-TERM RESULTS AND NEW WAYS TO COPE WITH PROBLEMS

All but one of our late failures were related to the development of new endoleaks. Only one case of late migration of an 'Extralarge' Palmaz stent was detected in our series. This latter case deserves special consideration. The proximal stent was placed 1.8 mm distally to the renal arteries and the proximal neck had only 15 mm in length. That means that the complete proximal end of the device was placed in contact with thrombus which was initially compressed and served as a temporary attachment site. As soon as the thrombus dissolved, the device migrated distally. We have not had any case of device-migration caused by proximal neck dilatation. We did find, however, one case in which the proximal neck enlarged significantly. The proximal stent was placed so far from the renal arteries that this enlargement caused a proximal endoleak.

In this chapter, we should consider two aspects of proximal neck dilatation since we believe strongly that this is one of the crucial problems which affect the durability of the endovascular treatment of aneurysms. Studies of the architecture of the proximal infrarenal aorta have demonstrated the presence of adventitial crossing fibres in the aorta at the level of the renal arteries. These fibres come from the adventitia of the branches and make the aorta more resistant to dilatation. It is the same mechanism that preserves the visceral sector of the aorta without dilatation. The Crawford technique takes advantage of this, allowing suture of all four visceral branches together to the side-opening created on the tubular polyester graft used to replace a thoracoabdominal aneurysm. Our own studies disclosed that the pressure applied to a balloon to dilate the infrarenal aorta is much lower than the pressure needed to dilate the visceral segment of the aorta. These observations tell us that the end of the device should be placed flush with the renal ostia where dilatation is less likely to occur. The second possibility that should be explored is to place the bare stent part of the device in the suprarenal position. The advantages are twofold: first, at that level the aorta decreases in diameter, thus the difference in diameter creates an additional mechanism of anchoring the device; second the aorta is stronger at that level allowing treatment of patients with short proximal necks. A theoretical drawback is the potential occlusion or embolization of the renal arteries caused by applying wires crossing the renal artery ostium. New devices can easily be constructed with orifices for renal arteries ostia. In our small experience of eight cases covering the renal arteries, no negative consequences were detected.

The lack of neck dilatation in most of the cases analysed after more than 5 years compares favourably with the changes found in a recent study of the proximal neck after conventional abdominal aortic aneurysm resection.[5] We should wait until other studies with more patients are available. We tentatively suggest that the presence of bare stent creates a tissue reaction mostly directed to cover the metal with a dense layer of myointimal hyperplasia. In our studies, after a variable period of time, the metal formed part of the architecture of the artery creating a 'reinforced' arterial wall which could be more resistant to dilatation in the long term. In the few specimens we were able to study the proximal bare stent could not be removed from the artery without literally destroying it. These findings are very encouraging in terms of long-term results as there is such a paucity of good basic research in the field.

Late endoleaks were frequent, most of them arose from the distal end of an aorto–aortic system. Only two endoleaks occurred at the proximal end. The first case is described above and the second case was similar to the first. The stent was placed far from the renal arteries in contact with thrombus, at the level of the thrombus. After some time, a perigraft flow was detected, which did not fill the aneurysm but a small pocket around the proximal stent. Distal endoleaks resulted mainly from lysis of thrombus interposed between the device and the artery and in some few cases by a defined dilatation of the distal neck. Only two of the aorto–uni–iliac cases resulted in late endoleak. Both of these resulted from dilatation of a small ring which was located in an aneurysmal iliac artery. These rings were the temporary attachment-sealing of the distal end until the ring dilated and allowed flow around the graft.

In summary, most of the late endoleaks came from the distal end of an aorto–aortic procedure and were caused by lysis of thrombus interposed or by dilatation of the artery.

CONCLUSIONS

Small and medium size aneurysms usually have a long proximal neck. Most small aneurysms also have a distal neck although shorter than the proximal one and they have a straight axis. Calculations of diameters, lengths and angles are easily accomplished; implantation of stent–grafts are usually performed without difficulty, and access problems are only related to the small sizes of iliac arteries in some female patients.

Microembolization was not seen in our series in this subgroup of patients. No significant dilatation of the necks were seen during a mean follow-up of 5 years and 2 months. The most significant feature in those cases was the high frequency of open lumbar and inferior mesenteric arteries. Consequences of these open branches in the long term should still be determined. Initial and late success on treating small and medium size aneurysms are very high. If the long-term follow-up continues to show good results (decrease in size of aneurysms and lack of complications) small aneurysms will be the main indication for endovascular treatments. A bifurcated endoluminal device is applicable for most of the small and medium size aneurysm and for us, is the first choice. We were discouraged by the distal neck dilatation and high failure rates of the aorto–aortic devices and we no longer use tubular grafts.

Large aneurysms pose a distinct problem. They usually have a shorter and wider proximal neck and the distal neck is absent in most of them. Iliac arteries and aortic axes are usually not straight and calculations of diameters, lengths and angles are difficult to perform. Access is inconvenient due to tortuosity, and embolization can be caused by instrumentation inside the sac. Initial and late leaks were more frequently seen after treating large aneurysms. Dilatation of the proximal neck was not significant after a mean follow-up of 5 years and 2 months after stent–graft implantation. An isolated case of proximal neck dilatation was seen in our series in a patient affected by a large aneurysm, with a neck of 28 mm in diameter. Distal neck dilatation was detected in a significant number of cases. Common iliac dilatation was seen infrequently. Causes of late leaks in our experience were related to the presence of thrombus interposed between the artery and the device.

Very large aneurysms often have an angulated neck and very tortuous iliac arteries. Sometimes iliac arteries are aneurysmatic. For those large aneurysms, an aorto–uni–iliac or a bifurcated device should be implanted as soon as the patient is selected for endoluminal repair.

In the near future an extraluminal (laparoscopic) and endoluminal treatments could be combined to solve some of the problems still pending when an endoluminal treatment is undertaken. Branches will be interrupted and bands placed around arteries by direct vision using laparoscopic techniques.

REFERENCES

1. Parodi JC, Palmaz JC, Barone HD: Transfemoral intraluminal graft implantation for abdominal aortic aneurysms. *Ann Vasc Surg* **5**: 491–9, 1991
2. Parodi JC: Endovascular repair of abdominal aortic aneurysms and other arterial lesions. *J Vasc Surg* **21**: 549–55, 1995

3. Blum U *et al.*: Endoluminal stent-grafts for infra-renal aortic aneurysms. *New Engl J Med* **336**: 13–20, 1997

4. Laborde JC, Parodi JC, Clem MFC *et al.*: Intraluminal bypass of abdominal aortic aneurysm: Feasibility study. *Radiology* **184**: 185–90, 1992

5. Illig KA, Green RM, Ouriel K *et al.*: Fate of the proximal aortic cuff: Implications for endovascular aneurysm repair. *J Vasc Surg* **26**: 492–501, 1997

6. Eton D, Warner D, Owens C *et al.*: Results of endoluminal grafting in an experimental aortic aneurysm model. *J Vasc Surg* **23**: 819–31, 1996

7. Shah DM, Chang RB, Paty PK *et al.*: Treatment of abdominal aortic aneurysm by exclusion and bypass, an analysis of outcome. *J Vasc Surg* **13**: 15–22, 1991

8. Yusuf SW, Whitaker SC, Chuter TAM *et al.*: Early results of endovascular aortic aneurysm surgery with aortouniiliac graft, contralateral iliac oclusion, and femorofemoral bypass. *J Vasc Surg* **25**: 165–72, 1997

9. Armon MP, Yusuf SW, Whitaker SC *et al.*: The fate of the aneurysm sac following endovascular aneurysm repair. XI Annual Meeting, p. 70. Lisbon: European Society for Vascular Surgery, 1997

10. Broeders IAMJ, Blankensteijn JD, Eikelboom BC: Are patent side branches predictive of endoleaks after transfemoral endovascular aneurysm management (TEAM)? XI Annual Meeting, p. 64. Lisbon: European Society for Vascular Surgery, 1997

Editorial comments by B.R. Hopkinson

Dr Parodi has the greatest experience of endovascular stenting in the world. He has certainly seen all the snags and hazards as they have arisen and has alerted the rest of us to them so that we can beware of them. It is salutary that only 2 years after the beginning of their experience his team changed from a simple aorta–aortic device to the much more widely applicable aorto–uni–iliac device. It is emphasized that the fundamental principle of endovascular surgery is just the same as any other bypass graft surgery in that the fixation points of the graft have to go from sound artery above to sound artery below with no evidence of aneurysm or clot lining at the points of fixation.

We would support Dr Parodi in his emphasis on accurate measurement. No method of measuring the shape and size of aneurysms is perfect, certainly the measuring angiogram catheter alone can give wildly variable results and it is hoped that the new three-dimensional reconstructions give much better forecasts of the shape and size of graft required. The problem is not so much one of large aneurysms but of a large lumen within aneurysms. We can never be quite sure within a large lumen exactly where the endoprosthesis will lie.

Dr Parodi rightly emphasizes the embolization problems in the early part of their and other people's series. This is probably a complication of excessive instrumentation disturbing the clot within the aneurysmal sac. Catheters and wires should be passed across the aneurysm sac as expeditiously and carefully as possible to avoid this happening. Clamping of the femorals, which is used in Chuter system, also prevents the problem of leg emboli.

I would agree with Dr Parodi that patients with circumferential clot around the aneurysm are very unlikely to develop leaks from lumbar branches. Endoleaks are most troublesome in patients with little or no clot covering large areas of the aneurysm sac. In Nottingham we have taken to filling up the aneurysm sac with gelatin sponge after the aorta–uni–iliac artery has been deployed, before the contralateral common iliac artery is occluded. This seems to have abolished the problem of branch endoleaks in a small series of about 25 patients. Pre- or intraoperative coil embolization of lumbar arteries is much more difficult and more likely to be the cause of microemboli. The greater use of the suprarenal portion of aorta for stent–graft fixation may well have benefits especially as the aorta at that level appears to be much stronger than the infrarenal aorta.

We would agree with Dr Parodi that large aneurysms are more likely to be more difficult to deal with than small ones but in any individual it is the summation of adverse factors which makes the final decision for the appropriateness of endovascular treatment.

What Are the Indications for Endovascular Stent–Graft Repair of Abdominal Aortic Aneurysms: Present Status

Evan C. Lipsitz, Takao Ohki and Frank J. Veith

INTRODUCTION

The enthusiasm for including endovascular stent–grafts in the armamentarium for repair of abdominal aortic aneurysms is growing rapidly as experience at many centres increases and with ongoing technical improvements in the devices used. The exact indications and contraindications for these procedures have yet to be defined and are evolving rapidly. Indications may be quite variable depending on which device has been chosen and its suitability for a given patient's anatomy. A number of commercial and 'home-made' devices are presently under investigation. These devices can be categorized based on design, anatomic variations that are treatable, and patient risk status. This chapter will review the general inclusion and exclusion criteria for the endovascular repair of abdominal aortic aneurysms with reference to the general endovascular graft types which are currently available.

PREOPERATIVE EVALUATION

The evaluation of patients for endovascular abdominal aortic aneurysm repair includes a screening abdominopelvic computed tomomgraphy (CT) scan. This study should be performed with intravenous contrast on a spiral scanner using 3–5 mm cuts. Aneurysm length, diameter, and quality are evaluated as are the dimensions of the proximal and distal necks.[1] The presence or absence of mural thrombus at the necks, which is of paramount importance, can only be ascertained on CT scan. If it appears that the patient may be a candidate for endovascular grafting based on the CT findings then an angiogram of at least the aortoiliac segment is performed. This permits assessment of the renal, inferior mesenteric, and iliac arteries. The mesenteric circulation as a whole, lumbar arteries, and any aberrant vessels are evaluated. Tortuosity or kinking of the iliac vessels, which has implications for device insertion and deployment, is noted.[2] The study is performed with a calibrating catheter which contains radiopaque markers at 1 cm intervals allowing for precise measurement of the vessels by minimizing the effects of parallax and magnification.[1]

GENERAL INDICATIONS

Regardless of the type of endovascular graft used, there are several anatomic criteria that must be fulfilled prior to attempting endovascular graft placement for abdominal aortic aneurysms. If these criteria are not fulfilled, the procedure is generally contraindicated.[2-5] These criteria include the following points:

1. The presence of a normal aortic segment at least 1.5–2 cm in length (Fig. 1A, length a) and not more than 25–30 mm in diameter (Fig. 1A, diameter b) distal to the renal ostia and proximal to the aneurysm (proximal neck) for the proximal fixation of the graft. This area should be free of thrombus and not conical in shape (no more than 3–4 mm widening from the proximal to distal ends of the neck). Depending on which device is chosen the angle between proximal neck and the aorta may preclude endovascular repair. (Fig. 1B, angle 1). The Vanguard and Talent devices, for example, require that this angle not be greater than 60 degrees, and Corvita requires that it not be greater than 30 degrees.

2. If a straight or tube graft is to be employed, the presence of a normal aortic segment approximately 2 cm in length (Fig. 1A, length d) and not greater than 25 mm in diameter (Fig. 1A, diameter e) without thrombus proximal to the aortic bifurcation (distal neck).

3. If the site selected for distal implantation is the common or external iliac artery, its morphology must be adequate for seating an attachment system. Patients with tortuosity of more than 90 degrees at any point (Fig. 1B, angle 2), significant dilatation to 16–20 mm (Fig. 1A, diameter g), or severe iliac artery calcification are generally not candidates. The presence of a short (<30 mm) common iliac (Fig. 1A, length f) or the use of the external iliac as the target vessel requires embolization of the internal iliac(s), if patent, to prevent back filling of the aneurysm.

4. The common and external iliac, and femoral arteries must be of sufficient caliber to allow passage of the introducer sheath or must be amenable to balloon dilatation to facilitate passage (Fig. 1A, diameter h). This is an important factor in the selection of patients for stent–graft repair. The size of the recipient vessel determines not only whether or not the patient is a candidate for endovascular repair but which devices may be used. The outer diameter (OD) of the delivery sheath for each devices varies. The size of the introducer systems are as follows: Talent (24-27 Fr OD), Vanguard (20.5 Fr OD), EVT (23-27 Fr OD), Corvita (21 Fr OD), and Montefiore Endovascular Graft system (18-20 Fr OD).

5. The femoral and iliac vessels must demonstrate limited tortuosity after arterial straightening manoeuvers, e.g. use of superstiff guide-wires or dissection and caudal traction on the external iliac artery, are completed.

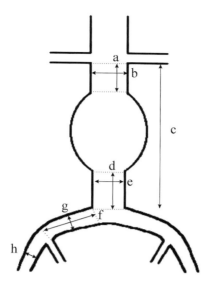

Fig. 1A. Measurements used in determining suitability for endovascular abdominal aortic aneurysm repair. Lines a, d, and f represent the lengths of the proximal neck, distal neck, and common iliac artery respectively. Line c represents the length of aorta from the renal arteries to the bifurcation. Lines b, e, g, and h represent the diameters of the proximal neck, the distal neck, the common iliac artery, and the external iliac and/or femoral arteries respectively. (Adapted from ref. 13.)

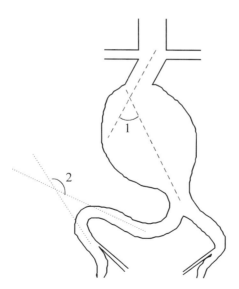

Fig. 1B. Shows some of the essential angles used in determining suitability for endovascular abdominal aortic aneurysm repair and device selection. The dashed lines represent the angle (1) created by the neck of the aneurysm and the aneurysm itself. The dotted lines represent an angle (2) created by tortuosity of the iliac artery.

6. Aberrant vessels, particularly an indispensable accessory renal artery, must not be present in the segment of aorta to be excluded from the circulation.

7. The patient cannot be dependent on the inferior mesenteric artery for perfusion of the intestine, since that artery will be excluded from the circulation.

8. The patient must have the ability to comply with whatever follow-up regimen is required.[2-5]

CLASSIFICATION OF DEVICES

Endovascular grafts can be categorized into two types based on whether their fixation stents are self-expanding or balloon-expandable. Self-expanding devices are somewhat easier to deploy and can accommodate a certain amount of aortic neck enlargement. Most manufactured grafts, including the EVT graft, the Talent graft, the Vanguard graft, the Corvita graft (Fig. 2), and the AneuRx graft, utilize a self-expanding stent. A 'surgeon-made' device with self-expanding stents is the Chuter graft. The White-Yu Endovascular GAD graft has a specially made, self-expanding stent which is called the graft attachment device (GAD). The most frequently used balloon-expandable stent is the large Palmaz stent (Cordis, Johnson and Johnson, Warren, NJ, USA). Although this stent may be technically more demanding to deploy

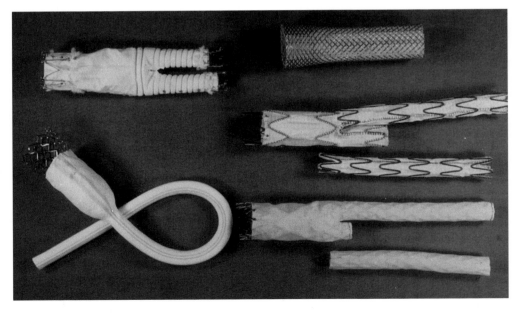

Fig. 2. Bifurcated EVT graft (top left), Corvita graft (top right), Talent modular bifurcated graft (middle right), Vanguard modular bifurcated graft (bottom right), and Montifiore aorto-uni-femoral graft (bottom left).

accurately, it has a stronger radial (hoop) strength than self-expanding stents. This may be important considering the high aortic pressure to which these grafts are exposed. The Palmaz stent has been used for many surgeon-made devices, including the Parodi graft, the Montefiore graft and the Leicester graft (Fig. 3).

Since the anatomy, length, and diameter of abdominal aortic aneurysms varies significantly from patient to patient, it is advantageous for an endovascular graft to have a certain dimensional adaptability to accommodate this variability. With the use of modular grafts, variability in length between the proximal and the distal landing points can be managed by changing the amount of overlap between each of two

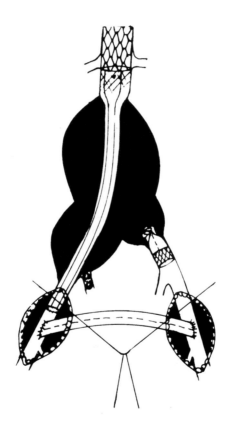

Fig. 3. Repair of aortoiliac aneurysm using an aorto-uni-femoral device with contralateral occlusion of the common iliac artery and coil embolization of the ipsilateral internal iliac artery followed by femorofemoral bypass grafting. The distal portion of the device can be trimmed and endoluminally anastomosed to the femoral artery. Note that the bare portion of the proximal stent is placed above the orifice of the renal arteries to achieve maximum contact between the stent and the native aorta and to provide secure leak-free fixation.

components. This concept was first described by the Sydney group and was called the 'Trombone' graft.[6] In most bifurcated grafts the additional limb of a modular bifurcated graft and extenders serve to achieve dimensional adaptability. The distal landing zone of the limb can be adjusted by changing the amount of overlap between the main body and the limb. In addition, the length of the main limb can be extended with an extender stent graft. These types of endovascular grafts include the Vanguard graft, the Talent graft, the Corvita graft, and the AneuRx graft.

Another approach to achieve length adaptability is demonstrated by the Montefiore device,[7] and the Leicester graft.[8] These grafts have enough length so that the distal end of the graft will always emerge from the insertion arteriotomy site, thereby allowing the physician to customize the length of the graft during the procedure.

SELECTION OF PATIENTS

Some device protocols select patients whose general health is good and who have favourable anatomy for endovascular repair. The rationale in these protocols is that if the endovascular procedure fails, these patients are the most likely to tolerate conversion to an open procedure. Although a reduction in the already low mortality rates of standard abdominal aortic aneurysms repair would be a welcome result of any new procedure, the primary goal of endovascular repair in these good risk patients is to improve quality of life by reducing postoperative pain, sexual dysfunction, and complications resulting from an intra-abdominal operation as well as to reduce costs by decreasing the need for intensive care unit care and the postoperative length of stay. Most of the manufactured devices, including the EVT, Vanguard, AneuRx, and Corvita grafts, are currently being evaluated in the USA, in good-risk patients. In addition, some of the 'surgeon-made' devices such as the Chuter bifurcated graft[5] and to some extent the White-Yu Endovascular GAD graft[9] were used for good-risk patients.

Although the morbidity and mortality rates of standard abdominal aortic aneurysm repair has proven to be excellent in good-risk patients, these rates increase with the presence of associated diseases. Mortality rates as high as 60% have been reported in high-risk patients.[10] Furthermore, standard repair may be difficult in patients with severe cardiopulmonary disease or a 'hostile' abdomen secondary to such factors as multiple abdominal operations complicated by extensive scarring or infection. Selection of these high-risk patients for endovascular repair is justified on a 'compassionate need' basis. The goal of the endovascular grafting in this group of patients is not only to reduce costs and improve the postoperative quality of life, but also to broaden the indications for repair by providing treatment for those patients who might otherwise be deemed untreatable. The devices made for these indications are primarily 'home-made' devices which include the Parodi graft, the Montefiore Endovascular Graft system[7,11] and the Nottingham graft.[12] In the USA, the Talent graft is the only manufactured graft that has a Food and Drug Administration (FDA) investigational device exemption which permits usage in high-risk cases.

ANATOMICAL CLASSIFICATION OF ABDOMINAL AORTIC ANEURYSMS

The type and morphology of the aneurysm as well as the characteristics of the device determine whether endovascular repair is feasible and if so, which type of device may be used (Fig. 4).

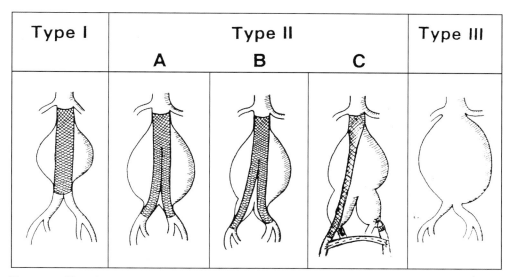

| Type I | Type II | | | Type III |
| | A | B | C | |

Fig. 4. Morphometric classification of abdominal aortic aneurysms and possible endovascular graft configurations.
Type I: Abdominal aortic aneurysm with sufficient proximal (>15 mm) and distal (>10 mm) aortic neck (tube graft).
Type IIA: Proximal neck (>15 mm), absence of distal aortic neck (bifurcated graft).
Type IIB: Proximal neck (>15 mm) with proximal common iliac artery involvement (bifurcated graft).
Type IIC: Proximal neck (>15 mm) with Iliac artery involvement to the iliac bifurcation (aorto-uni-iliac graft with contralateral iliac occlusion, femorofemoral bypass and coil embolization of hypogastric arteries).
Type III: Proximal neck <15 mm – requires grafts that permit suprarenal stent placement, e.g. in patients on haemodialysis. We have accomplished this successfully in patients with renal failure on haemodialysis.
Adapted from ref. 14.

CONCLUSIONS

Presently there are no universally agreed upon indications or contraindications for endovascular repair in patients deemed suitable by the criteria outlined above. Current indications for endovascular repair are highly variable and depend on which device is chosen. At this time an estimated 40–70% of abdominal aortic aneurysms are amenable to endovascular grafting again depending on which device is being used. While our preferred procedure for good risk patients is a standard repair using a transabdominal or occasionally a retroperitoneal approach, the ability to perform endovascular repair successfully is increasing on an almost daily basis spurred by technological advances and the accumulation of experience with these procedures. With continued improvements in the flexibility and durability of endovascular grafts as well as advances in the delivery systems of endovascular grafts and with greater proficiency and experience of the surgeons inserting them, the majority of patients with infrarenal abdominal aortic aneurysm may become candidates for endovascular graft repair.

REFERENCES

1. Moore WS: Transfemoral endovascular repair of abdominal aortic aneurysm: Feasibility study of the EGS system. In: Parodi JC, Veith FJ, Marin ML (Eds), *Endovascular Grafting Techniques*. St Louis: Quality Medical Publishing 1996
2. Faries PL: Clinical experience with endovascular grafts for aneurysmal arterial disease. In: Marin ML, Veith FJ, Levine BA (Eds), *Endovascular Stented Grafts for the Treatment of Vascular Diseases*. Austin: R.G. Landes Company, 1995
3. Chuter TAM, Nowygrod R: Bifurcated endovascular grafts for aortic aneurysm repair. In: Parodi JC, Veith FJ, Marin ML (Eds), *Endovascular Grafting Techniques*. St Louis: Quality Medical Publishing 1996
4. Moore WS: The EVT tube and bifurcated endograft systems: Technical considerations and clinical summary. *J Endovasc Surg* **4**: 182–94, 1997
5. Chuter TAM, Risberg Bo, Hopkinson BR *et al.*: Clinical experience with a bifurcated endovascular graft for abdominal aortic aneurysm repair. *J Vasc Surg* **24**: 655–66, 1996
6. Schumacher H, Eckstein HH, Kallinowski F, Allenberg JR: Morphometry and classification in abdominal aortic aneurysms: Patient selection for endovascular and open surgery. *J Endovasc Surg* **4**: 39-44, 1997
7. Wain RA, Marin ML, Veith FJ *et al.*: Endoleaks complicating endovascular graft treatment of aortic aneurysms: Classification, risk factors, and outcome. *J Vasc Surg* (in press)
8. Thompson MM, Sayers RD, Nasim A *et al.*: Aortomonoiliac endovascular grafting: Difficult solutions to difficult aneurysms. *J Endovasc Surg* **4**: 174–81, 1997
9. White GH, Yu W, May J *et al.*: Three year experience with the White-Yu endovascular GAD graft for transluminal repair of aortic and iliac aneurysms. *J Endovasc Surg* **4**: 124–36, 1997
10. McCombs RP, Roberts B: Acute renal failure after resection of abdominal aortic aneurysm. *Surg Gynecol Obstet* **148**: 175–9, 1970
11. Marin, M.L., Veith, F.J., Cynamon, J *et al.*: Initial experience with transluminally placed endovascular grafts for the treatment of complex vascular lesions. *Ann Surg* **222**: 1–17, 1995
12. Yusuf SW, Whitaker SC, Chuter TAM *et al.*: Early results of endovascular aortic aneurysm surgery with aortouni-iliacaortouniiniac graft, contralateral iliac occlusion, and femorofemoral bypass. *J Vasc Surg* **25**: 165–72: 1997
13. Bhum U: The Mintech system. In: Hopkinson B, Yusef W, Whitaker S, Veith J (Eds), *Endovascualar Surgery for Aortic Aneurysms*. London: WB Saunders Company, 1997
14. Schumacher H, Allenberg JR, Eckstein HH: Morphological classification of abdominal aortic aneurysm in selection of patients for endovascular grafting. *Br J Surg* **83**: 949–50, 1996

Editorial comments by B.R. Hopkinson

The authors emphasize the importance of the computed axial tomography (CAT) scan for assessing mural thrombus at the site of implantation in the neck. It is also important for excluding thrombus at the potential distal site of implantation of the graft. Their system seems to have changed slightly from a 'one size fits all', to 'two sizes fit nearly all'. We would agree that iliac tortuosity in itself is not a particular contraindication but iliac tortuosity combined with the calcification may well make introduction of the device very difficult. In Nottingham we have found that magnetic resonance imaging (MRI) can also be a very good indicator of the quality of the aorta and its lining and we no longer do preoperative angiograms as a routine. We find that the information from the reconstruction of the spiral CAT scan or MRI gives us sufficient information about the renals, the inferior mesenteric and the iliac arteries as well as the lumbars to go ahead and choose the appropriate graft. We always do a calibrating angiogram on the table to check that the device we have chosen is going to be of reasonable length. We agree entirely with their general indications for endovascular graft. Not only must the patient have the ability to comply with the follow-up regime so that we know what has happened to these grafts, but the patients and relatives must also understand that the endovascular device is relatively experimental and untried and that we do not have long-term results to give them.

The claimed advantages of the Montefoire device is that the length is not important and that it is always brought out through the distal arterotomy. The disadvantage of this is that the internal iliac is always sacrificed on that side and must reduce the pelvic perfusion. Also the smaller diameter of the vessel coming down to the femoral artery must decrease the amount of blood available to enter the legs and will make claudication more likely postoperatively. It is of interest that the Leicester device always uses a conduit where as the Montefoire device does not.

This chapter makes a very valid point that the EVT, Vanguard, AneuRx and Corvita grafts apparently are only available in the USA for good risk patients. The Talent graft is the only one with FDA approval for use in high-risk patients. This must always be borne in mind when reviewing results from different systems.

We would agree that some 70% of abdominal aortic aneurysms are amenable to endovascular grafting, in fact, using the Nottingham system we find 90% could theoretically be dealt with endovascularly. Just because something is possible does not always mean to say that it is right or wise. In the more difficult cases it is not usually a single adverse factor that may decide on suitability or not. It is often the addition of various slightly unfavourable factors each of which in themselves would not necessarily constitute a complete contraindication. In future with better devices for delivery and fixation, the majority of patients with infrarenal abdominal aortic aneurysms will become candidates for endovascular repair provided long-term outcomes are satisfactory.

In the future it may be that narrower introducer systems will allow a truly percutaneous treatment of aneurysms but in order to achieve this a new generation of thin or exceedingly thin walled grafts will have to be introduced and their longevity will have to be proven in comparison with the standard Dacron grafts that we have used since the 1950s. In fact until the new-generation thin-walled grafts have proved satisfactory in the long term in the arterial system, there is not much point trying to get smaller delivery systems. An 18 or 20 French introducer seems capable of delivering standard proven grafts through an arteriotomy which is best sealed by direct suturing techniques.

How Much Does an Aorto–Uni–Iliac Stent–Graft Increase the Endovascular Options for Abdominal Aortic Aneurysm Repair?

Matthew P. Armon and Brian R. Hopkinson

INTRODUCTION

Open abdominal aortic aneurysm repair has traditionally been performed with either a straight or bifurcated graft. Following Parodi's initial report of endovascular repair using straight aorto–aortic grafts[1] it soon became apparent that only a handful of aneurysms had the requisite distal aortic neck in which to implant the distal stent. Attention naturally turned to the production of a bifurcated endovascular graft, and the first successful implantation of such a device took place in 1993.[2] These remain the focus of most of the research and development in this field. Bifurcated grafts undoubtedly increased the options for endovascular abdominal aortic aneurysm repair but our experience was that a high proportion of aneurysms remained unsuitable for the available bifurcated systems because of adverse anatomy. The development of custom-built, aorto–uni–iliac stent grafts in Nottingham, and elsewhere, was thus born out of some frustration with the anatomical constraints of the early commercial bifurcated grafts coupled with a desire to treat a higher proportion of aneurysms by endovascular means. This chapter aims to review the evidence for the anatomical advantages of the aorto–uni–iliac system.

AORTO–UNI–ILIAC STENT GRAFT

The construction, delivery system and deployment of the aorto–uni–iliac stent graft used in Nottingham has been fully described previously.[3] The basic device consists of a thin-walled Dacron graft (Vascutek, Glasgow) with a proximal diameter of 18–34 mm, tapered to a distal (iliac) diameter of 12–24 mm. A modified 45 mm Gianturco stent (William Cook, Europe) with cranial hooks and caudal spikes is sutured to the proximal end of the graft, the graft is supported by a number of additional stents, and a final Gianturco stent (16, 20 or 30 mm) is sutured to the distal end of the graft (Fig. 1). The precise diameters and length of the aorto–uni–iliac graft are determined preoperatively by spiral computed tomographic (CT) angiography. The device is delivered via a femoral arteriotomy using a 20 French sheath introduced under fluoroscopic guidance. The procedure is completed by a femorofemoral crossover graft with an occluding device placed in the contralateral common iliac artery.

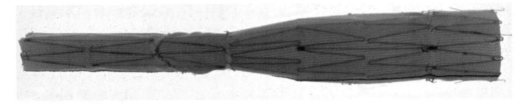

Fig. 1. An aorto–uni–iliac stent graft before deployment.

ADVANTAGES

The availability of the constituent parts of the aorto–uni–iliac stent-graft make it a relatively simple graft to construct once the dimensions of the abdominal aortic aneurysm are known. It can be put together at short notice in the emergency situation and this gives it a flexibility that is not readily available with commercial grafts. However, its main advantage is its ability to deal with the complex variety of aorto–iliac anatomy.

Aortic aneurysms come in a wide range of shapes and sizes. The dimensions that determine the size of an endovascular graft are the diameters of the proximal aortic neck and the common iliac arteries and the distance from the lowest renal artery to the common iliac artery bifurcation(s). The proximal aortic neck diameter varies from 16 to 30 mm, common iliac artery diameters range from 6 to 24 mm and the distance from the lowest renal artery to the common iliac artery bifurcation can be anything from 90 to 210 mm.[4] To complicate matters further, there is very little correlation between any of these variables[5] so that an aneurysm with a wide proximal neck may have narrow iliac arteries and vice versa. We have calculated previously that there are over 1500 potential combinations of these three anatomical variables. Ninety-nine of these combinations were present in a series of 131 abdominal aortic aneurysms.[4]

An aorto–uni–iliac stent graft can deal with all of these anatomical configurations.

ALTERNATIVE DEVICES

There are three alternative endovascular options; aorto–aortic grafts, non-modular bifurcated grafts and modular bifurcated grafts.

Aorto–aortic grafts are not serious alternatives in the majority of abdominal aortic aneurysms, as few aneurysms have the requisite distal cuff of normal aorta below the aneurysm. In the first 154 aneurysms of the Nottingham series less than 5% had a distal cuff.[6] There has been a high incidence of distal endoleak where these grafts have been used[7] and it is generally accepted that they have only a minor role to play in the endovascular management of abdominal aortic aneurysms. Where they are more useful is in the treatment of thoracic aneurysms.

Non-modular bifurcated grafts such as the Chuter–Gianturco and EVT extended the endovascular options by fixing the distal stents in the common iliac arteries. These are important grafts in a historical context but their delivery systems are complicated and by present standards cumbersome. Though they are able to treat more abdominal aortic aneurysms than straight grafts, their fixed dimensions severely limit their applicability to around 10% of patients.[5,6]

Modular bifurcated grafts are the focus of most current commercial development and these are the main rivals to an aorto–uni–iliac system. The subsequent analysis will therefore concentrate on the comparability of these two approaches. Grafts which fall into this category include the Mintec Stentor and its successor the Vanguard, the Talent, Corvita and AneuRx grafts as well as 'in-house' devices such as the Perth and Sydney systems.

AORTO-UNI-ILIAC VS MODULAR BIFURCATED STENT GRAFTS

Both types of system require a segment of 'normal' aorta between the renal arteries and the onset of the aneurysm (proximal aortic neck) in which to secure the proximal end of the stent–graft. How long a neck is required varies from device to device but most recommend a minimum length of 1.0–1.5 cm. Based on experimental work and a growing experience of intravascular stents, a number of centres have started to deploy uncovered stents across the renal arteries[8] and this practice, if proved to be safe in the long-term, would allow shorter necks to be used. Maximum neck diameter restrictions are more variable, ranging from 2.4 cm (Vanguard) to 3.0 cm (Nottingham). Nevertheless, there is no intrinsic advantage of one system over the other with regard to requiring a safe proximal implantation site. Whilst the Nottingham aorto–uni–iliac system does allow a wider range of proximal necks to be treated than all of the current commercial bifurcated systems, this is more a reflection of its in-house, customized nature rather than its uni–iliac characteristics. Further developments will rapidly narrow this particular gap.

The major area of difference is the ability of the two systems to deal with common iliac artery anatomy, and it is in this area that the aorto–uni–iliac graft significantly extends the endovascular options. All of the current modular bifurcated grafts require a normal segment of common iliac artery bilaterally in contrast to an aorto–uni–iliac approach which only requires a single good common iliac artery. The extent to which this extends the endovascular options depends on the precise limitations of each system. We have analysed 215 abdominal aortic aneurysms with spiral CT angiography. Using multiplanar reconstructions, measurements of the maximum and minimum diameters of the aneurysm, proximal aortic neck and both common iliac arteries were made. Sixty-eight patients (32%) had unsuitable proximal aortic necks that were less than 1 cm long, greater than 3 cm in diameter or angulated to greater than 90° with the axis of the aneurysm. A further 17 patients (8%) had bilateral common iliac artery diameters greater than 2.4 cm. A total of 85 patients (40%) were therefore unsuitable for either system. The aorto–uni–iliac stent graft can deal with all of the remaining anatomical variations (Fig. 2). The degree to which this extends the options over a modular bifurcated graft depends on the limitations of the particular system as illustrated in Figs 3–5. Those commercial systems which can deal only with iliac diameters up to 1.4 cm are limited to 18% of the abdominal aortic aneurysms in our study population – only a third as many as the Nottingham aorto–uni–iliac system. However, a modular bifurcated graft that could fit any combination of iliac diameter up to 2.4 cm would fit 50% of abdominal aortic aneurysms in this study. Only an extra 10% of aneurysms, with unilateral common iliac artery aneurysms greater than 2.4 cm could only be treated by an aorto–uni–iliac graft. Indeed, if one limb of a modular bifurcated graft could be extended into the external iliac artery on one side, even this advantage would be lost.

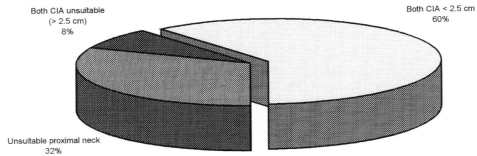

Suitability for an aorto-uni-iliac stent graft

Both CIA unsuitable
(> 2.5 cm)
8%

Both CIA < 2.5 cm
60%

Unsuitable proximal neck
32%

Fig. 2. Pie chart illustrating the distribution of 215 abdominal aortic aneurysm patients with unsuitable proximal necks and bilaterally unsuitable common iliac arteries (CIA). The remainder have at least one common iliac artery <2.5 cm and are therefore suitable for an aorto–uni–iliac graft with an iliac limb up to 2.4 cm.

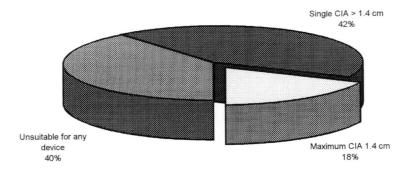

Suitability for a modular bifurcated graft with limbs up to 1.4 cm

Single CIA > 1.4 cm
42%

Unsuitable for any
device
40%

Maximum CIA 1.4 cm
18%

Fig. 3. Pie chart illustrating the proportion of patients with one common iliac artery (CIA) diameter greater or less than 1.4 cm; 18% have a maximum common iliac artery diameter of 1.4 cm and are therefore suitable for a bifurcated graft with iliac limbs up to 1.4 cm.

Suitability for a modular bifurcated graft with limbs up to 1.6 cm

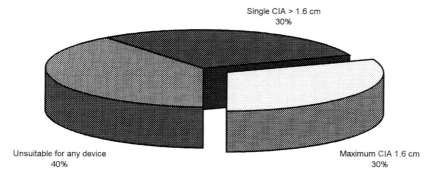

Single CIA > 1.6 cm
30%

Unsuitable for any device
40%

Maximum CIA 1.6 cm
30%

Fig. 4. Pie chart illustrating the proportion of patients with one common iliac artery (CIA) diameter greater or less than 1.6 cm; 30% have a maximum common iliac artery diameter of 1.6 cm and are therefore suitable for a bifurcated graft with iliac limbs up to 1.6 cm.

Suitability for a modular bifurcated graft with iliac limbs up to 2.4 cm

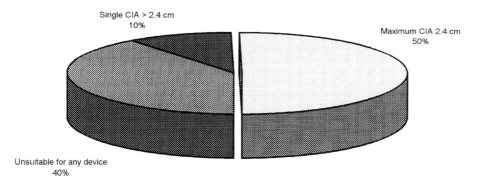

Single CIA > 2.4 cm
10%

Maximum CIA 2.4 cm
50%

Unsuitable for any device
40%

Fig. 5. Pie chart illustrating the proportion of patients with one common iliac artery (CIA) diameter greater or less than 2.4 cm; 50% have a maximum common iliac artery diameter of 2.4 cm and are therefore suitable for a bifurcated graft with iliac limbs up to 2.4 cm.

The anatomical advantages of the aorto–uni–iliac system are easy to define based on this evidence. The comparability of results with the two systems in terms of safety and complications is less clear. A number of centres have used both systems but none have conducted a formal randomized comparative study. The Sydney group has published their results with a number of devices and achieved higher success rates with aorto–uni–iliac grafts, but much of their early experience, and therefore learning curve, was with straight and bifurcated graft.[9] Some have raised objections to the aorto–uni–iliac system because it is aesthetically unappealing compared with the more anatomically correct bifurcated graft. Whilst this argument may have some artistic merit it is scientifically weak. The addition of a femorofemoral crossover graft raises the theoretical possibility of increased risks of graft infection and thrombosis. Crossover grafts were found to have lower patency rates than aortobifemoral grafts when used for iliac occlusive disease but only when runoff was poor. In the presence of good runoff, patency rates were equivalent.[10] There is little evidence as yet regarding their use in aneurysmal disease. Both groins are exposed and foreign material introduced via the femoral vessels with both systems and there remains no evidence that wound infections are more or less common with either approach. In Nottingham, there have been two cases of crossover graft infection, after 162 endovascular repairs.

FURTHER STUDIES

Assuming that the UK population is representative of the abdominal aortic aneurysm population as a whole, the anatomical data presented here allows accurate comparison of different stent–graft systems. Advocates of modular bifurcated grafts have claimed that higher proportions of patients than those found here are suitable for endovascular repair, but as yet these claims are unsubstantiated by anatomical data. Pre-selection of patients from referral sources will affect such figures. Further anatomical studies using high quality imaging such as magnetic resonance angiography or spiral CT are required, but must include comprehensive detail pertaining to population demographics, aneurysm size and sources of referral.

It is hoped that prospective comparative studies of endovascular vs open surgery will commence in the not too distant future. Inevitably, randomized comparison of different devices will be the next step. In the meantime, systematic audit of results with the various devices and systems is likely to be the best source of information about long-term patency and complication rates.

CONCLUSIONS

In conclusion, we have demonstrated that the aorto–uni–iliac graft stent is able to deal with between two and three times as many abdominal aortic aneurysms as current modular bifurcated grafts. This advantage falls to only an extra 10% when these systems are able to add iliac extensions with diameters up to 2.4 cm and may disappear altogether with further developments. With present technology however, the aorto–uni–iliac stent graft remains a step head of its bifurcated counterparts and significantly extends the endovascular options for abdominal aortic aneurysm repair.

REFERENCES

1. Parodi JC, Palmaz JC, Barone HD: Transfemoral intraluminal graft implantation for abdominal aortic aneurysms. *Ann Vasc Surg* **5**; 491–9, 1991
2. Chuter TAM, Donayre C, Wendt G: Bifurcated stent-grafts for endovascular repair of abdominal aortic aneurysm: Preliminary care reports. *Surg Endosc* **8**; 800–2, 1994

3. Yusuf SW, Baker DM, Hind RE *et al.*: Endoluminal transfemoral abdominal aortic aneurysm repair with aorto-uni-iliac graft and femorofemoral bypass. *Br J Surg* **82**; 916, 1995
4. Armon MP, Yusuf SW, Whitaker SC *et al.*: The anatomy of abdominal aortic aneurysms: implications for endovascular repair. *Eur J Vasc Endovasc Surg* **13**; 398–402, 1997
5. Armon MP, Yusuf SW, Whitaker SC *et al.*: Influence of abdominal aortic aneurysm size on the feasibility of endovascular repair. *J Endovasc Surg* **4**; 279–83, 1997
6. Armon MP, Yusuf SW, Latief K *et al.*: The anatomical suitability of abdominal aortic aneurysms for sizing of endovascular grafts. *Br J Surg* **84**; 178–80, 1997
7. May J, White GH, Yu W *et al.*: Endoluminal repair of abdominal aortic aneurysms: strengths and weaknesses of various prostheses observed in a 4.5 year experience. *J Endovasc Surg* **4**; 147–51, 1997
8. MacSweeney STR, Lawrence-Brown MMD: The Perth bifurcated system. In: Hopkinson, Yusuf, Whitaker, Veith (Eds) *Endovascular Surgery for Aortic Aneurysms* pp. 231–9. London: WB Saunders Co Ltd, 1996
9. White GH, Yu W, May J *et al.*: Three-year experience with the White–Yu endovascular GAD graft for transluminal repair of aortic and iliac aneurysms. *J Endovasc Surg* **4**; 124–36, 1997
10. Piotrowski J, Rutherford RB, Jones DN *et al.*: Aortobifemoral bypass: the operation of choice for unilateral iliac occlusion. *J Vasc Surg* **8**; 211–6, 1988

Editorial comments by P.R.F. Bell

Armon *et al.* correctly point out that the restrictions on endovascular aneurysm repair imposed by anatomical restraints are much greater than many of those inserting stents care to say. The authors rightly point out that the aorto–uni–iliac system allows more patients to be treated but even this system excludes a number of patients who have dilatation of the common iliac artery. Their comments about the likely long-term results of a crossover graft are entirely reasonable, they should, however, mention other techniques which take the lower end of the uni–iliac–graft right down to the groin and allow even more patients to be treated in this fashion.

Aorto–Uni–Iliac Endovascular Aneurysm Repair Utilizing ePTFE and Balloon-expandable Stents – The Leicester Experience

M.M. Thompson, J.R. Boyle, G. Fishwick and PRF Bell

INTRODUCTION

Aorto–uni–iliac endovascular aneurysm repair involves the placement of a tapered aortic endograft together with femorofemoral crossover bypass and occlusion of the contralateral common iliac artery (Fig. 1). This chapter reviews our experience of this technique and attempts to provide a rationale for incorporating tapered aortic endografting in the management of abdominal aortic aneurysms.

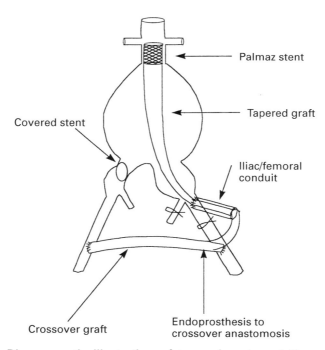

Fig. 1. Diagrammatic illustration of tapered aorto–uni–iliac endo-vascular aneurysm repair. The graft is inserted through a femoral or iliac conduit and is anchored in the proximal aneurysm neck using a balloon expandable Palmaz stent (Cordis, Brentford, UK). The graft is passed through the conduit and anastomosed to the crossover graft at the groin. The contralateral common iliac artery is occluded by use of a covered stent, detachable balloon or a ligature.

Patient selection

Patients with either symptomatic aneurysms or asymptomatic aneurysms of more than 5.5 cm diameter are considered for endovascular aneurysm repair in our institution. Patients are assessed with duplex ultrasound examination, axial computerized tomography and aortic arteriography utilizing a marker catheter. The criteria for aorto–uni–iliac aneurysm repair have been published previously[1,2] but

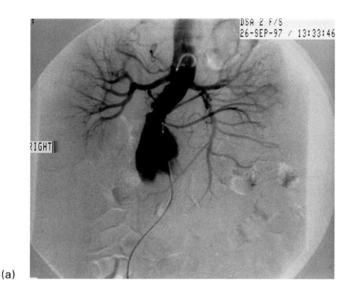

(a)

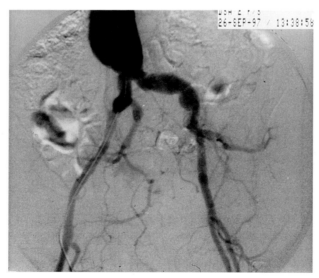

(b)

Fig. 2. Preoperative marker catheter demonstrating infrarenal abdominal aortic aneurysm with a long proximal neck, accessory left renal artery and bilateral iliac aneurysms (CT).

basically entail a proximal aortic neck length of more than 18 mm and a diameter less than 28 mm (Fig. 2). The extent of iliac artery aneurysms, turtuosity or calibre do not play a large part in the selection procedure, as most difficulties in these regions are surmountable with additional surgical or endovascular procedures. Due to the doubts surrounding durability of endovascular aneurysm repair, aortic endografts are not considered for patients under 65 years of age unless secondary indications are present (medical co-morbidity, inflammatory aneurysms, hostile abdomen).

Graft manufacture and design[1,2]

The tapered endograft has been modified from the initial descriptions of Parodi and Palmaz,[3-6] and consists of a tapered expanded polytetrafluoroethylene (ePTFE) graft (Impra, Worcs, UK) attached to an 'Extralarge' Palmaz stent (Cordis, Brentford, UK), which is in turn mounted on a balloon angioplasty catheter and packaged inside a 21F teflon sheath (Cook, Letchworth, UK). The graft is manufactured by stretching an 8 mm ePTFE graft to 30 mm proximally and tapering this to 13 mm at the distal end. The graft is manufactured to the same dimensions irrespective of the diameter of the proximal aortic neck.

Graft insertion and deployment[1,2]

Procedures are performed under balanced general anaesthetic in the operating theatre, which is equipped with mobile fluoroscopic equipment. Initially a standard femorofemoral crossover graft is constructed using a 10-mm Dacron prosthesis. It is our practice to insert the endograft through a temporary iliac or femoral conduit which is anastomosed above the crossover graft. Femoral access is utilized wherever possible, but in the presence of a highly tortuous or narrowed iliac artery, an iliac approach is utilized. The conduit comprises a 10-mm Dacron graft which is anastomosed to the front of the common femoral or iliac artery.

Following construction of the access conduit, the internal iliac artery on the side of graft insertion is embolized to prevent retrograde bleeding into the aneurysm sac after deployment of the endograft (Fig. 3). Access is then gained to the aorta from both sides. On the side contralateral to graft insertion, a pigtail catheter is positioned cephalad to the renal arteries. On the side for endograft insertion, a Lunderqvist wire (Boston Scientific Corp, St Albans, UK) is passed into the suprarenal aorta by an exchange technique. A 25F introducer sheath is then passed over this wire, through the access conduit, into the suprarenal aorta (Fig. 4). Following arteriography, the position of the renal arteries is marked and the mandril removed from the 25F sheath. The endograft, packaged inside a 21F sheath is then inserted through the introducer sheath and positioned at the level of the renal arteries.

At this stage, both sheaths are removed and the graft/stent combination is deployed just below the renal arteries by inflation of the angioplasty balloon to 2 atm pressure, under strict manometric control. No contrast is used to inflate the balloon as this allows excellent visualization of stent position. This is important as the Palmaz stent may shorten as much as 10 mm during deployment.[7]

To stop caudal displacement of the stent, the ePTFE endograft is then anastomosed to the crossover graft with the balloon inflated. Following partial completion of this anastomosis, the balloon is deflated and withdrawn. The anastomosis is then completed

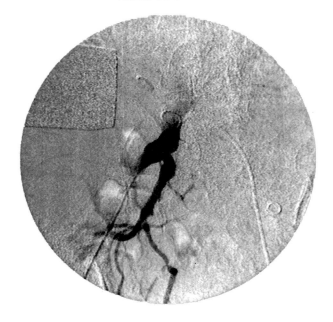

Fig. 3.   Coil embolization of right internal iliac artery.

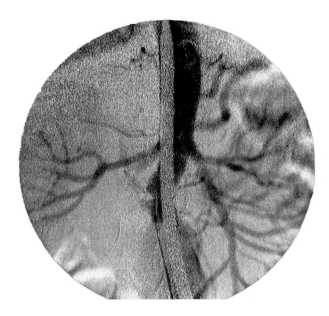

Fig. 4.   A 25F introducer sheath positioned in the suprarenal
aorta prior to endograft insertion.

and flow restored. The procedure is completed by occlusion of the contralateral common iliac artery with a covered Gianturco stent (Cook, Letchworth, UK), detachable balloon or a ligature (if the iliac diameter exceeds 20 mm). Arteriography is performed at the termination of the procedure to visualize stent position, the body of the graft, and retrograde perfusion of the contralateral internal iliac artery (Fig. 5).

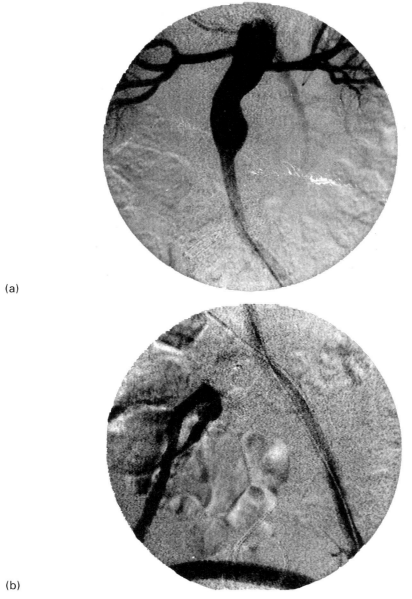

(a)

(b)

Fig. 5. Completion arteriogram demonstrating tapered aorto–iliac graft (a) with crossover graft and retrograde filling of left internal iliac artery (b). The left common iliac artery is occluded with a covered stent.

Quality control during endovascular aneurysm repair

To reduce the likelihood of intraoperative complications, we now routinely utilize both intra-aneurysmal sac pressure monitoring and monitoring of superficial femoral artery flow velocity. Intra-aneurysmal sac pressure falls during successful exclusion of the aneurysm sac,[8] and a diminution of this response gives early warning of an endoleak. Similarly, poor flow in the superficial femoral artery following tapered aorto-uni-iliac aneurysm repair may be diagnostic of an anastomotic problem or a distal endoleak. Since employing these techniques we have identified minor technical problems in 30% of cases, and all were corrected intraoperatively using endovascular techniques (Fig. 6).

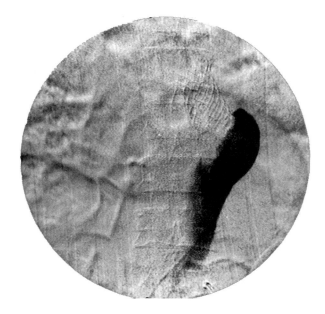

Fig. 6. Arteriogram performed through an intra–aneurysmal pressure monitor demonstrating failed occlusion of the right common iliac artery. This was associated with a rise in intra-aneurysmal pressure and poor flow in the ipsilateral superficial femoral artery. Formal ligation of the iliac artery was required to abolish this distal endoleak.

Results of aorto–uni–iliac endovascular aneurysm repair

To date (10/97), we have attempted aorto–uni–iliac endovascular aneurysm repair in 60 patients (median age 72 years [range 57–89], median aneurysm diameter 5.7 cm [4.8–7.9 cm]) using the ePTFE/Palmaz stent endograft. Eighteen patients had severe co-existing medical co-morbidities (American Society of Anesthesiologists grading: ASA IV), and 12 had 'hostile abdomens' (two inflammatory aneurysms, two horseshoe kidneys, one polycystic kidney, one hereditary haemorrhagic telangectasia, one post-radiotherapy and five with multiple previous laparotomies).

Initial success has been obtained in 87%, with eight technical failures. The temporal distribution of these failures is illustrated in Fig. 7, but it is interesting to note that four of these occurred within our first eight patients. In general terms the early failures we encountered were due to technical problems during the procedure, including low deployment of the Palmaz stent due to inadequate visualization during deployment,[7,9] perforation of the iliac system and balloon malfunction. In contrast the 'conversions' that occurred in the latter half of the series represented poor or overambitious case selection.

The 30-day mortality was 3% (two deaths – one massive microembolization and one iatrogenic small bowel perforation). There were seven serious early systemic complications (12%) of which three appeared to be due to microembolization affecting the lower limbs and kidneys. Late complications included one serious graft infection which was treated conservatively, and a 15% incidence of buttock claudication related to ligation of the internal iliac artery.

There was a low incidence of endoleak during this series, although three patients underwent intraoperative correction of large proximal endoleaks. There were no proximal endoleaks at discharge, and three distal endoleaks. All three distal leaks were related to incomplete 'occlusion' of the contralateral common iliac artery and have been successfully treated with retrograde coil embolization some time after their initial endovascular surgery.

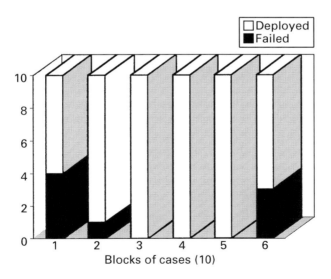

Fig. 7. Graph illustrating the number of technical failures in each succeeding block of ten cases throughout the 60-patient series.

ALTERNATIVES TO AORTO–UNI–LIAC ENDOVASCULAR ANEURYSM REPAIR

There are clear alternative procedures to aorto–uni–iliac endovascular aneurysm repair, namely conventional surgery or the use of commercially available aorto–aortic or aorto–bi–iliac endovascular systems.

Conventional surgery

The role of conventional surgery in the treatment of abdominal aortic aneurysms is well defined and obviously represents the gold standard by which endovascular techniques must be judged. Selected single-centre series of conventional aneurysm repairs have reported very low mortality rates,[10] but community based figures often suggest mortality approaching 10%.[11] One of the difficult problems in evaluating the results of endovascular aneurysm repair is to account for the high proportion of patients with severe co-morbidities who are preferentially referred for endovascular repair. Changing referral patterns and patient population may have an effect on reported mortality rates for conventional aneurysm repair. Since commencing our endovascular programme we have observed a large increase in tertiary referrals, especially in patients who are considered 'unfit' for conventional surgery. This has manifest in an increased workload, but also in a dramatic rise in elective surgical mortality (6.7–12%), which has been largely attributable to patients with severe ischaemic heart disease, renovascular disease or respiratory failure.[12]

Aorto–aortic and bifurcated endovascular grafts

The feasibility of straight and bifurcated endovascular aneurysm repair has been established by many centres.[13–16] In general, results have been acceptable although no direct comparative studies have been reported either with conventional surgery or with aorto–uni–iliac endovascular procedures.

The main advantage of the tapered graft over straight or bifurcated endovascular systems is their flexibility and relatively lax morphological requirements. Current studies have suggested that only 3–7% of patients will be suitable for straight endografts whilst 20–40% may be treated by bifurcated systems. These limitations are lessened with tapered grafts, and at present, approximately 60% of all infrarenal aneurysms may be treated by aorto–uni–iliac grafts. Additionally, it remains possible that tapered grafts may be utilized for emergency cases,[17] as it is possible to repair the majority of aneurysms with one size of aorto–uni–iliac graft, whereas commercially available grafts have to be accurately sized to specific aortic dimensions.

The disadvantages of tapered aorto–iliac endografting relate to the non-anatomical nature of the procedure. A crossover graft is required to revascularize the contralateral limb and this may have a lower patency than anatomical reconstructions. Additionally, performing anastomoses in both groins could lead to graft infections or false aneurysms, although we have not encountered these problems to date. Finally, elective occlusion of the internal iliac artery may lead to buttock claudication, but this does appear to be self-limiting.

EVIDENCE TO SUPPORT AORTO–UNI–ILIAC GRAFTING

There are no randomized studies to support the use of aorto–uni–iliac grafts over either conventional surgery or commercially available straight or bifurcated endografts.[18,19] To determine whether the theoretical advantages of endovascular aneurysm repair are observed in practice, we performed a concurrent cohort study of aorto–uni–iliac vs conventional surgery, looking specifically at physiological parameters.

Physiological studies

Preliminary observations on the cardiovascular system have suggested that there was little difference in cardiac output, pulmonary artery occlusion pressure, or systemic vascular resistance between conventional and endovascular procedures; principally due to pharmacological manipulation of the circulation before and after aortic cross-clamping. However, respiratory spirometry has demonstrated that patients undergoing endovascular aneurysm repair return to normal respiratory function significantly sooner than patients undergoing conventional surgery, a finding which may be related to differences in analgesic requirements.[20] Additionally, metabolic studies have revealed that the ischaemia/reperfusion response that characterizes conventional aneurysm repair is largely attenuated by endovascular techniques, which also manifest a lower level of inflammatory cytokines.[21]

By contrast, quantification and characterization of lower limb embolization during aneurysm repair has demonstrated significantly higher numbers of particulate emboli during endovascular techniques.[22,23] Massive microembolization is a significant problem following endovascular aortic surgery, and further research is required in this area to minimize embolization to renal and visceral beds.

Registry for endovascular treatment of aneurysms (RETA)

Although no randomized trials of endovascular aneurysm repair exist, some multicentre data is starting to appear from centralized registries of treatment (RETA/Eurostar). Results from RETA for 1996 have demonstrated that 46% of endovascular repairs were performed with aorto–uni–iliac grafts and that mortality, operative time and blood loss were significantly greater than for straight of bifurcated endografts. However, these data may be somewhat misleading as approximately 50% of patients undergoing uni–iliac grafting were ASA 4, compared with less than 20% for the straight/bifurcated group.

FUTURE TRIALS

Clearly, the first priority in any future trial of endovascular aortic surgery is to establish the long-term efficacy and durability of endovascular repair, compared with conventional surgery in fit patients. Further trials will need to assess the place of 'minimally invasive' aortic procedures in unfit patients and also in patients with small aneurysms. It is unlikely that aorto-uni-iliac techniques will be directly compared with straight or bifurcated endovascular techniques, as all have different morphological requirements, and will probably be used to treat differing proportions of aneurysms. One of the most interesting aspects may be to investigate the place of aorto-uni-iliac grafts in emergency aneurysm repair, as this scenario may offer the greatest potential for endovascular surgery to reduce surgical mortality.

REFERENCES

1. Thompson MM, Sayers RD, Nasim A *et al.*: Aortomonoiliac endovascular grafting: difficult solutions to difficult problems. *J Endovasc Surg* **4**: 174–81, 1997
2. Thompson MM, Nasim A, Bell PRF: The Leicester experience. In: Hopkinson BR, Yusef SW, Whitaker SC, Veith FJ (Eds), *Endovascular Surgery for Aortic Aneurysms* pp. 240–53. London: WB Saunders Co. Ltd, 1997
3. Parodi JC: Endovascular repair of abdominal aortic aneurysms and other arterial lesions. *J Vasc Surg* **21**: 549–55, 1995
4. Parodi JC: Endovascular repair of abdominal aortic aneurysms. In: *Advances in Vascular Surgery* Vol 1, pp. 85–106. St Louis, USA: Moseby, 1993
5. Parodi JC, Palmaz JC, Barone HD: Transfemoral intraluminal graft implantation for abdominal aortic aneurysms. *Ann Vasc Surg* **5**: 491–9, 1991
6. Richter GM, Palmaz JC, Allenberg JR, Kauffmann GW: Die transluminale stentprosthese beim bauchaortenaneurysma. *Radiologie* **34**: 511–8, 1994
7. Boyle JR, Thompson MM, Nasin A *et al.*: Proximal stent deployment without contrast during endovascular aneurysm repair: An improved technique. *J Endovasc Surg* **3**: 380–1, 1996
8. Chuter T, Ivancev K, Malina M *et al.*: Aneurysm pressure following endovascular exclusion. *Eur J Vasc Endovasc Surg* **13**: 85–7, 1997
9. Nasim A, Thompson MM, Sayers RD *et al.*: Initial experience with endovascular aneurysm repair. *Br J Surg* **83**: 516–9, 1996
10. Sandison AP, Panayiotopoulos Y, Edmondson RC *et al.*: A 4-year prospective audit of the cause of death after infrarenal aortic aneurysm surgery. *Br J Surg* **83**: 1386–9, 1996
11. Berridge DC, Chamberlain J, Guy AJ, Lambert D: Prospective audit of abdominal aortic aneurysm surgery in the northern region from 1988 to 1992. *Br J Surg* **82**: 906–10, 1995
12. Boyle JR, Thompson MM, Sayers R *et al.*: Changes in referral practice, workload and operative mortality following the establishment of an endovascular abdominal aortic aneurysm programme. *J Endovasc Surg* (in press) 1998
13. Balm R, Eikelboom BC, May J *et al.*: Early experience with transfemoral endovascular aneurysm management (TEAM) in the treatment of aortic aneurysms. *Eur J Vasc Endovasc Surg* **11**: 214–20, 1996
14. Blum U, Voshage G, Lammer J *et al.*: Endoluminal stent-grafts for infrarenal abdominal aortic aneurysms. *New Engl J Med* **336**: 13–20, 1997
15. White GH, Yu W, May J *et al.*: A new nonstented balloon-expandable graft for straight or bifurcated endoluminal bypass. *J Endovasc Surg* **1**: 16–24, 1995
16. Mialhe C, Amicabile C: Experience with the Stentor system for AAA treatment. *J Endovasc Surg* **2**: 405, 1995
17. Yusef SW, Whitaker SC, Chuter TAM *et al.*: Emergency endovascular abdominal aortic aneurysm repair. *Lancet* **344**: 1645, 1995
18. Thompson MM, Sayers RD, Bell PR: Endovascular aneurysm repair [editorial]. *Br Med J* **314**: 1139–40, 1997
19. Porter JM: Endovascular arterial intervention: expression of concern. *J Vasc Surg* **21**: 995–8, 1995
20. Boyle JR, Thompson JP, Thompson MM *et al.*: Improved respiratory function and analgesia control after endovascular AAA repair. *J Endovasc Surg* **4**: 62–5, 1997
21. Thompson MM, Nasim A, Sayers RD *et al.*: Oxygen free radical and cytokine generation

during endovascular and conventional aneurysm repair. *Eur J Vasc Endovasc Surg* **12**: 70–5, 1996

22. Thompson MM, Smith J, Naylor AR *et al.*: Ultrasound based quantification of emboli during conventional and endovascular aneurysm repair. *J Endovasc Surg* **4**: 33–8, 1997

23. Thompson MM, Smith J, Naylor AR *et al.*: Microembolisation during endovascular and conventional aneurysm repair. *J Vasc Surg* **25**: 179–86, 1996

Editorial comments by B.R. Hopkinson

This chapter describes the experience of one centre with a system which is very similar to the Montefoire graft described in the chapter by Lipsitz and Veith (pp. 211–220). This system is applicable to a wide range of patients for whom the commercially made aorto–aortic and aortic bifurcation devices are not available. It has always worried me that a graft is made by pre-dilatating an 8mm PTFE graft to 30mm. However, the results seem to be satisfactory so far with no evidence of further aneurysmal dilatation or graft damage resulting from this treatment.

It has also mystified me as to why the Leicester group put a femorofemoral crossover graft in first and then use a separate arterotomy for a femoral or iliac conduit to introduce the endograft. The few occasions I have done so were earlier in our own experience in Nottingham but have not found this necessary for a very long time now. The determining factor as to whether one can get an introducer and an endograft around a tortuous iliac is more to do with its calcification than its innate tortuosity and once one has got the Lundaquist wire up (it is very stiff indeed) there should be no difficulty getting the introducer system to follow it from the femoral.

I also wonder why they use a 25 French introducer sheath which is rather large and then introduce a 21 French sheath through it. The Montefoire system, which is very similar, does not seem to need the extra 25 French sheath.

I presume that the distal end of graft is routinely placed in the external iliac which seems a shame as it means that the internal iliac has to be sacrificed every time. Placing the distal end in the common iliac when it is suitable, as it so often is, would seem to be the better idea but would probably need a graft much bigger than 13mm diameter in many cases. I am sure the buttock claudication that is described is more likely to occur with a narrower graft put into the external iliac than a larger one in the common iliac.

Monitoring the intra-aneurysmal sac pressure is certainly of interest. I am not quite sure how it is measured after successful exclusion of the aneurysm sac unless the catheter is left alongside either the graft or the occluder in the opposite iliac. The presence of a catheter alongside the graft or going alongside the occlusion device would to my mind interfere with the completion of exclusion of the aneurysm sac by allowing leakage along its track. I think these particular measurements should be interpreted with caution. We would all agree that poor flow in the superficial femoral artery would indicate a problem with the run-in and be either due to excessive narrowing of the iliac system or to kinking. Using unsupported aorta–uni–iliac

Dacron grafts in Nottingham we found that roughly 50% of them required the addition of a wall stent to correct kinking. It is good to know that the early technical failures have been corrected. It also makes sense that the conversions in the latter half of their series probably represent overambitious case selection. Once one has an option of treating patients by a more gentle method than open surgery, pressure is often on from the relatives, patient and the referring surgeons for something to be done.

I would totally agree with the Leicester experience that with the introduction of an endovascular programme a high proportion of patients with severe co-morbidities are preferentially referred for endovascular repair. I think it is very important to note that pressure from these tertiary referrals actually increased the workload in Leicester and that there has been a dramatic rise in elective open surgical mortality from 6.7 to 12%. I am sure that this is largely attributable to more patients with severe ischaemic heart disease and endovascular respiratory failure being offered surgery. This again emphasizes the need for better risk stratification so that we can more truly compare like with like when comparing different methods of repairing aneurysms in patients with differing levels of physiological fitness.

Does Size of Aneurysm Affect Our Choice of Management of Abdominal Aortic Aneurysm?

D. Raithel, P. Heilberger and C. Schunn

INTRODUCTION

In the following chapter we will delineate our diagnostic and therapeutic concept for minor (< 4 cm) and small aortic aneurysms (< 5 cm) at Nuremberg Southern Hospital.

AUTHORS' CHOICE OF PROCEDURE

Because of the significant risk of rupture we treat patients with small aortic aneurysms aggressively.

Minor aneurysms (< 4 cm) are followed closely at 6-month intervals using duplex scans. Only when specific morphologic or clinical conditions call for it (i.e. back pain, sackiform aneurysm morphology, false aneurysm or suspected mycotic aneurysm) will these be reconstructed by endovascular or conventional surgical techniques.

In our opinion small aneurysms (4–5 cm diameter) are a clear indication for reconstruction, particularly in low risk patients with expected long-term survival. For these patients we prefer endovascular reconstruction to minimize perioperative risk and avoid sexual dysfunction.

1. Aneurysms with transverse or sagittal diameter of more than 5 cm are considered an indication for reconstruction even in patients with significant co-morbidities, associated with higher perioperative risk. If aneurysm morphology permits, this is preferably achieved by endovascular aortic exclusion (Fig. 1). This therapeutic strategy is based on the following thoughts and observations of aneurysm patients.
2. As aneurysms continue to grow the patient will not be younger or healthier at the projected time of treatment.[1]
3. Following these patients conservatively we may very well miss the time for an elective operation due to unexpected rupture.[1] Perioperative risk for elective aneurysm repair increases with advancing age due to worsening of co-morbid conditions like coronary artery disease, lung disease and others.[1]
4. Minor and small aneurysms lend themselves to endovascular repair more frequently and with less risk than larger aneurysms.[2]
5. The risk of rupture of small aneurysms is real and not insignificant as clearly delineated in the literature.[3–5]
6. Perioperative mortality of small ruptured aneurysms is no different from perioperative mortality of large ruptured aortic aneurysms.[1]

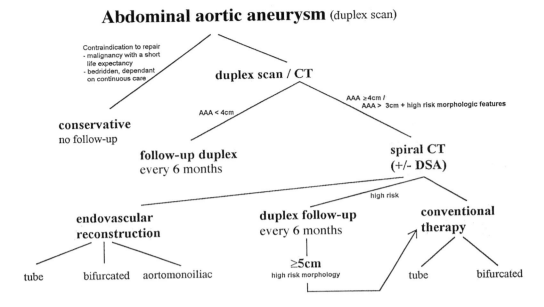

Fig. 1.

ALTERNATIVES AVAILABLE

There are divergent opinions regarding two major points of our treatment strategy.

Opposition to endovascular aortic grafting as a suitable option to treat infrarenal aortic aneurysms

Several European authors are opposed to endovascular reconstruction of aortic aneurysms claiming that this is still an experimental modality, lacking long-term results. Due to the high rate of endoleaks and thrombotic complications this therapeutic option is viewed as inferior to conventional aortic repair.[6]

Opposition to the need to correct minor and small aneurysms

Several authors adhere to the view that aneurysms of less than 5 cm diameter run a low risk of rupture and therefore should be followed clinically rather than treated aggressively with surgery.

Kremer *et al.* observed 35 patients with aortic aneurysms of less than 5 cm diameter as determined by ultrasound. Mean follow-up was 3.1 years. During this time no aneurysm rupture occurred.[7] For aneurysms of less than 4 cm diameter Michaels reported an annual risk of rupture of 0.5%. This is less than the current perioperative mortality after elective aneurysm surgery of 2.8–6.2% as reported in the literature.[8,9]

Nevitt et al. followed 176 patients with aortic aneurysms. During the first 5 years of follow-up no rupture was seen in the group with aneurysms less than 5 cm diameter.[5]

Glimåker observed a 2.5% rupture rate after 7 years of follow-up of 111 patients with aneurysms less than 5 cm in diameter. At time of rupture, however, all aneurysms had increased to a diameter greater than 5 cm.[3]

Thus the major argument to support expectant therapy of aneurysms with less than 5 cm diameter is the unfavourable risk–benefit ratio between reported perioperative mortalities (2.8–6.2%) and the small or non-existent risk of aneurysm rupture of minor and small aneurysms.[1,8,9]

EVIDENCE FOR AUTHORS' CHOICE

Analysing our own patient population we come to the following conclusions:

The risk of rupture of minor and small infrarenal aortic aneurysms is significant

At our institution 3418 patients with infrarenal aortic aneurysms were reconstructed surgically during the past 13 years. Of 278 patients with ruptured aneurysms 41 or 14.7% demonstrated a diameter of less than 5 cm at surgery. In all, 13 (31.7%) of patients with ruptured minor or small aneurysms died during the perioperative period (Table 1).

Table 1. Results of conventional abdominal aortic aneurysm (AAA) reconstructions (8/84–8/97)

		AAA <5cm	Mortality AAA < 5cm (%)
Non-ruptured	2140	696	11 (1.6)
Ruptured	278	41	13 (31.7)
Total	2418	737	24 (3.3)

Six patients with an aneurysm diameter of less than 5 cm were advised to undergo elective therapy but declined surgery. All six patients returned with an acute rupture and had to undergo emergent surgery (Figs 2 and 3).

Patients with minor and small aneurysms may be treated with low (≤ 1%) mortality

Since August 1994 122 patients with infrarenal aortic aneurysms with a mean diameter of 43.6 mm (28–67 mm) were treated with a straight endovascular graft. The perioperative 30-day mortality was 0%.

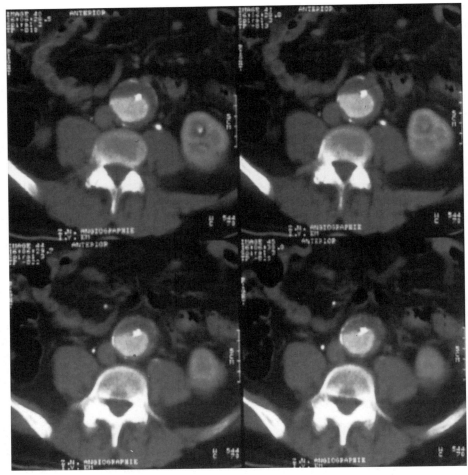

Fig. 2. Small infrarenal aortic aneurysm. Patient refused recommended surgical repair

During the same time period 71 bifurcated endografts were used to treat aneurysms with a mean diameter of 49.1 mm range (30–79 mm). There was one postoperative death due to faulty implantation technique (mortality 1.4 %). This was our 21st endoluminal reconstruction using a bifurcated MinTec^R endograft. Due to faulty puncture technique a retroperitoneal haemorrhage occurred to which the patient succumbed. Since changing our implantation technique (surgical access to the groin and arteriotomy) no further patient has been lost. The current 30-day perioperative mortality after endovascular infrarenal aortic reconstruction at Nuremberg Southern Hospital is 0.5% (one of 193 patients).

During the past 3 years our perioperative 30-day mortality after elective conventional reconstruction of aortic aneurysms of less than 5 cm diameter using a tube graft has been 1.6% (Tables 1, 2). Using endovascular techniques we have thus been able to lower our perioperative hospital mortality to less than 1 %.

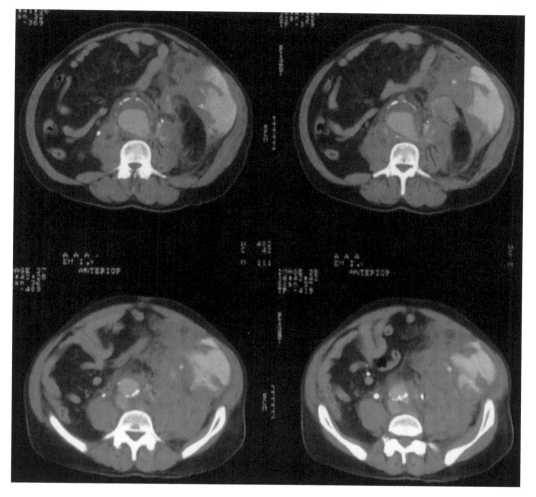

Fig. 3. Contained rupture of small infrarenal aortic aneurysm, 4 months after diagnosis

What trials support authors' view?

The current literature was analysed to define recent hospital mortality after endovascular reconstruction of infrarenal aortic aneurysms. Using adequate patient selection criteria and preferential endovascular reconstruction of small aneurysms four other study groups have demonstrated a mortality of 0–0.7% (Table 3).

The quoted authors performed endovascular repairs similar to our own approach, using predominantly the modular system of MinTec[R] and Vanguard[R] design as well as the EVT system.[10–13]

Conventional surgical reconstruction also may be performed with a perioperative mortality as low as 1–2%. Dryjski *et al.* reported surgical treatment of 37 patients

Table 2. Results of endovascular abdominal aortic aneurysm reconstructions (8/94–8/97)

	Diameter (mm) Mean (range)	n	Mortality (< 30 days) (%)
Tube	43.6 (28–67)	122	0 (0)
Bifurcated	49.1 (30–79)	71	1 (1.4)
Total	45.6 (28–79)	193	1 (0.5)

Table 3. Current results after endovascular aortic reconstruction

	Blum et al.[10] (1997)	Düber et al.[11] (1996)	Malina et al.[12] (1997)	Moore et al.[13] (1996)
Mean diameter (mm)	54	53	52	52
Device	MinTec/Vang.	MinTec	homemade	EVT
n	154	19	35	46
Mortality (%)	0.7 (1)	0	0	0/46 (<30 T)

(mean 64 years) with aortic aneurysms of less than 5 cm diameter achieving a 0% mortality.[14] Moriyama *et al.* report a 1.9% mortality (two patients) in 103 aortic reconstructions. They found a significant positive correlation between perioperative mortality, aneurysm size, operative time and blood loss.[15]

Risk of rupture of small aortic aneurysms

In patients with aneurysms greater than 5 cm and concurrent chronic obstructive pulmonary disease as well as elevated diastolic blood pressure, Cronenwett *et al.* calculated the risk of rupture to be 98% within 3 years.[16] Patients with 3-cm aneurysms and presence of significant pulmonary disease as well as arterial hypertension had a risk of rupture of 54% within 3 years of diagnosis.[16] In a later publication of 1992 the same authors quote the risk of rupture or acute expansion for aneuryms of less than 4 cm in diameter to be 0. Aneurysms between 4 and 5 cm displayed a risk of 3.3% per year. At a perioperative mortality risk of 4.6% these patients would clearly benefit from early elective correction.[17]

In a postmortem examination of 265 aneurysm patients Darling *et al.* found 12.8% of ruptured aneurysms to be less than 5 cm.[18]

Jensen *et al.* experienced a 38% mortality rate in eight ruptured aortic aneurysms that were measured to be less than 5 cm.[19] In a series of 42 aneuryms smaller than 5 cm who were treated expectantly a 7% rupture rate (three patients) was observed by Johansson *et al.*[4] Katz *et al.* found a positive risk-benefit ratio for patients with small aneurysms (less than 5 cm) at a projected rupture rate of 3.3% per year provided that a perioperative lethality of less than 5% could be achieved.[20]

Limet *et al.* described a 12% rupture rate in 34 patients who were diagnosed by duplex scan to have an infrarenal aortic aneurysm of less than 50 mm.[21]

As small aneurysms continue to grow at a projected growth rate of 3.7 mm per year we also may risk missing the point in time when they have reached the critical 5 cm margin.[22,23] Nevitt *et al.* demonstrated that small aneurysms did not rupture during the first 5 years of follow-up. However, he observed a 5% rupture rate during the subsequent 4 years.[5]

In 111 patients with aneurysms less than 5 cm in diameter Glimåker *et al.* demonstrated a 2.5% rupture rate during a 7-year follow-up. At the time of rupture, however, all of these aneurysms, had passed the margin of 5 cm.[3] Also the three ruptures reported by Johannsen on closer scrutiny had passed the 5-cm margin at the time of rupture.[4]

Another factor that needs to be considered is the ratio of the infrarenal aortic diameter and the suprarenal aortic diameter. A 5-cm aneurysm in a female with normal aortic diameter of 1.4 cm is a different entity than a 5-cm aneurysm in a male with a suprarenal aortic diameter of 2.5 cm.[24]

As a consequence Ouriel *et al.* introduced the ratio of aneurysm diameter compared with diameter of the third lumbar vertebrae to determine aortic aneurysm size. In his series none of the aneurysms with a ratio of less than 1.0 ruptured during follow-up.[25]

These data in our opinion are sufficient to support an aggressive therapeutic approach towards small aortic aneurysms.

WHAT FUTURE TRIALS WOULD BE HELPFUL?

Repair of small aneurysms using endovascular or conventional surgical techniques may be performed with less than 1% perioperative mortality as demonstrated above. Future trials should focus on the risk of rupture of minor and small aneurysms in a large patient population. The United Kingdom Small Aneurysm Trial of 1995 may be able to answer this question in the future.[26]

May *et al.* report a 4.4% mortality in 43 patients with aneurysms of less than 5 cm diameter and called for a randomized study comparing endoluminal with open conventional therapy of small aneurysms expecting a lower complication rate after endovascular repair.[27]

Follow-up studies need to demonstrate the long-term durability of the endoluminal aortic repair. Aneurysms must be safely excluded for decades preventing aneurysm growth and rupture. In this context retrograde perfusion of the aneurysm sack via side-branches (inferior mesenteric artery, lumbar arteries) may be of clinical significance as these side-branches usually remain open in small aortic aneurysms.[28]

In conclusion we have been able to demonstrate both in our own patient population as well as in reviewing the world literature that aneurysms less than 5 cm in diameter incur a significant risk of rupture. Using endovascular techniques we may treat these aneurysms with a perioperative mortality that is approaching 0% (Fig. 1).

REFERENCES

1. Schröder A, Imig H, Riepe G, Braun St: Das kleine Bauchaortenaneurysma - Frühzeitige Operation oder Beobachtung? In: Maurer P, von Sommoggy S (Eds), *Gefäßchirurgie im Fortschritt* pp. 92–101. Berlin: Blackwell Wissenschafts-Verlag
2. Allenberg JR, Schumacher H, Kallinowski F *et* al.: Klassifikation des infrarenalen Aortenaneurysmas: endovaskuläre oder konventionelle Chirurgie ? *Gefäßchirurgie* **1**: 21–6, 1996
3. Glimåker HL, Holmberg AE, Nybacka O *et al.*: Natural history of patients with abdominal aortic aneurysm. *Eur J Vasc Surg* **5**: 125, 1995
4. Johansson G, Nydahl S, Olofsson P, Swedenborg J: Survival in patients with abdominal aneurysms. Comparsion between operative and nonoperative management. *Eur Vasc Surg* **4**: 497–502, 1990
5. Nevitt MP, Ballard DJ, Hallett JW: Prognosis of abdominal aortic aneurysms. *New Engl J Med* **124**: 419, 1989
6. Sandmann W: Endovaskuläre Therapie des infrarenalen Aortenaneurysma. *Gefäßchirurgie* **2**: 1–4, 1997
7. Kremer H, Weigold B, Dobrinski W *et al.*: Sonographische Verlaufsbegutachtung von Bauchaortenaneurysmen. *Klein Wochenschr* **62**: 1120, 1984
8. Michaels JA: The management of small abdominal aortic aneurysms: a computer simulation using Monte Carlo Methods. *Eur J Vasc Surg* **6**: 551, 1992
9. Cappeler WA, Hinz MH, Lauterjung L: Das infrarenale Aortenaneurysma – 10-Jahres-Verlauf nach Ausschaltungsoperation mit Kostenanalyse. *Der Chirurg* **67**: 697–702, 1996
10. Blum U, Voshage G, Lammer J *et al.*: Endoluminal stent-grafts for infrarenal abdominal aortic aneurysms. *New Engl J Medicine* **336**: 13–20, 1997
11. Düber VC, Schmiedt W, Pitton M *et al.*: endovaskuläre Therapie aortaler Aneurysmen: erste klinische Ergebnisse. *RöFo* **164**: 1–94, 1996
12. Malina M, Ivancev K, Chuter TA *et al.*: Changing aneurysmal morphology after endovascular grafting: Relation to leakage or persistent perfusion. *J Endovasc Surg* **4**: 23–30, 1997
13. Moore WS, Rutherford RB: Transfemoral endovascular repair of abdominal aortic aneurysm: Results of the North American EVT phase 1 trial. *J Vasc Surg* **23**: 543–53, 1996
14. Dryjski M, Driscoll JL, Blair *et al.*: The small abdominal aortic aneurysm: the eternal dilemma. *J Cardiovasc Surg (Torino)* **35**: 95–100, 1994
15. Moriyama Y, Toyohira H, Saigenji H *et al.*: A review of 103 cases with elective repair for abdominal aortic aneurysm: an analysis of the risk factors based on postoperative complications and long-term follow-up. *Surg Today* **24**: 591–5, 1994
16. Cronenwett JL, Murphy TF, Zelenock GB *et al.*: Actuarial analysis of variables associated with rupture of small abdominal aortic aneurysms. *Surgery* **98**: 472, 1985
17. Cronenwett JL, Katz DA, Littenberg B: Management of small abdominal aortic aneurysms. Early surgery vs watchful waiting. *J Am Med Assoc* **268**: 2678–86, 1992
18. Darling RC.,Messina CR, Brewster DC, Ottinger LW: Autopsy study of unoperated abdominal aortic aneurysms. *Circulation* **56** (Supp 2): 161, 1977
19. Jensen BS, Vestersgaard-Andersen T: The natural history of abdominal aortic aneurysm. *Eur J Vasc Surg* **3**: 135, 1989
20. Katz DA, Cronenwett JL: The cost-effectiveness of early surgery versus watchful waiting in the management of small abdominal aortic aneurysms. *J Vasc Surg* **19**: 980–90, 1994
21. Limet R, Sakalihassan N. Albert A: Determination of the expansion rate and incidence of rupture of abdominal aortic aneurysms. *J Vasc Surg* **14**: 540, 1991
22. Bengtsson H, Bergqvist D, Ekberg O, Ranstam J: Expansion pattern and risk of rupture of abdominal aortic aneurysms that were not operated on. *Eur J Sug* **159**: 461–70, 1993
23. Brown PM, Pattenden R, Vernooy C *et al.*: Selective management of abdominal aortic aneurysm in a prospective measurement program. *J Vasc Surg* **23**: 213–22, 1996
24. Katz DJ. Stanley JC, Zelenock GB: Abdominal aortic aneurysms. *Semin Vasc Surg* **8**: 289, 1995

25. Ouriel K, Green RM, Donayre C *et al.*: An evaluation of new methods of expressing aortic aneurysm size: Relationship to rupture. *J Vasc Surg* **15**: 12–20, 1992.
26. The UK Small Aneurysm Trial: Design, methods and progress. The UK Small Aneurysm Trial participants. *Eur J Vasc Endovasc Surg* **9**: 42–8, 1995.
27. May J, White GH, Yu W *et al.*: Concurrent comparison of endoluminal repair vs. no treatment for small abdominal aortic aneurysms. *Eur J Vasc Endovasc Surg* **13**: 472–6, 1997.
28. Heilberger P, Schunn C, Ritter W *et al.*: Postoperative color flow duplex scanning in aortic endografting. *J Endovasc Surg* **4**: 262–71, 1997.

Editorial comments by P.R.F. Bell

This chapter looks at a personal series of aneurysms in a single centre in Germany. The authors have undoubtedly achieved excellent mortality statistics and because of these they claim that all aneuryms between 4 and 5 cm in diameter should be operated on. They quote selectively a number of references to prove their point ignoring the fact that the mortality for aneurysm repair is on average 4% and the recent Small Aneurysm Study supported by the Medical Research Council and to be reported on next year, will tell us what we should do with small aneurysms. Although the results of this study have not yet been published it was not stopped by the monitoring committee which leads me to the conclusion that there is no different mortality between surgery and regular screening for small aneurysms. Having stated that small aneuryms should be operated on the authors then say that patients with small aneuryms should be treated by endovascular reconstruction because it is better, avoiding sexual dysfunction and minimizing perioperative risks. Sexual function and operative risks can of course be best avoided by not operating at all! The authors fail to consider the obvious question of whether endovascular repair is effective and what the long-term outloook is in such patients. They never at any stage mention a trial. They make the point that if the lesion is dealt with when it is smaller, the patient is younger and fitter and will do better. This is certainly a possibility but remains to be proven in my view. I do not believe that the authors have made a case for operating upon small aneuryms.

What is the Case for the Bifurcated Modular Stent–Graft for Abdominal Aneurysms?

Andrew S. Brown, John D.G. Rose and Michael G. Wyatt

INTRODUCTION

The advent of endovascular techniques in abdominal aortic aneurysm surgery has meant that a previously extremely invasive procedure can now potentially be carried out with minimal surgical trauma to the patient. This should allow a higher risk group of patients to be treated. There are currently a number of devices and techniques available for endovascular abdominal aortic aneurysm repair and each may have a role in patient management.

The simplest and original device for endovascular repair was the tube graft.[1] This required the presence of a segment of distal as well as proximal aneurysm neck and in practice only about 4% of abdominal aortic aneurysms are suitable for this type of procedure.[2]

The remaining 96% of abdominal aortic aneurysms have either insufficient distal neck or extend into the iliac vessels thus requiring extension of the graft into the common or external iliac artery. This can be achieved in one of two ways: a) aorto–uni–iliac graft requiring an additional femorofemoral crossover graft, or b) a bifurcated stent–graft combination.

By definition an aorto–uni–iliac graft uses only one side of the iliac bifurcation necessitating occlusion of the contralateral iliac system and insertion of an extra-anatomic femorofemoral crossover graft.[3] Although this extra procedure can be carried out with minimally increased morbidity[4] and little risk of producing a 'steal' phenomenon in the donor limb,[5] it does carry with it inherent problems of possible anastomotic stricture and graft occlusion. Indeed, even in the most favourable situation of a patient without previous surgery and good runoff, a primary patency of 58% and secondary patency of 80% at 5 years can be expected for a femorofemoral crossover.[6]

The gold standard of open abdominal aortic aneurysm repair attempts to return the arterial blood flow, as near as possible, to anatomical normality. The introduction of a crossover graft requires changes in direction of blood flow. Anastomotic intimal hyperplasia occurs because of smooth muscle cell proliferation within the intima of the vessel wall.[7] Although the pathogenesis is not fully understood, it may be promoted by flow change at the distal anastomosis, which causes low wall shear stress at the toe and heel of the anastomosis and high shear stresses on the native arterial wall opposite the anastomosis.[8,9]

A bifurcated endovascular stent–graft maintains normality of blood flow, does not sacrifice a potentially normal iliac system and does not require an extra-anatomic bypass.

THE MODULAR BIFURCATED STENT–GRAFT SYSTEM

Three modular bifurcate aortic stent–grafts are presently available for repair of abdominal aortic aneurysm. These are the AneuRx (Medtronic), Vanguard (Boston Scientific) and Talent (World Medical) devices. Each consists of two or more components which can be used to 'build' a stent–graft combination to fit a pre-measured arterial tree in order to exclude the aneurysm sac from the systemic arterial circulation. The main body and one iliac limb are built as one component and carried in the main delivery sheath. The contralateral limb is packaged separately. In addition, extension limbs and proximal cuffs are available if required (Fig. 1).

Our experience primarily involves the Boston device. This is constructed from a heat labile self-expanding Nitinol[10-12] (Nickel Tantalum alloy) wire stent and an outer Dacron graft. Each component is packaged within its own delivery system, allowing for separate deployment, and these interlock at the graft bifurcation. The nitinol stent is heat sensitive. It expands at body temperature and assumes its original shape, holding the stent–graft combination *in situ* within the native vascular tree.

The AneuRx system is similar, but is constructed with a Dacron graft attached to the inner aspect of a nitinol stent. It is only now becoming available for use on the UK market and will not be considered further. The Talent device also comprises a fully (nitinol) stented graft, but with the stent embedded in the graft material. We have as yet no experience with this system.

PATIENT SELECTION

Aneurysms are initially assessed using a conventional contrast enhanced computed tomography (CT) scan. If this suggests that the aneurysm is suitable for aortic stenting,

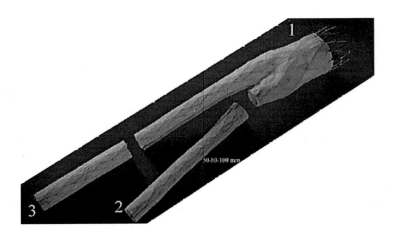

Fig. 1. The Stentor device which became the Vanguard. 1: Main body + iliac limb; 2: contralateral limb; 3: iliac limb extension.

a calibrating arteriogram is performed (Fig. 2). This allows for accurate biplanar assessment of the internal dimensions of the aneurysm, proximal neck and iliac vessels.

Our current criteria for treatment of aortic aneurysms with the bifurcated stent–graft are detailed in Table 1.

Table 1. Current criteria for treatment of aortic aneurysms with bifurcated stent–graft

	Length (mm)	Diameter (mm)	Angulation (°)
Proximal neck	>13	<26	<75
Common iliacs	N/A	8–12[a]	<90

[a]8–16 with AneuRx device

METHOD OF DEPLOYMENT

With the patient under general anaesthetic, a cut-down is made in the appropriate groin to expose the femoral artery. The main body of the aortic stent is usually deployed via the least tortuous and largest iliac artery as shown on the preoperative calibration angiogram (Fig. 2). A radio-opaque ruler is placed beneath the patient to assist in the real time localization of the renal vessels. An angiogram is performed percutaneously through the contralateral femoral artery in order to guide initial placement of the device.

With the exposed femoral vessel clamped an arteriotomy is performed. The main body and ipsilateral limb of the device within a 21F introducer (approximately 7mm in diameter), is flushed with ice cold saline to minimize the tendency of the nitinol stent to expand.[10] The assembly is then inserted over a 'superstiff' guide-wire into the iliac artery. The introducer is gently advanced through the iliac system into the lumen of the aorta until it lies at the level of the renal vessels. The stent–graft is deployed by withdrawing the outer sheath of the introducer over a coaxial 'pusher'. As the device is exposed and unconstrained, it expands but tends to migrate caudally by a few millimetres. This effect is anticipated by releasing the stent slightly high and the device will then attach to the proximal neck by virtue of the diameter of the proximal end of the stent as well as by hooks. A low pressure balloon is then inflated to secure this attachment. Momentary occlusion of the lumen of the aorta causes minimal haemodynamic upset with an increase of the systolic blood pressure of only 5–10 mmHg. The remainder of the main body of the graft and the ipsilateral limb is then allowed to deploy as the delivery sheath is gradually removed.

The contralateral limb is inserted percutaneously over a guide-wire via the contralateral femoral vessel. It is guided through a small 'stump' at the distal end of the main body of the graft adjacent to the ipsilateral limb. When the superior aspect of the contralateral limb is deployed a seal is formed as it expands against the surrounding stump.

Following deployment, a biplanar arteriogram (Fig. 3) is performed to ensure correct graft positioning and the absence of endoleak (extraluminal flow). The groin wound is closed, the percutaneous catheter removed and, following recovery from the anaesthetic, the patient is returned to the ward.

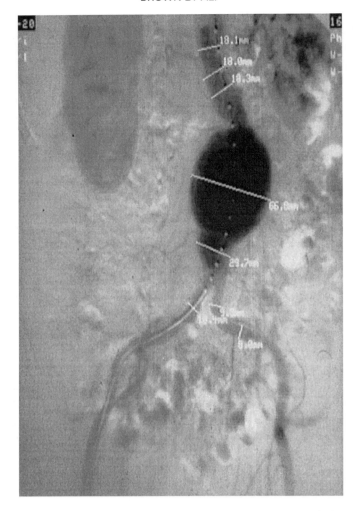

Fig. 2. A calibrating angiogram of a typical infrarenal abdominal aortic aneurysm. This allows accurate assessment of the proximal neck, the aneurysm and the iliac vessels.

RESULTS

Over an 18-month period 200 patients with abdominal aortic aneurysms have been assessed using contrast enhanced CT scans. Of these, 81 (40.5%) went on to have calibration angiograms. Thirty-five were repaired using a modular bifurcated stent–graft combination (Vanguard, Boston Scientific). The median aneurysm diameter was 55 mm (range 45–84 mm) and the median proximal neck length, 24 mm (range 14–100 mm). Although the overall use of stent–grafts is 17%, this is skewed by progression along the learning curve. Over the last 12 months 32% of abdominal aortic aneurysms have been treated using bifurcate modular grafts.

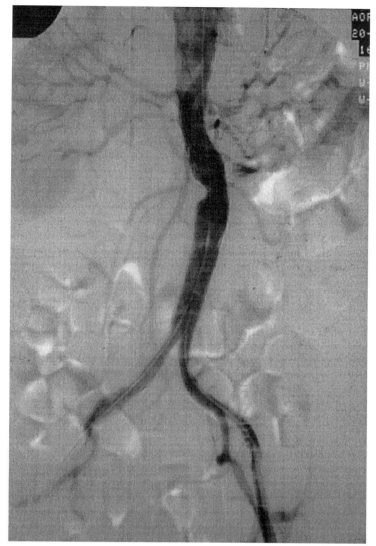

Fig. 3. Completion angiogram showing complete exclusion of the aneurysm (Fig. 2) with no evidence of contrast leakage into the sac. The upper extremity of the nitinol stent can be seen just below the renal vessels.

All deployments were successful. The median age of patients treated was 69.5 years (range 45–89 years) and 18 patients were in the high risk group ASA (American Society of Anesthesiologists) grades III and IV.

Table 2 shows the relationship between ASA grade and the patient's age, postoperative stay, operative blood loss and operative time. Results are presented as median values with ranges. Analysis with a Fisher's exact test and Mann-Whitney U test shows there to be no significant difference in any of these operative parameters between the low and high risk groups.

Table 2. Relationship between patient's age, postoperative stay, operative blood loss and operative time

ASA		Age (years)	Postop stay (days)	Blood loss (ml)	Operative time (min)
II	(n=17)	70 (62–81)	3 (2–13)	200 (50-800)	100 (70–195)
III–IV	(n=18)	68 (45-89)	4 (3–19)	300 (60–800)	120 (100–270)

Where stenosis or tortuosity of the iliac arteries has been identified on the preoperative angiogram, iliac wallstents have been deployed to allow for smoother delivery of the aortic device. This has been carried out in nine patients with no significant increase in radiographic time or dose of contrast used. There have been four unilateral iliac limb occlusions all occurring in patients who had not received pre-deployment iliac stents. Three required a femorofemoral crossover graft as a secondary procedure and the fourth was treated successfully with thrombolysis. One patient developed a false femoral aneurysm requiring surgical repair and a further patient suffered a transient femoral nerve palsy. This gives a perioperative morbidity of 17%.

There were two perioperative deaths (mortality rate 5.7%). One occurred following problems in stent deployment resulting in a proximal endoleak. Despite sealing the leak by external aortic banding at laparotomy, the patient died on day 6 post-stent from a myocardial infarct. The second patient died of congestive cardiac failure 2 days after the procedure.

Follow-up is with contrast enhanced CT scans at 1, 6, 12, 18, 24 months. Scans have demonstrated three small distal endoleaks, two of which have sealed spontaneously. One patient has a persistent endoleak into the distal aspect of the aneurysm sac (due to a patent iliolumbar vessel) but the aneurysm has continued to decrease in diameter. Two aneurysms (Fig. 4) have increased by more than 5% of their immediate postoperative diameter. No endoleaks have as yet been identified in these patients, but previous data[13] suggests that small leaks are probably present and further angiography may be required.

DISCUSSION

In an ideal world a minimally invasive procedure will reduce the perioperative morbidity and mortality rates[14] of the standard open procedure while maintaining the long-term patency of the grafts and exclusion of the aneurysm from the arterial circulation.

The modular bifurcated stent–graft system is perhaps the least invasive of the current devices available while still allowing treatment of aorto–iliac disease. It maintains the normal anatomical blood flow and does not involve the additional risk of an extra-anatomic graft with two peripheral arterial anastomoses. It is a fully stented device, which may have the advantage of preventing distal migration in the event of any continued expansion of the aortic neck. The modular nature of the device ensures that it can be assembled from several parts at the time of operation to fit precisely the aneurysm to be treated.

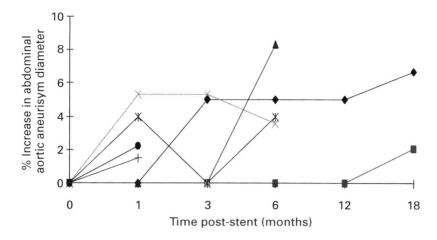

Fig. 4. Those abdominal aortic aneurysms that have increased in diameter since stent deployment.

Stenotic or tortuous iliac arteries can lead to difficulties in stent–graft deployment. If it is felt preoperatively that this is likely to be a problem, iliac wallstents can be inserted prior to stent–graft deployment allowing for smoother delivery of the device.

This device does not have to be confined to the common iliac arteries. Following transcatheter coil occlusion of the internal iliac artery, the limbs can be taken well into the external iliac system to allow treatment of more distal aneurysmal involvement of the iliac vessels.

There have been reports of devices failing 18 months following deployment resulting in significant endoleak.[15] We believe that this fully stented device may be more durable but our median follow-up is currently 6 months with only four patients having reached 18 months. A multicentre blind prospective trial is required to fully assess the incidence of long-term graft failure.

As to the type of endovascular device used, perhaps efforts should be directed at further refining a bifurcated system. This would leave the aorto–uni–iliac with a femorofemoral crossover for cases where the iliac arteries are too large, or their endovascular negotiation is impossible. In addition, the patency rates for femoro-femoral crossover grafts in aneurysmal patients is unknown, but occlusion of the single donor iliac artery or crossover graft may require more extensive revascularization such as an axillobifemoral graft.

It is apparent that a significant number of aneurysms will remain treatable by open repair alone. However, those that can be managed endovascularly are likely to pose a variety of deployment problems and it will be essential that various devices are available to the interventionalist. The modular system combines the versatility required for successful stenting of abdominal aortic aneurysms, while still conforming to the traditional principles of open repair.

REFERENCES

1. Parodi JC, Palmaz JC, Barone HD: Transfemoral intraluminal graft implantation for abdominal aortic aneurysms. *Ann Vasc Surg* **5**: 491–9, 1991
2. Armon MP, Yusuf SW, Latief K *et al.*: Anatomical suitability of abdominal aortic aneurysms for endovascular repair. *Br J Surg* **84**: 178–180, 1997
3. Yusuf SW, Hopkinson BR: Endovascular repair of aortic aneurysm. *Br J Surg* **82**: 289–91, 1995
4. Fahal AH, McDonald AM, Marston A: Femorofemoral bypass in unilateral iliac artery occlusion. *Br J Surg* **76**; 22-25: 1989
5. Sumner DS, Stradness DE: The hemodynamics of the femorofemoral shunt. *Surg Gynecol Obstet* **134**: 629–36, 1972
6. Brener BJ, Brief DK, Veith FJ: Extraanatomic bypasses. In: Veith FJ, Hobson RW, Wilson SE (Eds), *Vascular Surgery; Principles and Practice*. New York: McGraw-Hill Inc., 1994.
7. O'Malley MK: The development of intimal hyperplasia and its possible prevention. In: Greenhalgh RM, Hollier LH (Eds), *The Maintenance of Arterial Reconstruction*. London: WB Saunders Co Ltd, 1991
8. Ojha M, Cobbold RSC, Johnston KW: Hemodynamics of a side to end proximal arterial anastomosis model. *J Vasc Surg* **17**: 646–55, 1993
9. Lei M, Archie JP, Kleinstreuer C: Computational design of a bypass graft that minimizes wall shear stress gradients in the region of the distal anastomosis. *J Vasc Surg* **25**: 637–46, 1997
10. Cragg AH, De Jong SC, Barnhart WH *et al.*: Nitinol intravascular stent: results of preclinical evaluation. *Radiology* **189**: 775–78, 1993
11. Vinograd I, Klin B, Brosh T *et al.*: A new intratracheal stent made from nitinol, an alloy with "shape memory effect". *J Thorac Cardiovasc Surg* **107**: 1255–61, 1994
12. Miahle C, Amicabile C, Becquemin JP: Endovascular treatment of infrarenal abdominal aneurysms by the Stentor system: Preliminary results of 79 cases. *J Vasc Surg* **26**: 199–209, 1997
13. Armon MP, Yusuf SW, Whitaker SC *et al.*: The fate of the aneurysm sac following endovascular aneurysm repair (abstract). Portugal: European Society for Vascular Surgery, 1997
14. Blum U, Voshage G, Lammer J *et al.*: Endoluminal stent–grafts for infrarenal   aortic aneurysms. *New Engl J Med* **336**: 13–20, 1996
15. Coppi G, Moratto R, Silingardi R *et al.*: The Italian trial of endovascular AAA exclusion using the Parodi endograft. *J Endovasc Surg* **4**: 299–306, 1997

Editorial comments by P.R.F. Bell

These authors have set the scene against a crossover graft by quoting a paper about patency and results in a totally different group of patients. The patients they are quoting are in fact ischaemic patients and not those with aneurysms. The results of crossover grafting in an aneurysm patient is unknown. The comments they make about intimal hyperplasia and shear stress being equal are also unfounded. However, the comments about the preferability of a bifurcated system are well made. The authors' experience relates to the Vanguard system almost entirely and exposes the limitations of the bifurcated system. The common iliacs have to be no more than 12 mm in diameter or 15 mm with the AneuRx device and the angulation has to be less than 90 degrees. The authors have found a higher percentage than usual, numbering 32% of patients who have been dealt with by bifurcated grafts. Four of their patients have required crossover grafts, the mortality was 5.7%, there was one persistent endoleak, and two further patients have an increase in the aneurysm sac. This chapter is an audit of the learning curve of one unit using a modular graft which shows the standard results of that procedure.

Should an Anchor Stent Cross the Renal Artery Orifices When Placing an Endoluminal Graft for Abdominal Aortic Aneurysm?

M. Lawrence-Brown, K. Sieunarine, D. Hartley, G. Van Schie
and J. Anderson

INTRODUCTION

Endoluminal grafting for abdominal aortic aneurysm is an attractive alternative to open aneurysm repair because it is much less invasive, with reduced stress upon the patient – if it is successful and durable. This latter factor is relevant because we know that open aneurysm repair has a good track record for durability and prophylaxis against rupture, with life expectancy close to the peer group. This has been confirmed in Western Australia by data obtained for the past 15 years, through a linked database.[1,2] For the period 1980–1995, the 30-day mortality for all age groups for open elective aneurysm repair was 4.4%; 70% of males aged 70 years are expected to survive for 5 years and 50% will survive 10 years, with a life expectancy within 7% of the normal life survival curve of the Western Australian population. Endoluminal grafting, as a minimally invasive procedure, has been offered primarily to the elderly, frail and to those with higher co-morbid risk factors. However, endoluminal grafting as a prophylactic procedure for ruptured abdominal aortic aneurysm fails if it does not prove to be durable. This includes mortality figures for open intervention as a salvage procedure after primary endoluminal grafting.[3]

THE NEED FOR SECURE PROXIMAL FIXATION WITH ENDOLUMINAL GRAFTING FOR ABDOMINAL AORTIC ANEURYSM

Success and durability of endoluminal grafting depends primarily on a proximal secure attachment and seal. Endoleaks,[4] especially proximal endoleaks, are not only evidence of failure, but also increase the risk of rupture.[5] An endoleak with significant in-flow and no out-flow may create a higher mean pressure in the aneurysm chamber than in the lumen of the aorta, and the increase in mean pressure increases the potential for expansion and rupture of the aneurysm. Secure proximal attachment and seal are dependent on patient selection (aneurysmal anatomy) and graft design. Patient selection is not the topic of this chapter but it is the foundation on which to proceed. Distal migration of the endoluminal device will result in an endoleak if the aneurysm chamber is exposed, and the aneurysm will be re-pressurized.

Resistance to migration is dependent upon three factors.

1. The force required to overcome the friction against migration.
2. The amount of strain that can be withstood by the wall.
3. The pillar strength of the device. Each factor is independent, but equally important in maintaining position of the stent graft within the neck of the aneurysm. Friction is dependent on the coefficient of friction and the radial (normal) force applied, according to the equation is $F = \mu N$.

F = Force required to overcome resistance
μ = Co-efficient friction
N = Normal force (radial force).

It is important that the equation for strain involves the parameter for area in the denominator and this is pertinent to patient selection with adequate length of neck to absorb the strain. If the wall or inner layers of the neck of the aneurysm are weak, loosely attached or composed of pultaceous atheroma or thrombus then they are unlikely to withstand the strain, particularly in the shorter necks.

$$Strain = \frac{Force}{Area}$$

Woven Dacron does not adhere or incorporate into tissues, and is even less likely to incorporate into intima. Metal stent placement on the outside of the Dacron may increase the ability of the device to embed itself into the wall of the neck of the aneurysm, but may reduce the ability to seal and possibly potentiate the risk of endoleak. Hooks alone within the neck of the aneurysm may provide an initial secure attachment, but the area of contact for each will be small, the strain therefore great and the constant pulsation subjects each hook to fatigue.

The strain relates to the strength and cohesion of the layers in the wall of the neck to resist breakages and shearing within the wall which would allow the device to break away. Strain is equal to Force divided by Area of contact or Force $\div 2\pi r \times$ Length of wall contact. The length of wall contact, or aneurysm neck, is related to strain.

Pillar strength is related to the rigidity of the device, when it is unsupported in the aneurysm chamber and any part of the arterial wall acting as a structural support to maintain position. An example of this would be a rigid device, lodged distally which resisted buckling, thereby maintaining the proximal position. A second example would be the lodgement of part of the structure within a recess, for example, a stent lodged behind the waist formed by lumbar vessels or by some other such ledge in the arterial wall.

Pillar strength based upon distal lodgement is appealing for reliable maintenance of position through an aneurysm chamber and stability in the neck of the aneurysm. The difficulty with providing sufficient pillar strength to hold a device in position is that flexibility is required to negotiate the curved, and often the tortuous iliac access pathway to the aneurysm. The flexibility compromises the pillar strength where it is most needed within the aneurysm chamber where the device is unsupported. Flexibility which could be converted to rigidity would be an answer – for example a material which was flexible for insertion and then sets rigid when in position.

Bare metal in contact with the arterial wall, particularly with some radial force is known to become incorporated or embedded. Stainless steel Z-stents were placed in growing pigs and adult dogs for periods of up to 9 months. Single stent struts across normal renal orifices have not been associated with the growth of intima along a wire strut beyond a millimetre (Fig. 1). For a 6-mm diameter renal orifice the cross-sectional area compromised by a wire strut across the diameter of the orifice causes approximately 6% cross-sectional area loss. This should not cause a haemodynamic reduction in flow. Potential drawback of 'jailing'[5-7] the orifice is offset by the security provided by placing the metal stent within an artery which has a more normal surface and wall and provides a secure anchor, particularly if also associated with hooks.

The likelihood of intimal hyperplasia across an orifice is related to the proximity of the struts of the stent to each other. Those that are close together, such as in braided or small aperture expanded mesh stents, will provide a scaffold upon which intimal hyperplasia may link across. Whereas with the widely separated single wires of a Z-stent with relatively few crowns, occlusion is unlikely. Experience with 90 cases over 4 years, with a mean follow-up period of 18 months has not shown any deterioration in biochemical renal function measured by creatine levels, and no renal artery occlusions following the procedure. The argument therefore for placing open stents across the renal arteries is that the risk of renal impairment when the renal artery orifices are normal are less than the risks to the patient of an insecure proximal fixation or an open operation.[8]

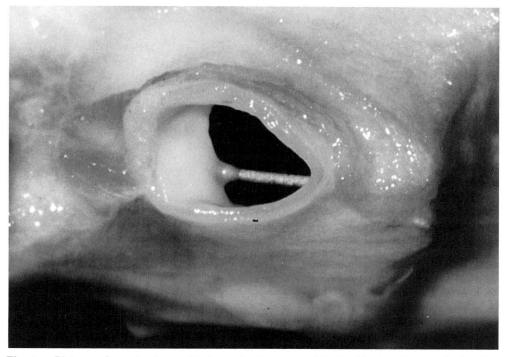

Fig.1.   Picture of renal artery with bare stent strut and limit of intimal hyperplasia after 9 months in aorta of growing pig.

RENAL ARTERY STENOSIS AND ENDOLUMINAL GRAFTING FOR ABDOMINAL AORTIC ANEURYSM

Problems may arise when anchoring stents across the renal arteries in patients with renal artery stenosis.[9] There is good evidence in the literature to support the treatment of renal artery stenoses greater than 80%, and possibly greater than 60%, to preserve renal function and size.[10–13] The natural history is for severe stenoses (>80%) to progress to occlusion with a consequence of ischaemic atrophy of the kidney. A degree of renal artery stenosis is present in up to 30% of cases of abdominal aortic aneurysm. In view of current opinion to treat asymptomatic renal artery stenosis to preserve renal function,[12] and the risk of causing problems with a strut across a stenosed renal orifice, other strategies may be employed with endoluminal grafting.

Treatment of renal artery stenosis in this age group has been conservative if the renal function is sufficient to give normal, or acceptable, levels of urea and creatinine, and if the blood pressure can be controlled by medical therapy to an acceptable level. Biochemically measured renal function may be 'normal' despite atrophy of one kidney as a result of renal artery stenosis, because of renal reserve and the function of the contralateral kidney. Bilateral renal artery stenosis is even more relevant to the potential for renal failure when a patient is undergoing treatment of abdominal aortic aneurysmal disease. Severe renal artery stenosis

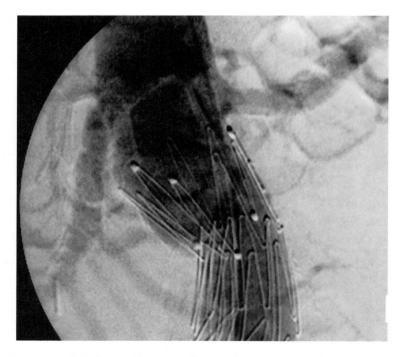

Fig. 2.   A stent graft below solitary renal artery in aneurysm with proximal neck 3 cm (previous right nephrectomy for carcinoma).

therefore warrants treatment in its own right to preserve renal tissue where there is renal artery orifice stenosis. When there is renal artery orifice stenosis in association with an abdominal aortic aneurysm for which endoluminal grafting is indicated, it may not be associated with the same expectation of renal artery preservation, particularly if the stenosis is severe and over 80%, when a further 6%+ may accelerate or significantly increase the impediment to flow for the compromised orifice. A proximal secure attachment is still required with the arguments for this necessity unchanged. The strategies we have employed to ensure secure attachment and preserve renal vessels (Fig. 2) have been the following:

1. Attach the stent below the renal arteries if the neck of the aneurysm is longer than usual and exclude the possibility of the stent contributing to renal artery occlusion.
2. Place an anchor stent above the renal and mesenteric vessels in the descending thoracic aorta, and suspend the covered stent via suspension wires (Fig. 3). These wires may be sited so as to avoid the major vessel orifices.
3. Pre-treat the renal artery stenoses with balloon dilatation and stent placement and then place an uncovered stent, as for a normal renal artery orifice (Fig. 4).

Fenestrated stents (Fig. 5) are being developed and have been inserted experimentally. Fenestrated stents require precise construction and deployment and the use of intraluminal imaging for guidance. They may, however, hold promise for the future.

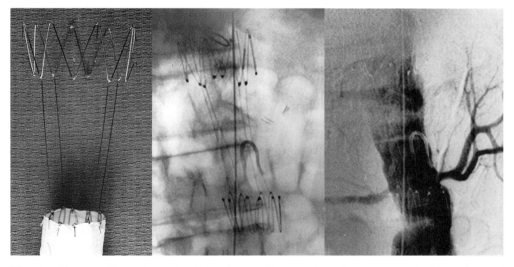

Fig.3. 'Carousel' anchor stent in descending aorta, above mesenteric and renal vessels.

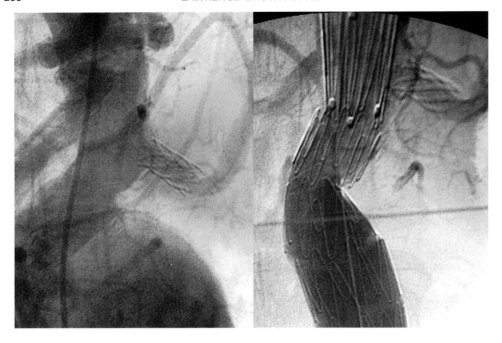

Fig. 4.   Pre- and postendoluminal grafting of abdominal aortic aneurysm with Palmaz
stent in left renal artery.

EMPLOYING THESE TECHNIQUES

The proximal stent migration rate is 3% (four in 140 cases). On review poor patient
selection accounted for three of these. Filling defects in the wall of the aneurysm
neck, implicating thrombus or soft atheroma were clearly apparent in two, and in the
third the stent was placed within a neck that was affected by aneurysmal disease
which further expanded.

Initially endoluminal grafting was only offered to patients with significant co-
morbidity or reduced life expectancy due to recent malignancy or age over 80 years.
With reassuring results of a 30-day mortality of 3.7% for all cases since conception of
programming, low migration rates with proximal security, and better patient
selection with clearer guidelines, the procedure is offered to more patients. The
indications are therefore more liberal than they have been during the earlier part of
the programme. The increasing support for dilating and stenting renal arteries as
prophylaxis against progressive renal artery occlusion and renal atrophy means that
in a person with an abdominal aortic aneurysm for endoluminal grafting, the
possibility of renal artery stenosis should be looked for and if the stenosis is greater
than 80%, or possibly 60%, then angioplasty and stenting should be considered if it is
planned to place the open stent across the renal arteries. Follow-up of these patients
will need to be compared with the current trends towards re-stenosis of treated renal
arteries.[10]

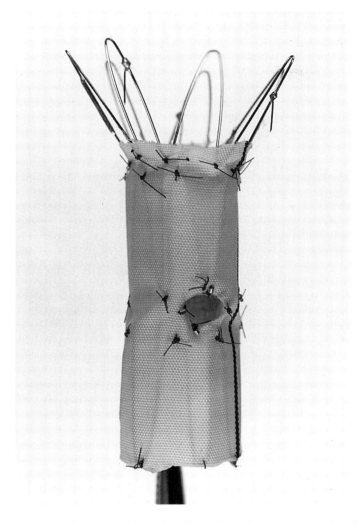

Fig. 5. Experimental fenestrated graft with gold radioopaque marker beads around the fenestration.

In summary the need for proximal secure fixation of an endoluminal graft for abdominal aortic aneurysm outweighs the risks of impairing renal function when the renal artery orifice is normal. For stenosed renal artery orifices, pre-dilatation and stent placement should be performed before inserting an endoluminal graft and consideration given to a carousel anchor stent, or restricting anchoring to below the renal arteries, and in the future consideration for using fenestrated covered stents.

ACKNOWLEDGMENTS

The members of the Vascular and Radiology Departments of Royal Perth Hospital.

REFERENCES

1. Semmens JB, Norman PE, Lawrence-Brown MMD *et al.*: A population-based record linkage study: The incidence of abdominal aortic aneurysm in Western Australia for 1985–94. *Br Med J* (accepted for publication)
2. Semmens JB, Lawrence-Brown MMD, Norman PE *et al.*: The quality of surgical care project: Benchmark standards for open repair of abdominal aortic aneurysms in Western Australia. *Austr NZ J Surg* (accepted for publication)
3. Gosset J, Olin JW: Atherosclerotic renovascular disease: Clinical clues and natural history. *J Endovasc Surg* **4**: 316, 1977
4. Beebe HG, Bernhard VM, Parodi JC, White GC: Leaks after endovascular therapy for aneurysm: Detection and classification. *J Endovasc Surg* **3**: 445, 1996
5. Lawrence-Brown MMD, Hartley D, MacSweeney STR *et al.*: The Perth endoluminal bifurcated graft system. Development and early experience. *Cardiovasc Surg* **4**: 706–12, 1996
6. Whitbread, P, Birch S, Rogers ID *et al.*: The effect of placing an aortic wallstent across the renal artery. Origins in an animal model. *Eur J Vasc Endovasc Surg* **14**: 154, 1997
7. Malina M, Brunkwall J, Ivancev K *et al.*: Renal arteries covered by aortic stents. Clinical experience from endovascular grafting of aortic aneurysms. *Eur J Vasc Endovasc Surg* **14**: 109, 1997
8. May J, White GH, Yu W *et al.*: Conversion from endoluminal to open repair of abdominal aortic aneurysm. A hazardous procedure. *Eur J Vasc Endovasc Surg* **14**: 4, 1997
9. Harden PN, Macleod MJ, Rodger RSC *et al.*: Effect of renal artery stenting on progression of renovascular renal failure. *Lancet* **349**: 1133, 1997
10. Choudhri AH, Cleland JGF, Rowlands PC *et al.*: Unsuspected renal artery stenosis in peripheral vascular disease. *Br Med J* **301**: 1990
11. Strandness DE, Jr: Natural history of renal artery stenosis. *Am J Kidn Dis* **24**: 630–5, 1994
12. Tollefson DFJ, Ernst CB: Natural history of atherosclerotic renal artery stenosis associated with aortic disease. *J Vasc Surg* **14**: 327, 1991
13. Eugene Zierler R, Bergelin RO *et al.*: Natural history of atherosclerotic renal artery stenosis. A prospective study with duplex ultrasonography. *J Vasc Surg* **19**: 250, 1994

Editorial comments by P.R.F. Bell

This paper discusses an important problem but should I think concentrate more on the difficulties facing us with suprarenal stenting. The paper goes into much detail about proximal fixation of endoluminal graft pointing out that incorporation does not necessarily occur and discusses precisely the forces required to maintain a stent in place. It would be better to provide some facts about whether or not suprarenal stenting is a valuable thing to do. The authors have used it in a number of patients and have made the point that using a Z stent is the only safe way of doing this. They should also commment about other stents that have been used and also animal work which has shown that putting other than Z stents across renal arteries leads to their occulsion. Perhaps they should also produce some of their data telling us exactly what the renal functions etc is in patients following this procedure. The paper is, however, interesting and will be a source for discussion and may expand the horizons of this technique further.

INTERMITTENT CLAUDICATION
QUESTIONS AND INDICATIONS

Has the Endovascular Management of Aorto–iliac Disease Buried the Need for Open Surgery?

P.A. Gaines and S.M. Thomas

The answer is a resounding 'maybe' (see Fig. 1).

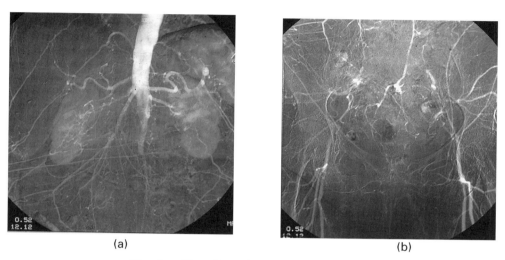

(a)   (b)

Fig. 1a, 1b.   Complete aortoiliac occlusion

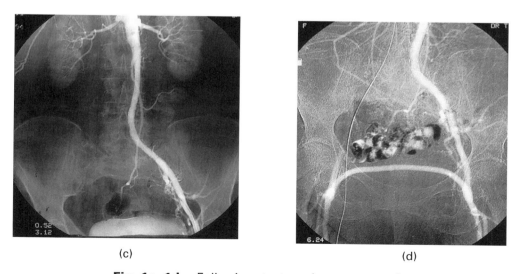

(c)   (d)

Fig. 1c, 1d.   Following stents and crossover graft.

INTRODUCTION

Chronic occlusive arterial disease of the lower limbs is common. In the Western world 5% of the population over the age of 50 have claudication.[1] In a survey of the Edinburgh population 25% of the population aged 55-74 years had objective evidence of atherosclerosis although only 5% were symptomatic.[1-3] The distal aorta and iliac arteries are amongst the most common sites involved[4] and when the disease is limited to this segment it is most unlikely to result in leg threatening ischaemia but can be responsible for disabling buttock, thigh and calf claudication, and impotence. Very occasionally unstable plaque will embolize distally resulting in the blue digit syndrome. Young smoking females with small main vessels appear to be particularly prone to develop severe occlusive disease at the aortic bifurcation. When this aorto–iliac disease is coupled with infrainguinal disease then flow is limited sufficiently to present a threat to limb viability. Whilst intervention is clearly indicated, where possible, to prevent limb loss, claudication may severely interfere with quality of life. In such instances it would be a useful health system that could respond to these patients needs also. Over the last 10–20 years the endovascular management of occlusive arterial disease has provided an alternative to the conventional, more invasive surgical bypass. This article reviews the data to investigate whether these new techniques can indeed totally replace traditional surgery.

ENDOVASCULAR TECHNIQUES IN THE AORTO–ILIAC SEGMENT

In 1964 Dotter described the use of a coaxial catheter to treat peripheral occlusive disease. The technique was innately limited because the size of the channel was the same as the percutaneous puncture and limited to the diameter of the catheter. Like all truly great inventions the Gruentzig concept of a balloon dilatation catheter was simplicity itself. Through the ingenuity of clinical practitioners, and the technical skills of industry, the basic balloon design has been miniaturized and developed with such limits of safety that it has been used in virtually all arterial and venous territories throughout the body.

The currently available stents are metallic and either self-expanding or balloon expandable. The self-expanding designs are either interwoven spring steel filaments (e.g. Schneider Wallstent) or based on Nitinol technology. In general they offer less crush resistance than the balloon expandable designs and are more difficult to place precisely, but they take curves well and are available in a long length (upto 11 cm). The balloon expandable systems have the advantages described but are not particularly flexible and are only available in shorter lengths.

The spread of clinical expertise has been so efficient that arterial dilatation is available to a variable extent throughout most health care systems around the world. Its perceived advantage over conventional surgery is that it offers acceptable levels of efficacy and safety whilst being inexpensive, quick, and cosmetically acceptable to patients.

The quality of reporting has not always matched the quality of the treatment, and because this is a relatively new area compared with surgery the volume of data does not compare. However, some generalizations can be made.

ANGIOPLASTY

Aortic stenoses

The dilatation of aortic stenoses is usually undertaken using the kissing balloon technique. Two recent reports of a total of 115 patients described a 94% technical success rate with an 80% 3–5 year clinical success rate. A review of the literature reveals 70–89% are symptom free at 5 years. Significant complications are rare.[5,6]

Iliac stenoses

There are extensive data pertaining to angioplasty of iliac stenosis since this was an early lesion to be tackled by interventionalists and it is a relatively common pattern of disease. However, data presentation has been bedevilled by different reporting standards, the problems of defining technical and clinical success, and how long-term patency should be defined using non-invasive techniques given the inaccuracy of femoral wave-form analysis and the limitations of the ankle brachial index in the presence of distal disease. In addition, the patient is more likely to be interested in his quality of life rather than patency, something that has received scant attention.

The initial technical success (however that is defined) of 94-96% is very high for short (<5 cm) iliac stenoses. Long-term patency in those studies that present life-table analysis is a mean of 84% at 1 year, 76% at 3 years, and 74 % at 5 years.[7-10] The much revered data from Wayne Johnston[11] presents pessimistically low patency rates because of the need for both clinical success and maintenance of ankle brachial index on follow-up as the definition of patency, even in the presence of distal disease. The procedural complication rate is excellent with an overall death rate of 0.3%. Only 0.9% of patients require surgery for ischaemic complications and there are no complications related to anaesthesia.[7-11] Where angioplasty eventually fails, 85% return to baseline, 5.5% remain clinically improved and only 9.5% are worse than at presentation.[12] Even where amputation is required this is due to progression of disease rather than failure of the angioplasty site. Poor outcome is related to the treatment of diffuse disease, external iliac stenoses, critical ischaemia, patients with superficial femoral artery occlusions and women. Each variable adds approximately 10% to the drop in patency.[13]

Iliac occlusions

The enthusiasm for approaching occlusions with balloons was initially tempered because of concerns regarding the bulk of disease, distal embolization and vessel rupture. Thankfully most of these problems have not been realized. In this country chronic iliac occlusion is not initially managed with thrombolysis because of the extra risks involved. Colapinto[14] published a large series of 64 patients with occlusions treated by balloon angioplasty and recorded different success according to the length of disease treated. If the occlusion was less than 5cm then the initial technical success was 90% and the 4-year patency 72%. If the lesion was greater than 5 cm then the technical success was 70% and the 5-year patency 86% (excluding primary failures). They did have a 3.1% embolization rate treated by surgery, and this significant complication has previously been reported to affect 20–50% of long iliac occlusions treated by balloon dilatation.[7,15] Since Colapintos' report in 1986 there have been advances in catheter and guide-wire technology. Despite that, Gupta,[16] in a series from 1993 only had a 71.4% technical success rate in 56 occluded arteries. The 4-year patency rate was 63% overall, 76% including primary failures. In addition there was one iliac rupture and four episodes of distal embolization. Clearly any technology that can improve the primary success in iliac occlusions and reduce the distal embolization has much to offer.

STENTS

Endovascular stents offer the tantalizing prospect of providing internal support to the treated segment and resist recoil. This has the potential to improve the primary success, improve long-term patency and prevent distal embolization. The down side is that although the initial lumen gain is better, the overall long-term benefits may be offset by a more aggressive restenosis reaction. My own concern is that stents may also hinder the beneficial effects of re-modelling. So what of the data? Unfortunately combining different clinical groups, and both stenoses and occlusions, confuses many of the data. I will attempt to detail some of the highlights.

Iliac stenoses

There have been many non-randomized uncontrolled studies published in the literature. The as yet unpublished data from Richter (Table 1) offers some insight into stenting all iliac stenoses. The group randomized 286 short segment (less than 50% of the iliac artery) symptomatic iliac stenoses or recent (< 6 months) occlusions to either balloon dilatation or the Palmaz stent. Occlusions were reduced back to a stenosis using thrombolysis. They apparently have demonstrated a significant improvement in primary success, complications, initial clinical success, and 5-year clinical and

Table 1.   Richter data

	Angioplasty	Stent	Significance
Technical success	92%	99%	
Major complications	8 of 145 patients	5 of 141 patients	
Mean residual gradient	6.7mmHg	1.4mmHg	$p < 0.001$
Initial clinical success	88%	98.6%	
5-year angiographic patency	64.6%	91.6%	$p < 0.001$–0.005
5-year clinical success	72.7%	90.7%	

angiographic patency in favour of stents. Given the financial constraints of the Health Service it is not possible to blindly treat all iliac stenoses in this way. The Dutch Iliac Stent Trial (in press) was designed to investigate whether it was possible to obtain benefit by selective stenting. Patients were divided randomly into two groups: either primary stenting, or placement of a stent only where there was a significant residual gradient following balloon angioplasty. There was no difference in eventual residual stenosis, complications, clinical success and patency, and quality of life. The only difference was the reduced cost of elective stenting. The problem is that there are no data to show that a residual gradient is associated with a poor outcome and it would have been more beneficial to compare selective stenting against no stenting in that cohort of patients. Death from the procedure is extremely uncommon but there is a local major complication rate of 2-3.4%.[17]

Iliac occlusions

Iliac occlusions fair less well than stenoses when treated by balloon dilatation, and stents may therefore have more to offer (Fig. 2). Vorwerk[18] treated 127 patients with an overall primary success rate of 81%. Their learning curve was nicely demonstrated with a technical success in the first 70 and second 57 patients of 71% and 93% respectively. Primary patency at 1,2,3 and 4 years was 87, 83, 81 and 78% respectively. This increased with secondary patencies of 94, 90, 88 and 88% at the same time intervals. This is very similar to our own data[19] and those of Blum[20] who prior treated the lesions with thrombolysis. No procedure-related deaths were recorded. The embolic complications are interesting. Blum and Vorwerk recorded peripheral embolization in 6 and 4 % although only occasionally were they clinically significant. We have abolished distal embolization by transferring from balloon dilatation prior to stent, to stent placement followed by balloon dilatation.[19] With current endovascular techniques those emboli considered significant can usually be treated by the Radiologist.

There are presently no completed randomized trials looking at the management of iliac occlusions. We are in the middle of a multicentre randomized trial comparing balloon dilatation or stent placement in the management of symptomatic iliac occlusions less than 6 cm long. The interim report will soon be prepared. There is a proposal presented to the NHS Health Technology Assessment Programme committee seeking for funding to support a randomized trial of surgery vs stent in the management of long iliac occlusions.

Meta-analysis

Bosch and Hunink[21] recently published the results of a meta-analysis of percutaneous transluminal angioplasty (PTA) and stent placement in the management of aorto–iliac disease. Whilst they reviewed six PTA studies and eight stent studies they could only include one paper of sufficient quality that dealt specifically with iliac occlusion. Their data must necessarily reflect the management of iliac stenoses and they concluded that stent placement and angioplasty yield similar complications but the technical success rate and long-term success was improved by stent placement.

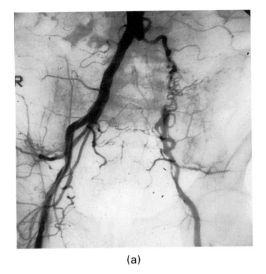

(a)

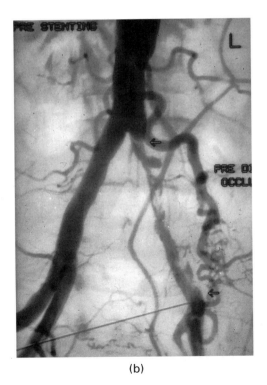

(b)

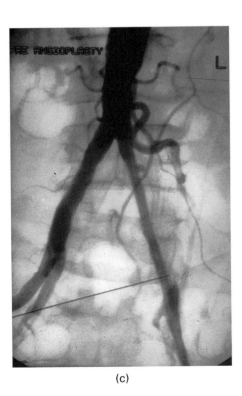

(c)

Fig. 2. (a) Left common iliac angioplasty; (b) Poor result following balloon dilatation, 20 mm Hg residual gradient; (c) Good result following stent placement, no residual gradient.

Current indications for stent placement

Iliac occlusions

In the absence of randomized data the current feeling is that stents reduce complications, and probably increase the primary success and long-term patency. We await the results of our Trent-funded randomized trial with baited breath.

Iliac stenoses with residual disease following PTA

The determination of residual disease is open to debate. Angiography is unreliable, residual pressure gradient should be the gold standard but lacks science, and both techniques ignore the potential benefits of late remodelling.

Iliac dissection

Iliac dissection usually following catheter manipulation en-route to the coronary circulation, or occasionally following angioplasty is an indication.

The presence of diffuse disease, superior femoral artery occlusions, a stent diameter of less than 8cm, and the use of multiple stents adversely affect long-term patency of stents.[22,23] Use should reflect this.

SURGERY IN THE MANAGEMENT OF AORTO–ILIAC DISEASE[24–26]

Surgery has long been the mainstay of managing aorto–iliac occlusive disease. In our unit, with the alternative endovascular therapies available, the number of cases performed has fallen remarkably. In the light of the alternative therapies available, and the natural history of peripheral vascular disease, the results and indications deserve review.

Aorto–iliac endarterectomy has durable results in very localized disease and is not associated with infection of prosthetics, but is technically demanding, not practised widely, and is suitable for those patients who may best be treated by endovascular techniques.[27]

The aortobifemoral graft is probably the most common technique for managing this pattern of disease where considered technically suitable. The procedure results in effective treatment of ischaemia in 70-80% of cases and the long-term patencies are 85-90% at 5 years, and 70-75% at 10 years. Unfortunately, 25-30% of patients are dead at 5 years and 50-60% at 10 years, usually from coexistent cardiac disease. The short-term complications are not trivial. The perioperative mortality is around 3%. Other complications include; acute thrombosis in 1-3%, acute renal failure 4-6%, intestinal ischaemia 2%, and spinal cord ischaemia 0.25%. One percent of grafts become infected, impotence occurs in 25%, and late thrombosis usually results in deterioration in the level of ischaemia. Patients who develop aortoenteric fistulas suffer a high mortality.

In patients with a hostile abdomen alternative 'non-anatomical' by-pass may be preferred. The axillobifemoral graft carries an overall 30-day mortality of 2-18% presumably reflecting the high co-morbidity of these patients. However, even when

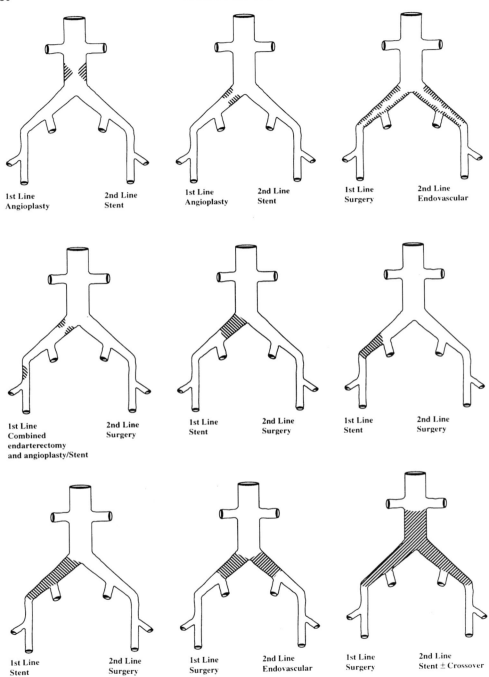

Fig. 3. Proposed preferred treatment options for various disease morphology.

this technique is used to treat claudicants the mortality is still 5%. The long-term patency is reduced compared with aortobifemoral grafting with a 3-year patency of approximately 50%. The femorofemoral crossover graft may be used for unilateral iliac disease with good run-off. The operative mortality is 0-15%, on the lower side of this range for claudicants. The long-term patency is 44-81% at 5years, and is adversely affected by associated superior femoral artery occlusions.

RANDOMIZED STUDIES COMPARING SURGERY AND ANGIOPLASTY

Sadly these are few, none if you wish to compare surgery vs stenting/combined interventional techniques.

Holm and colleagues[28] randomized 102 patients with claudication or critical limb ischaemia to surgery or angioplasty. The patients were required to have occlusions or stenoses <6 cm of the iliac or superficial artery to be included in the trial and comment was made that this represented only 5% of the vascular practice. Up to 1-year follow-up there was no difference in the success or complication rate.

Wolf and colleagues[29] randomized 236 patients with occlusions or stenoses of the iliac, superficial femoral or popliteal artery to either angioplasty or surgery. In both the iliac and infrainguinal groups, at 4 years, there was no difference in outcome (including the sickness impact profile).

CONCLUSIONS

The decision as to which technique to apply to a patient is tailored on an individual basis but some generalizations may be based on the above data. Consideration must not only be made of the morphology of the underlying disease process, but also on the natural history of the disease and cost implications. Unfortunately there is little comparative economic data focused on the aorto–iliac segment.

Claudication is not a benign process. Men have a 5-year mortality that is two to three times expected and this is primarily due to coronary disease and stroke.[2] Whilst less than 50% of claudicants will experience a deterioration in the severity of their leg ischaemia, only 5% ever require an amputation.[30] The principal problem therefore is one of premature death and not of limb loss. Any attempts to treat the claudication must involve little risk to life and limb, even if it fails, and very long-term patencies are a secondary issue. Endovascular intervention is probably the treatment of choice in the majority of situations. It has a low procedural complication rate. When the procedure is a technical failure, or the treatment fails in the long term, only rarely is limb viability threatened, and with the pursuit of day-case intervention it will be the cheapest form of treatment.

Patients with critical limb ischaemia have a 55% chance of death at 5 years. Revascularization is the principal objective and again long durability of therapy is a secondary issue. With this in mind the randomized and non-randomized data show acceptable clinical and long-term benefit with a low complication rate in this fragile group of patients.

Suggested treatment strategies are shown in the accompanying diagrams. The results of focal iliac and aortic stenoses treated by balloon dilatation are good and can be supported by adjunctive stenting if required. The published data on the treatment of iliac occlusions by angioplasty are sufficiently good to be used as first line therapy, although many would now prefer to primarily stent to reduce complications, and possibly improve patency. Poor patency is found with run-off disease but this applies to conventional surgery too. Iliac disease complicated by common femoral disease can be treated by combining femoral endarterectomy and angioplasty/stent. The results of stenting compared with conventional alternatives in very diffuse disease is unclear and deserves further scrutiny. The occasional pattern of bilateral common iliac occlusions with a patent distal aorta is technically difficult to manage by angioplasty/stenting and in the majority of cases is probably a surgical option.

Surgery should probably be restricted to those patients with severe symptoms and either bilateral diffuse disease, aorto–iliac occlusion, or failed endovascular therapy. Aortobifemoral grafting has good results and, given the correct distribution of disease, particularly when there is no co-existent superior femoral artery occlusion, the femorofemoral crossover graft is a useful alternative. Disease present on the donor side can be successfully treated by angioplasty or stenting without jeopardizing long-term patency.

THE WORK AHEAD

On-going or proposed trials are mentioned above. Further data is required on the relative merits of managing diffuse disease by surgery or endovascular disease. Much more effort is required in the field of quality of life and health economics. The battle against restenosis will one day be won and we can then look forward to a truely minimally invasive world.

REFERENCES

1. Fowkes FGR, Housley E, Cawood EHH *et al.*: Edinburgh Artery Study: prevalence of asymptomatic and symptomatic peripheral arterial disease in the general population. *Int J Epidem* **20**: 384–92, 1991
2. Dormandy J, Mahir M, Ascady G *et al.*: Fate of the patient with chronic leg ischaemia: a review article. *J Cardiovasc Surg* **30**: 50–7, 1989
3. Fowkes FGR (Ed): *Epidemiology of Peripheral Vascular Disease*. London: Springer Verlag, 1991
4. DeBakey ME, Lawrie GM, Glaeser DH: Patterns of atherosclerosis and their surgical significance. *Ann Surg* **201**: 115, 1985
5. Install RL, Loose HWC, Chamberlain J: Long-term results of double–balloon percutaneous transluminal angioplasty of the aorta and iliac arteries. *Eur J Vasc Surg* **7**: 31–6, 1993
6. Hedeman Joosten PphA, Ho GH, Breuking FA *et al.*: Percutaneous translumonal angioplasty of the infrarenal aorta: Initial outcome and long-term clinical and angiographic results. *Eur J Vasc Endovasc Surg* **12**: 210–16, 1996
7. Kumpe DA, Jones DN: Percutaneous transluminal angioplasty:radiological viewpoint. *Appl Radiol* **11**: 29–40, 1982

8. Van Andel GJ, van Erp WFM, Krepel VM *et al*.: Percutaneous transluminal dilatation of the iliac arteries: long term results. *Radiology* **156**: 321–3, 1985

9. Dalsing MC, Ehrman KO, Cikrit DF *et al*.: Iliac artery angioplasty and stents: a current experience. *In*: Yao JST, Pearce WH (Eds), *Technology in Vascular Surgery* pp. 373–86. Philadelphia: WB Saunders Company, 1992

10. Stokes KR, Strunk HM, Campbell DR *et al*.: Five-year results of iliac and femoropopliteal angioplasty in diabetic patients. *Radiology* **174**: 977–82, 1990

11. Johnston KW: Iliac arteries: Reanalysis of results of balloon angioplasty. *Radiology* **186**: 207–12, 1993

12. Kalman PG, Johnston KW: Outcome from a failed percutaneous transluminal dilatation. *Surg Gynecol Obstet* **161**: 43, 1985

13. Rutherford RB, Durham J: Percutaneous balloon angioplasty for arteriosclerosis obliterans: Long term results. *In*: Yoa JST, Pearce WH (Eds), *Technologies in Vascular Surgery* pp. 329–45. Philadelphia, WB Saunders Company, 1992

14. Colapinto RF, Stronell RD, Johnston WK: Transluminal angioplasty of complete iliac obstructions. *Am J Roent* **146**: 859–62, 1986

15. Ring EJ, Freiman DB, McLean GK *et al*.: Percutaneous recanalisation of common iliac artery occlusions: an unacceptable complication rate? *Am J Roent* **139**: 587, 1982

16. Gupta AK, Ravimandalam R, Rao VRK *et al*.: Total occlusion of the iliac arteries: Results of balloon angioplasty. *Cardiovasc Intervent Radiol* **16**: 165–77, 1993

17. Vorwerk D, Gunther RW, Schurmann K, Wendt G. Aortic and iliac stenoses: Follow-up results of stent placement after insufficient balloon angioplasty in 118 cases. *Radiology* **198**: 45–48, 1996

18. Vorwerk D, Guenther RW, Schurmann Wendt G, Peters I. Primary stent placement for chronic iliac occlusions: Follow-up results in 103 patients. *Radiology* **194**: 745–9, 1995

19. Dyet JF, Gaines PA, Nicholson AA *et al*.: Treatment of chronic iliac artery occlusions by means of percutaneous endovascular stent placement. *JVIR* **8**: 349–53, 1997

20. Blum U, Gabelmann A, Redecker M *et al*.: Percutaneous recanalization of iliac artery occlusions: Results of a prospective study. *Radiology* **189**: 536–40, 1993

21. Bosch JL, Hunink MG: Meta-analysis of the results of percutaneous transluminal angioplasty and stent placement for aortoiliac occlusive disease. *Radiology* **204**: 87–96, 1997

22. Sapoval MR, Chatellier G, Long AL *et al*.: Self expanding stents for the treatment of iliac artery obstructive lesions: Long-term success and prognostic factors *Am J Roent* **166**: 1173–9, 1996

23. Laborde JC, Palmaz JC, Rivera FJ *et al*.: Influence of anatomic distribution of atherosclerosis on the outcome of revascularization with iliac stent placement. *JVIR* **6**: 513–21, 1995

24. Brewster DC: Direct reconstruction for aortoiliac occlusive disease. *In*: Rutherford RB (Ed). *Vascular Surgery*. Philadelphia: WB Saunders Company, 1995.

25. Harrington ME, Harrington EB, Haimov M *et al*.: Axillofemoral bypass: compromised bypass for compromised patients. *J Vasc Surg* **20**: 195–201, 1994

26. Rutherford RB, Mitchell MB: Extra-anatomic bypass. *In*: Rutherford RB (Ed). *Vascular Surgery*. Philadelphia: WB Saunders Company, 1995

27. Steinmetz OK, McPhaill NV, Hajjar GE *et al*.: Endarterectomy versus angioplasty in the treatment of localised stenosis of the abdominal aorta. *Can J Surgery* **37**: 385–90, 1994

28. Holm J, Arfvidsson L, Jivegard F *et al*.: Chronic lower limb ischaemia. A prospective randomised controlled study comparing the 1-year results of vascular surgery and percutaneous transluminal angioplasty. *Eur J Vasc Surg* **5**: 517–22, 1991

29. Wolf GL, Wilson SE, Cross AP *et al*.: Surgery or balloon angioplasty for peripheral vascular disease: A randomised trial. *JVIR* **4**: 639–48, 1993

30. Lowe G: Can Claudicants be prevented from ever developing CLI. *Critical Ischaemia* **5**: 89–95, 1995

Editorial comments by C.V. Ruckley

The answer to the question in the title of this paper is 'no', for two principal reasons both of which are made clear by the authors. The first is that, despite technical advances, the radiologist in a proportion of cases is unsuccessful in achieving patency. The second is that the evidence for replacing surgery with endovascular intervention is, as yet, of poor quality.

Concerning the first reason, it is not known in published series to what extent the reported 'technical failure' rates reflect the true proportion of patients in whom endovascular management fails. Many factors obscure the true picture, not least of which is publication bias. In most units the process of selection which takes place in discussions between radiologist and surgeon eleminates a proportion of patients from the outset. This proportion is unknown and must vary widely. In the Lothian Vascular Surgical Audit, despite a fivefold increase in endovascular treatments for aorto-iliac occlusive disease in the last 10 years the annual number of open surgical reconstructions has remained constant. This suggests that the indications have changed. Until audits and trials define case mix in terms of indications, referral practices, selection processes, ratios of endovascular to surgical intervention etc. and analyse their populations on an 'intention to treat' basis the true role of each type of intervention will remain unclear.

The second reason, well emphasized by the authors, is the paucity of randomized trial data. Such trials are no small undertaking since, for credibility, they must incorporate long-term follow-ups. Until then the authors' statement that 'surgery should be restricted to those patients with severe symptoms and either bilateral diffuse disease, aorto–iliac occlusion or failed endovascular therapy' may be pragmatic, and widely practised, but it is not evidence-based.

Is Balloon Angioplasty Indicated for Intermittent Claudication? – Yes

Lars Norgren

INTRODUCTION

A generally accepted view has been that intermittent claudication does not require any invasive intervention, simply depending on a fairly good prognosis for the limb, with only a very limited proportion of patients progressing to severe ischaemia. As long as surgery was the only option, a majority of surgeons claimed they accepted this view, although quite a few patients were operated on due to what was usually called disabling claudication. Not only were reconstructions of the aortofemoral segment performed but also femoropopliteal procedures, and more astonishingly, even tibial bypasses were claimed to be useful.[1] There is, however, no consensus regarding either symptoms or haemodynamic parameters of what kind of therapy is required for intermittent claudication.

The development of endovascular procedures has changed this, and more liberal indications are accepted by most vascular surgeons. Some questions thereby arise: Is there evidence for such a liberalization, and what is the alternative, exercise - supervised or not, or surgery? To what extent do indications differ with regard to the location of the lesions?

The following are also major concerns. If a balloon angioplasty is indicated, but is not successful, should surgery be attempted or not? If a complication to a balloon angioplasty occurs, are there any limitations to what kind of secondary treatment should be allowed?

PERSONAL APPROACH

All patients suffering from intermittent claudication will be given advice regarding changing their lifestyle, especially stopping smoking, and other risk factors are taken care of as far as possible. In principle, exercise is my first option for a symptom-related treatment, irrespective of the suggested localization of the arterial lesion. If the patient wishes, he is offered initial supervision by a physiotherapist. As a rule, this kind of treatment is tried for a period of 3-6 months.

Should it appear that the patient is not improving or for other reasons claims that he needs another kind of treatment, a subsequent decision follows consideration of the patient's age, his needs to walk, his grade of disability, and not least the probable location of the occlusive disease.

A younger patient, claiming he cannot fulfill his work, or continue important leisure activities will in most instances be accepted for a further work-up, especially if he has a proximal lesion, indicated by a weak or absent femoral pulse. My requirements are rather more for older patients and for those with a femoropopliteal block as the clinical finding.

For those patients accepted, my next step is an angiography, at present preceded by an ultrasonography, which will probably replace many angiographies in the future. If a lesion suited for an angioplasty is found, an immediate decision is taken and the treatment follows during the same catheterization. The requirement is that the interventional radiologist and the vascular surgeon can communicate immediately, something which rarely fails. In principle, the decision to treat is easiest with a short iliac lesion, even an occlusion, and more difficult with a long (>10 cm) femoral lesion. I accept femoral stenosis and also occlusion, as long as I and the radiologist believe it might work. This kind of decision can only be taken when the vascular and radiology team know each other very well. A below knee-lesion will not be accepted in a claudicant, if it is not a secondary finding when a femoral block is treated and it is found that the runoff is severely restricted. This finding is extremely rare in a patient suffering only intermittent claudication.

A second question deals with the use of stents. Are they needed? From a practical point of view, it is most reasonable that they are used if a dissection, an intimal tear or any other local complication occurs with the angioplasty and is supposed to restrict the chance of a good outcome. Again, if it happens in the iliac artery this repair seems more reasonable than if it happens in the femoral artery.

If for any reason the outcome of an angioplasty is not what was expected, another question is raised: is the patient now a case for surgery? Again it depends. If a simple femorofemoral crossover bypass can be performed or any other limited procedure,it may be justified, while age and grade of disability now have an even greater impact. No doubt there are patients requiring an aortofemoral reconstruction, or a femoropopliteal bypass above the knee that will also be accepted. If a bypass to the below-knee popliteal artery is required I hesitate and a bypass to the crural arteries is in my view never indicated because of claudication.

WHAT EVIDENCE EXISTS?

To restate my view: the first choice for treatment of intermittent cludication is exercise; second, angioplasty is fairly often accepted, even below the groin, but above the knee. Surgery plays a limited role, but is an option if there are strong indications that the patient may benefit from this treatment.

There is little robust evidence to support any opinion concerning treatment of intermittent claudication. If only strong evidence is accepted, then possibly exercise treatment is justified. With reference to two reviews of the clinical effectiveness of exercise[2,3] a recent American Heart Association Medical/Scientific statement[4] claims that 'exercise therapy is the most consistently effective medical treatment' for intermittent claudication. Of 28 reviewed trials, nine were controlled or randomized controlled. The main outcome was an increase of the maximum walking distance by about 100%. These data are relevant as long as this increase also means a reasonable improvement of the patient's quality of life, which has rarely been discussed.

Only a few studies have been performed to compare angioplasty with other kinds of treatment in such large patient populations that reliable evidence might be achieved. Another drawback with most studies is that they combine outcomes for both severe ischaemia and claudication.

The following chapter on this subject by Andrew Bradbury includes studies negative to angioplasty. Most of these studies are concerned with the fact that secondary procedures are to some extent required and that recurrences during medium to long-term follow-up are not uncommon. Some other evidence exists, though not from randomized controlled studies. Johnston analysed 584 angioplasties for stenosis and 82 procedures for occlusion of the iliac arteries with a 1-year patency of 77% and 73% respectively.[5] The complication rate was low, 3-4%. After 3 years the primary patency rates were reduced to 61% and 59% respectively. In a recent study[6] Zeitler et al. treating 286 iliac stenoses also had a 3-year primary patency of 63%. It is not possible to evaluate the benefits to patients in these studies. Compared with the Oxford study[7,8] and the Edinburgh study[9] described by Bradbury, it might well be that although the treated lesion is patent, the walking ability had not changed or had been reduced again. On the other hand it seems to be taken for granted that a relapse of claudication symptoms necessarily implies a restenosis or reocclusion. It has been shown, in a small study, that a considerable proportion of recurrencies (80%) depends on a new lesion.[10] Whether this could be an explanation in the UK studies is not possible to interpret.

An interesting decision and cost-effectiveness analysis was made by Hunink et al.,[11] purely for femoropopliteal disease, but dealing with all reported studies for both intermittent claudication and severe ischaemia. One of the conclusions was that a 65-year-old man with intermittent claudication due to a femoropopliteal stenosis or occlusion gained quality adjusted life time with reduced expenditures if an angioplasty was performed.

Comparing surgery and angioplasty only a few studies are available and conclusive. Wolf and co-workers[12] randomized 252 patients with either iliac or femoropopliteal lesions, finding no differences in clinical outcome after 4 years. One-third of patients randomized to angioplasty required an additional procedure during the follow-up period. Also with an high initial success rate, the late outcome is frequently severely reduced. In the study by Johnston[5] the 5-year patency was 63% for iliac lesions with good runoff, and 51% with restricted runoff. Claudication also offers better long-term outcome than severe ischaemia with a 5-year patency of 76% vs 29% .[13]

Is there a difference between iliac and femoropopliteal angioplasty concerning the outcome? Only poor evidence exists for long-term results,[14] concluding better outcome for iliac lesions.

It is frequently said that there are two prerequisites for a good outcome from angioplasty; one is that the lesion should be less than 10 cm, and the second that a skilled radiologist is required, which is an understatement. It is not common to find any comment that a 'skilled vascular surgeon' is required.

A simple conclusion is that the early success rate for percutaneous transluminal balloon angioplasty used for claudication is good, both for iliac and femoropopliteal lesions, while the long-term patency does not have such a good rate of success. Common practice tells that angioplasty has replaced surgery and probably also extended the indications for invasive treatments of claudicants. This may be fully acceptable as long as complications are limited even though the long-term effect is not optimal. The Swedish Vascular Registry (Swedvasc) has helped to study time trends and obviously the use of angioplasty has increased dramatically during a 10-year period.[15] Table 1 shows the increase of angioplasty for intermittent claudication in a percentage of all procedures in the three various locations from 1987 until 1996. Apparently more distal angioplasties are also now performed. Table 2 also depicts complication rates, which have been reasonably low for the angioplasties. Swedvasc allows follow-up for 1 year, and for that reason any long-term outcome cannot be discussed.

Although it is generally seen that long-term outcome is not very good after angioplasty in any location, it is obvious that this treatment is frequently used. Does this mean that vascular surgeons, who in many health care systems are the only referring physicians, are misled? Maybe not everyone is aware of the long-term outcome, but on the other hand taking into consideration that claudicants have a limited life expectancy due to other manifestations of atherosclerosis, it may be very relevant to accept a treatment which gives relief for definitely 1 year, and to a great

Table 1. Percutaneous transluminal balloon angioplasty in percentages of all procedures

Year	Aorto–iliaco femoral	Femoropopliteal (above knee)	Distal (below knee)
1987	28.8	25.7	0
1988	37.7	38.4	10.4
1989	49.5	46.6	15.7
1990	40.3	45.0	17.8
1991	52.1	43.5	17.4
1992	55.3	38.5	8.2
1993	61.8	45.2	17.0
1994	65.2	46.3	21.4
1995	72.9	49.2	31.3
1996	73.5	50.0	35.3

Table 2. Outcome 30 days after 8372 procedures due to intermittent claudication

	Open reconstruction: 4436			Angioplasty: 3936		
	Aorto-iliaco-femoral	Femoro-popliteal (above knee)	Distal (below knee)	Aorto-iliaco-femoral	Femoro-popliteal (above knee)	Distal (below knee)
Procedures	1493	2018	925	2088	1637	211
Amputation and/or mortality (%)	2.2	1.4	2.0	0.4	0.6	1.0

extent for much longer. A problem is that angioplasty studies usually mix the indications of severe ischaemia and intermittent claudication and infrequently the impact on the quality of life is discussed. There is, however, data from Cook *et al.*, using the EuroQuol questionnaire, finding that the quality of life is significantly impaired in patients with intermittent claudication, but it is also significantly improved after an angioplasty.[16] The Edinburgh study also gave evidence for at least a short-term improvement of the quality of life after angioplasty.[9]

From the relevant literature and from personal experience, it is still my understanding that angioplasty is a treatment of choice for many claudicants, provided exercise has failed to give relief and risk factors have been carefully dealt with. A careful audit is required to make sure that the rate of complications and failures do not increase due to too liberal and possibly sliding indications. Some reports have pointed out that the proportion of lesions amenable for an angioplasty is very limited (around 10%), and theoretically this could imply that nine out of ten angiographies are not necessary, provided the next treatment recommendation is continued exercise. First, in patients with intermittent claudication it seems evident that the proportion of patients who in reality can be treated is higher, even though more prospective studies are required to prove this. Second, this specific group of patients may be investigated by a duplex scan and only those with a lesion, which apparently is suited for an angioplasty have to undergo an angiography. Whether this is cost-effective has to be proven.

Surgery has a more limited role, but is acceptable under certain conditions as earlier described. It is also most important to state that angioplasties should only be performed provided a vascular surgeon is available to take care of possible complications.

Stenting on the other hand has a very limited role, and should only be applied with complications such as dissection and intimal tearing, which is easier treated this way than by surgery. One study which is proposing to produce strong evidence,[17] has shown a significant benefit from the use of stents in iliac lesions. For femoropopliteal lesions few studies have discussed stents in an appropriate way. Some evidence exists, however,[18, 19] that the risk of intimal hyperplasia overwhelms the possible early benefit of the stent.

FUTURE STUDIES

There is little reason to compare surgery and angioplasty, as they are in most instances not used in the same situation. The important issue is whether angioplasty on top of exercise provides an improvement of the quality of life and if this improvement is cost-effective, considering return to work, less pension payments and a better social life. This kind of study can only be performed for intermittent claudication. Long-term follow-up is a prerequisite, although patency after 5 years may have little to do with the patient's impression of his life conditions. Again quality of life measures should be reported. The same study protocol may be used for both iliac and femoropopliteal lesions, although, results should be interpreted separately.

Second, the question has to be addressed of whether ultrasonography to find the lesions amenable to angioplasty, reducing the number of unnecessary angiographies, is cost-effective ?

The magnitude of reduction of the pressure gradient over a stenosis has not been sufficiently examined in studies of risk factors. It may well be that a less satisfactory outcome of a treatment depends on either a limited pressure decrease over the stenosis from the beginning, or that the gradient has not been adequately reduced by the angioplasty, although patency is achieved. It should therefore be a requirement to measure the initial gradient and its change in a prospective way, also in unrandomized studies to be planned. The best results would appear if all centres dealing with angioplasty agreed to perform and report pressure measurements.

CONCLUSIONS AND COMMENTS

Detailed prospective study protocols are needed to achieve the quality of evidence required to determine the role of angioplasty. On the other hand, common sense may sometimes be a relevant guide in decision-taking. Angioplasty of iliac arteries and to some extent the femoropopliteal segment has in practice been shown to be an acceptable treatment, such that scientific conclusive evidence may never be available. Guidelines, on the other hand, may be helpful to limit the role of angioplasty.

When purchasers of health care require that a treatment works, they have to realize that few fully accepted treatments have been accepted on first-grade evidence. Cost-effectiveness is important, but also short-term benefit of a treatment may be valuable. Not all positive outcome from any treatment can be easily transformed into economic terms.

It seems that angioplasty performed on strict indications, and after exercise has been tried, may be recommended, provided exercise continues afterwards and risk factors are properly reduced.

REFERENCES

1. Conte MS, Belkin M, Donaldson MC et al.: Femorotibial bypass for claudication: do results justify an aggressive approach? *J Vasc Surg* **21**: 873, 880; Discussion 880–1, 1995
2. Ernst E, Fialka V: A review of the clinical effectiveness of exercise therapy for intermittent claudication. *Arch Intern Med* **153**: 2357–60, 1993
3. Radack K. Wyderski RJ: Conservative management of intermittent claudication. *Ann Intern Med* **113**: 135–146, 1990
4. Weitz JI, Byhrne J, Clagett GP et al.: Diagnosis and treatment of chronic arterial insufficiency of the lower extremities: A critical review. *Circulation* **94**: 3026–49, 1996
5. Johnston KW: Iliac arteries: Reanalysis of results of balloon angioplasty. *Radiology* **186**: 207–12, 1993
6. Zeitler E, Lammer J, König J et al.: German-Austria Multicenter Study (GAMS): a randomized controlled trial of platelet inhibition therapy vs placebo after successful iliac PTA. (in prep.) 1998

7. Creasy TS, McMillan PJ, Fletcher EWL *et al.*: Is percuteneous transluminal angioplasty better than exercise for claudication? Preliminary results from a randomized controlled trial. *Eur J Vasc Surg* **4**: 135–40, 1990

8. Perkins J, Collin J: Balloon angioplasty versus exercise for intermittent claudication. *Critical Ischemia* **6**: 57–62, 1997

9. Whyman MR, Fowkes FGR, Kerracher EMG *et al.*: Randomized controlled trial of percutaneous transluminal angioplasty for intermittent claudication. *Eur J Vasc Endovasc Surg* 12: 167–72, 1996

10. Thorvinger B, Norgren L, Albrechtsson U: Patency after iliac and femoropopliteal angioplasty. *Acta Radiol* **33**: 29–30, 1992

11. Hunink MGM, Wong JB, Donaldson MC *et al.*: Revascularization for femoropopliteal disease. A decision and cost-effectiveness analysis. *J Am Med Assoc* **274**: 165–71, 1995

12. Wolf GL, Wilson SE, Cross AP *et al.*: for the principal investigators and their associates of Veterans Administration Cooperative Study Number 199. Surgery or balloon angioplasty for peripheral vascular disease: a randomized clinical trial. *J Vasc Interv Radiol* 4: 639–48, 1993

13. Stokes KR, Strunk HM, Campbell DR *et al.*: Five-year results of iliac and femoropopliteal angioplasty in diabetic patients. *Radiology* 174: 977–82, 1990

14. Casarella WJ: Noncoronary angioplasty. *Curr Probl Cardiol* **11**: 141–74, 1986

15. Swedvasc. The Swedish Vascular Registry. 10-year experience. (in press) 1997

16. Cook TA, O'Regan M, Galland RB: Quality of life following percutaneous transluminal angioplasty for claudication. *Eur J Vasc Endovasc Surg* **11**: 191–4, 1996

17. Richter GM, Noeldge G, Roeren T *et al.*: Further analysis of the randomized trial: primary iliac stenting vs PTA. In: Kollath J, Liermann D (Eds), *Stents* III. Schnetztor, Konstanz 1995

18. Gray BH, Sullivan TM, Childs MB *et al.*: High incidence of restenosis/reocclusion of stents in the percutaneous treatment of long-segment superficial femoral artery disease after suboptimal angioplasty. *J Vasc Surg* **25**: 74–83, 1997

19. Zdanowski Z, Albrechtsson U, Lundin A *et al.*: Percutaneous transluminal angioplasty and stenting versus angioplasty alone for femoropopliteal occlusions. A randomized controlled study. (in press) 1997

Editorial comments by C.V. Ruckley

The approach to claudication could be caricatured by saying that the radiologist is interested in the radiological lesion, the surgeon is interested in the limb, the physician in the whole patient and the public health doctor in outcomes for the population. All would protest at this oversimplification but there is a large enough grain of truth to account for the wide differences in published perspectives.

Norgren concedes that what clinical trial data do exist show no advantage for percutaneous transluminal balloon angioplasty (PTA) over conservative management, but rightly argues that further trials are required. In the meantime he describes an approach which most vascular teams would endorse (and currently practise) namely a broadly conservative i.e. non-interventionist approach to claudication with selective use of PTA in patients whose work or leisure is restricted. If PTA could be combined with effective control of risk factors and/or mechanisms determining restenosis its place would be secure even in claudicants.

The difficulties in everyday clinical practice are that patients do not find it easy to understand or accept the reasons for withholding treatment, that few surgeons are temperamentally suited to spending the considerable time required to explain in full the conservative rationale, to educate in the control of risk factors and influence life style and find it much simpler to request duplex scans and that the radiologist finds it difficult to resist a lesion which ostensibly is suitable for angioplasty. Few would disagree with Norgren's statement that the early success rate for PTA in claudication is good. The immediate response is usually technically impressive and symptomatically gratifying. In a group of patients with multifocal disease and high premature mortality from thrombotic events at other sites, late patency does not equate with symptomatic outcome or quality of life. There being no evidence that late outcome is superior after PTA the question currently boils down to whether short-term benefit is worthwhile and the debate focusses on the criteria for selection. Published series have commonly mixed mild and severe symptoms and proximal and distal disease.

Claudication is so common and the economic implications of interventionist policies are so great, in the context of increasingly limited health care resources, that one can only strongly endorse Norgren's search for first-grade evidence and his view that detailed prospective study protocols are required.

Is Balloon Angioplasty Indicated for Intermittent Claudication? – No

Andrew W. Bradbury

GENERAL APPROACH

The prognosis for claudication is benign in terms of local progression of ischaemia to a point where revascularization is required to avert amputation. However, as a marker for widespread arterial disease and a two- to threefold increase in mortality from cardiovascular and cerebrovascular events, intermittent claudication is anything but benign. Assuming history and examination findings support the diagnosis, and that there is no evidence of an unusual arterial cause such as cystic disease of the popliteal artery or an entrapment syndrome, the priorities are to:

1. Explain to the patient the natural history of the condition and reassure them that by following medical advice they can reduce the risk of losing their limb to a very low level.
2. Counsel the patient about how their lifestyle may have brought about their symptoms; how it places them at risk of heart attack and stroke, and how they can change it for the better. This would include advice about cessation of smoking and exercise. Unfortunately, I do not have the resources to offer a supervised exercise programme. Patients are routinely prescribed aspirin.
3. Screen and treat the patient for recognized risk factors such as hyperlipidaemia and diabetes.
4. Exclude the life and limb threatening manifestations of peripheral arterial disease that frequently accompany claudication; principally, aortic aneurysm and carotid artery stenosis.
5. Ensure that co-existent medical conditions are optimally managed.

I would normally review the patient again after 6 weeks to discuss the results of investigations and then at 3–6 months to monitor progress. If the patient's symptoms have stabilized or improved at this stage, and there are no other 'surgical' vascular problems such as aneurysm or carotid stenosis to monitor, then I would normally discharge the patient back to GP care. If the patients symptoms are deteriorating or they are in a high risk group then clinic review is continued.

The above approach maximizes collateralization and minimizes the risk of disease progression and the great majority of patients respond well. A proportion fail to improve and their symptoms impair their quality of life. A few patients will progress to critical limb ischaemia. It is in these patients that I consider intervention. Willingness to contemplate percutaneous transluminal balloon angioplasty (PTA) depends primarily upon whether disease is aorto–iliac or infrainguinal. The former responds better to both surgery and PTA and tends to affect younger patients who may be at risk of losing their livelihood. It may also be possible to remedy bilateral symptoms from aorto–iliac occlusion with a single procedure; and it is my impression that the body's ability to collateralize around aorto–iliac disease is less than at the femoropopliteal level.

AORTO–ILIAC DISEASE

I would arrange either an outpatient intravenous digital subtraction angiography (IV-DSA) or duplex ultrasound depending upon the build of the patient. If the investigation shows unilateral disease and the contralateral side looks adequate to support a crossover graft then I would perform this in preference to PTA. If the donor side were diseased and amenable to endovascular intervention then I would discuss PTA, and in most cases primary stent placement, with my radiological colleague. If there is bilateral disease and my radiological colleague felt it was amenable to PTA, with or without stent placement, either as two separate procedures or as a 'kissing' balloon or stent procedure then I would opt for endovascular treatment. If this were not possible then I would perform aortic surgery. Regardless of what intervention is chosen it is vital that the patient and the family are fully aware of all the risks and benefits of intervention and that this is recorded in the case-notes. Sooner or later a patient will die or lose a limb as a result of intervention for a condition which was not *per se* life- or limb-threatening and one does not want to be compromised morally, ethically or medico-legally when that occurs.

INFRAINGUINAL DISEASE

Infrainguinal PTA for claudication is almost never indicated. Occasionally in a patient with diminished but intact distal pulses and a bruit over the adductor hiatus IV-DSA will show a discrete (1–2cm), haemodynamically significant superficial femoral artery stenosis and in this circumstance I would contemplate PTA. There is no controlled evidence for this approach but I have seen good long-term patency from such procedures and I believe that it reduces the risk of superficial femoral artery occlusion.

I would also consider PTA in patients who present with 'blue toe syndrome' although, admittedly, this is not often associated with claudication. At the present time I do not think that infrapopliteal PTA for claudication is indicated and there appears to be no place for infrainguinal stent placement.

CRITICAL LIMB ISCHAEMIA

Only a small number of patients who are already consulting me for claudication progress to this. Even then, the critical ischaemia that these patients develop is often less severe, some might call it subcritical ischaemia,[1] than typically presents *de novo*. There are a number of reasons why this may be so. My view is that PTA has little to offer in full-blown critical ischaemia that meets the European Consensus haemodynamic criteria.[2] In subcritical ischaemia, early rest pain and small trophic lesions often respond to conservative therapy. In some patients there may be a place for PTA although at the present time there are no data on which to base definite practice and each patient must be considered on a case-by-case basis.

EVIDENCE FOR THE AUTHOR'S APPROACH

Complications and long-term patency

There have been numerous uncontrolled series documenting complication and patency rates after PTA for claudication. Although reported data vary widely an average would be a combined mortality and limb loss of 1–2%; major morbidity of <5%, minor morbidity of 5–15%, and a 3–5 year haemodynamic patency (usually determined by a fall of ABPI > 0.10–0.15) of 50% at 5 years.[3] Virtually all of these reports confirm the superiority of aorto–iliac over infrainguinal angioplasty.

Randomized controlled trials of PTA for claudication

The Oxford group[4] randomized 20 patients to PTA and 16 to exercise therapy. The two groups were well matched in terms of age, sex, smoking status, and arteriographic extent of disease. Two PTAs failed and two other patients required surgery for deteriorating symptoms. One patient in the exercise group had PTA. After PTA the ankle brachial pressure index (ABPI) was significantly improved at 3, 6 and 9 months but this haemodynamic improvement was not accompanied by any significant increase in mean maximum walking distance. By contrast, in the exercise group, despite no increase in mean ABPI, mean maximal walking distance increased progressively at 3, 6 and 9 months. In a follow-up report[5] 56 patients with unilateral stable, lower limb claudication were randomized to either PTA or exercise treatment and followed 3-monthly for 15 months. Thirty-seven patients were available for late follow-up up to 6 years. Although PTA was associated with a significant increase in ABPI, in terms of improved walking performance the patients undergoing exercise treatment again experienced a better clinical result in the long-term although the improvement following exercise lagged about 6 months behind that of the PTA group. Patients with superficial femoral artery disease did particularly well with exercise. The overall prognosis of the patients was good with only two undergoing amputation.

The most obvious conclusion to be drawn from this study would seem to be that PTA confers no advantage over best medical therapy in the medium to long term. However, it is interesting to read a discussion of this trial in a recent review article where Hunink,[3] a long-term advocate of PTA, implies that best medical therapy was only better because more patients in the exercise group may have stopped smoking and because it was actually contralateral disease that limited the walking distance of those patients treated by PTA.[3] Paradoxically, these comments in support of PTA, rather than suggesting the superiority of angioplasty, only serve to highlight the benefits of medical therapy, not least of which is that it refocuses attention away from the lesion and its haemodynamics on to the patient, their life-style, and their quality of life.

In Edinburgh, Whyman *et al*. 1996[6] randomized 62 claudicants with either short femoral stenoses or occlusions (n = 47) or iliac stenoses (n = 15) to best medical therapy (n = 32) or best medical therapy and PTA (n = 30). Medical therapy comprised aspirin and advice on exercise and smoking. At 6 months PTA patients had significantly higher ABPI, greater walking distance and less pain on the Nottingham Health Profile than the control group. However, at 2 years the two groups did not differ significantly in terms of reported or treadmill maximum walking distance or distance to onset of claudication. Although the PTA group had significantly fewer occluded arteries and a lesser degree of stenosis in patient arteries this did not translate into a significant advantage in terms of walking or quality of life as determined by the Nottingham Health Profile.

The Edinburgh data indicate that only a small proportion of patients with claudication have lesions amenable to angioplasty. Even in this highly selected and favourable group of patients with limited disease, PTA conferred no advantage over best medical therapy in the long term despite the fact that the medical therapy offered could be considered suboptimal by today's standards in that no formal exercise programme was available[7] and that hyperlipidaemia was not specifically sought and corrected.[8] Furthermore, with regard to identifying patients suitable for PTA it was clear that duplex was not as reliable as originally thought.[9] Thus of 600 claudicants initially assessed clinically, 425 were thought potentially suitable for randomization and underwent duplex. Of these, 94 were still thought to be suitable and underwent angiography. However, on the basis of angiography a further 32 patients were excluded leaving only 62 patients (10%) for randomization. Even if one were to argue that PTA might offer an advantage in the patients with even more limited disease than were included in this study, and there is no suggestion from these data that this is the case as these are the very patients who do best with medical therapy, then one would have to screen very many patients to identify them. This may not be priority in a struggling health service.

Randomized controlled trial of PTA in lower limb ischaemia of mixed severity

There have been two trials comparing PTA with surgery in series of patients with ischaemia of mixed severity, some of whom were claudicants.

Over a 6-year period, 102 patients with 'severe' lower limb ischaemia (rest pain and/or ulceration), or claudication 'resistant' to exercise therapy, were randomized to either PTA or surgery.[10] Only patients with occlusions or significant (> 75%) stenoses 6cm or less in length within the iliac, femoral or popliteal arteries were included. Patients had to be suitable for either therapy as judged by a surgical and radiological consensus. For these reasons, the study population comprised only 5% of their total patient population with lower limb ischaemia over the period of recruitment. The groups were well matched; 53 patients (23 claudicants) were randomized to PTA and 49 (18 claudicants) to surgery. Patients were reviewed at 1, 3 and 6 months and some underwent repeat angiography at 1 year. The primary and secondary patencies, analysed on an intention to treat basis, were for PTA (60% vs 62%) and surgery (77% vs 67%) respectively. There were four haematomas in the PTA group; two of which required surgical exploration. A further three patients developed limb-threatening ischaemia after PTA and underwent successful emergency vascular reconstruction. In the surgical group five patients required re-operation; two for bleeding and three for acute thrombosis. In the PTA group, ten interventions were required; four repeat PTAs and six vascular reconstructions. In the surgery group, four surgical re-interventions were required. Eleven amputations were necessary; three in the PTA group (one of whom presented initially with claudication) and eight in the surgery group (all of whom had presented with rest pain and/or ulceration). Six patients died in the PTA group and four in the surgery group. Patients treated by PTA had a significantly shorter hospital stay.

Wilson and colleagues[11] conducted a trial comparing PTA with surgery in the management of iliac, superficial femoral and popliteal occlusive disease of various anatomic and clinical severities through the Veteran's Administration Medical Centers (VAMC). An initial study had shown that 1320 angiograms were obtained annually for claudication, rest pain and/or tissue loss in VAMCs. Of these, it was estimated that 26% and 23% were suitable iliac and/or femoropopliteal PTA, respectively. Eligibility was determined by significant stenosis (>80%) or occlusion (<10cm); an ABPI of <0.9; and the presence of claudication (less than 'two blocks'), rest pain and 'impending gangrene'. Radiologists and surgeons independently assessed the arterial lesions to determine whether PTA and surgery were appropriate. Despite the apparently large number of cases available, over a 4-year period only 263 patients were randomized, 126 received surgery and 129 PTA. Although the two groups were well matched the authors specifically point out that, because the arterial lesions had to be suitable for both surgery and PTA, the severity of ischaemia was less than that of their general population. In fact, claudication was the principal indication for intervention (184/255, 72%). Of 163 patients with an iliac index lesion, 108 had claudication and 45 rest pain; and of 100 patients with femoropopliteal lesion, 73 had claudication and 27 rest pain. The immediate failure rate for PTA was 15.5%, the morbidity rate 17.1% but there was no mortality. The operative mortality was 0.8% and morbidity 13.5%. At a median (maximum) follow-up of 2 (4.5) years, there were 50 deaths (20%) (28 surgery, 22 PTA) and 24 major amputations (13 surgery, 11 PTA). If analysis is confined to only those patients who had a technically successful procedure then both PTA and surgery have a similar durability, both in iliac and femoropopliteal lesions, in terms of death, amputations, ABPI and late interventions. However, if results are analysed on an intention to treat basis, then the high immediate failure rate for PTA translates in to a significant late advantage for surgery in the iliac but not the femoropopliteal group. The authors concluded that PTA has a higher initial technical failure rate; in patients whose stage of disease permits a choice between PTA and surgery then both therapies (if PTA is technically successful) have similar haemodynamic results; and that an unsuccessful PTA does not appear to prejudice the results of surgical revascularization.

Despite small patient numbers and variable case mix, both in terms of clinical and anatomic severity and site of disease, it is probably safe to conclude from these studies that less than 5–10% of claudicants are suitable for conventional PTA and that the relatively good secondary patency rates observed for PTA were due largely to subsequent surgical intervention for technical failure, immediate complications or restenosis.

PTA for severe or critical limb ischaemia

There have been no prospective controlled trials addressing specifically the indications for PTA in patients with critical limb ischaemia. However, there have been a number of non-randomized, uncontrolled studies.[12–15] Most of these authors concluded that many patients with severe limb ischaemia are unsuitable for angioplasty and the number who benefit are small. However, some groups have taken the view that since PTA does not seem to prejudice subsequent bypass, rather than use PTA for the high risk cases unsuitable for surgery, why not use it routinely in the first instance wherever possible, reserving surgery for those cases in which PTA is either technically impossible or fails.

The Leicester group have published a number of papers examining the consequences of such a policy.[16,17] At a minimum follow-up of 1 year, they achieved a limb salvage of 79% for surgery, 81% for PTA, and 55% for non-intervention. These results lead them to conclude that 'a clinical management algorithm centred on the use of PTA produces durable results at 1 year in the majority of patients equivalent to surgery'. At first glance these data support a policy of treating patients with severe limb ischaemia with angioplasty rather than surgery wherever possible. However, patient survival was 90% for surgery and 78% for angioplasty; emergency surgery was required to deal with the complications of angioplasty in 6.2% of cases; and death from on-going ischaemia occurred in 11% of cases after angioplasty and not after surgery. The authors also point out that limb salvage rates were biased towards PTA because patients undergoing it subsequently underwent surgery in a significant number of cases.

Infrapopliteal angioplasty

Sivanathan and co-workers[18] from Leeds evaluated the results of tibial PTA in 38 patients who underwent crural angioplasty with an overall technical success rate was 96%. Patients were followed for a mean of 21 months. At last follow-up 58% had improved clinically, 43% had improvements in limb isotope blood flow studies, and 52% an increase in ABPI. The authors conclude that PTA should be the first treatment option in patients with infrapopliteal arterial disease needing intervention, whenever it is technically feasible. Buckenham[19] reported on 14 infrapopliteal angioplasties performed in 13 patients with critical limb ischaemia. Technical success was achieved in all patients with an average increase in ABPI of 0.5 above a median pre-procedure ABPI of 0.22 in non-diabetics. At an average follow-up of 8 (range 1–18) months, 11 patients showed early clinical improvement. In 40 consecutive infrapopliteal PTAs performed for claudication in 20 cases (50%) and critical limb ischaemia in the remainder there was one technical failure, no limb loss, no deaths and no complications requiring surgical intervention.[20] The primary and secondary symptomatic patencies at 24 months were 59% and 79% respectively. Subintimal PTA as pioneered by Bolia appears to be a major advance with regard to opening up long arterial occlusions both at femoropopliteal level and in the crural arteries but there are no controlled data.[21]

THE EDINBURGH EXPERIENCE

When PTA first came in to clinical practice it was directed almost solely at large, proximal, high flow vessels and towards stenoses rather than occlusions. Over the last 10 years, with the advent of new technologies, the growing technical competence and confidence of the interventional radiologists, and the increasing pressure on surgical resources, there has been a steady expansion in both the perceived clinical and anatomic indications for PTA.

Like several other vascular centres[22] the Edinburgh Unit has seen a tripling of PTA for lower limb ischaemia over the last 15 years;[23] although enthusiasm for PTA in patients with claudication has understandably waned following publication of our trial data indicating no long-term benefit (Fig. 1). This increase in endovascular

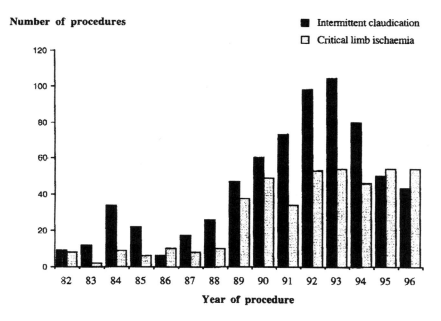

Fig. 1.   Percutaneous transluminal angioplasty performed in the Edinburgh Regional Vascular Unit for lower limb ischaemia, 1982–1996.

activity has not been associated with a reduction in surgical revascularization nor, regrettably, in major amputation rates.[24] It is also apparent from our own data that the proportion of PTAs being performed for critical limb ischaemia, as well as the proportion of PTAs in the distal leg, has increased significantly (Fig. 2). There is no doubt that these changes have been technology and circumstance driven and are not supported by any form of scientific evidence that this is the correct thing to do. Indeed, even in large calibre, high-flow vessels affected by limited disease confined to a single level, whenever PTA has been compared with other treatment modalities it has been found wanting.[25,26] The direct consequence of this policy has been an

Number of procedures

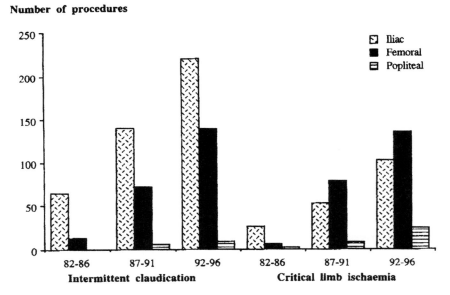

Fig. 2. Changes in the clinical indication and anatomical site of percutaneous transluminal angioplasty performed in the Edinburgh Vascular Unit between 1982 and 1986.

increasing technical failure and complication rate and an increasing proportion of patients who, despite an apparently technically successful procedure, gain no short- or long-term clinical benefit (Fig. 3).

WHAT FUTURE TRIALS WOULD BE HELPFUL?

Most patients being offered a particular treatment will assume, unless informed otherwise by their doctor, that it is of proven efficacy, has been compared with and found to be superior to the alternatives, and associated with a well defined and satisfactory level of risk. If these criteria are not met then the patient is essentially undergoing an experimental procedure. Despite the fact that a form of PTA was first described more than 30 years ago,[27] and that since then millions of procedures have been performed world-wide, it is immediately apparent from reviewing the available literature that in most respects PTA falls well within this 'experimental' category, and that the indications for PTA are far from clear.[28,29] This state of affairs is the result of an almost complete absence of properly conducted trials. Although attempts are currently being made to rectify this situation, at the present time vascular surgeons contemplating PTA for their patients have very little scientific data on which to base their judgements.

There is little doubt that PTA, with or without stent placement, has a valuable role to play in the management of peripheral vascular disease. Unfortunately, at the present time, it is not possible to state with any certainty or precision what

Number of procedures

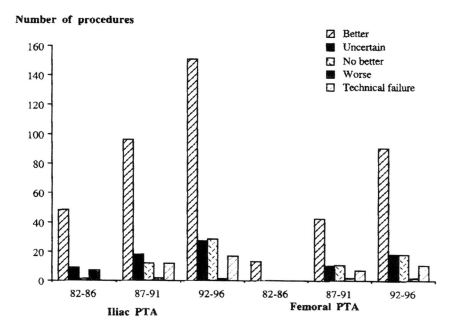

Fig. 3.   Clinical status at first post-procedure clinical visit following percutaneous transluminal angioplasty for lower limb ischaemia.

that role might be. In many areas of cardiovascular surgery and medicine, large randomized controlled trials have and are being conducted in order to determine best practice. There is an urgent need to do the same in the field of endovascular technology.

With regard to PTA and claudication, my own view is that infrainguinal angioplasty has been proven ineffective and that there is no need to perform yet more trials. Of much greater merit would be a trial specifically looking at aorto-iliac PTA and stent placement for claudication. In such a trial PTA should be compared with surgery and best medical therapy. Assessment of quality of life and cost-effectiveness should be included in any proposed trial together with late follow-up   data.   Patency   will   have   to   be   assessed   symptomatically, haemodynamically and anatomically by duplex or angiography as there is often little relationship between the three and merely choosing one will inevitably be misleading. Patients will have to be entered in sufficiently large numbers that subgroup analysis will be possible and statistical power acceptable. Such trials will almost certainly have to be multicentre. At the present time several trials of PTA in lower limb schaemia are in the early stages of preparation. One can only hope that government and charitable funding bodies appreciate the importance of such studies both in terms of clinical efficacy and in the interests of ensuring scarce clinical resources are used cost-effectively.

REFERENCES

1. Wolfe JHN, Wyatt MG: Critical and subcritical ischaemia. *Eur J Vasc Endovasc Surg* **13**; 578–82, 1997
2. Second European consensus on critical limb ischaemia. *Eur J Vasc Surg* **6** (Suppl A); 1–32, 1992
3. Hunink MGM, Meyerovitz MF: Infra-inguinal percutaneous transluminal balloon angioplasty. *Advances in Vascular Surgery* pp. 135–59. St Louis: Mosby Year Book, 1994
4. Creasy TS, McMillan PJ, Fletcher EWL *et al.*: Is percutaneous transluminal angioplasty better than exercise for claudication? Preliminary results from a randomised controlled trial. *Eur J Vasc Surg* **4**; 135–40, 1990
5. Perkins J, Collins J: Balloon angioplasty versus exercise for intermittent claudication. *Critical Ischaemia* **6**; 57–62, 1997
6. Whyman MR, Fowkes FGR, Kerracher EMG *et al.*: Randomised controlled trial of percutaneous transluminal angioplasty for intermittent claudication. *Eur J Vasc Endovasc Surg* **12**; 167–72, 1996
7. Patterson RB, Pinto B, Marcus B *et al.*: Value of a supervised exercise programme for the therapy of arterial claudication. *J Vasc Surg* **25**; 312–9, 1997
8. Haq IU, Yeo WW, Jackson PR, Ramsay LE: The case for cholesterol reduction in peripheral arterial disease. *Critical Ischaemia* **7**; 15–22, 1997
9. Whyman MR, Gillespie IN, Ruckley CV *et al.*: Screening patients with claudication from femoropopliteal disease before angioplasty using Doppler colour flow imaging. *Br J Surg* **79**; 907–9, 1992
10. Holm J, Arfvidsson B, Jivegard L *et al.*: Chronic lower limb ischaemia. A prospective randomised controlled study comparing 1 year results of vascular surgery and percutaneous transluminal angioplasty (PTA). *Eur J Vasc Surg* **5**; 517–22, 1991
11. Wilson SE, Wolf GL, Cross AP: Percutaneous transluminal angioplasty versus operation for peripheral arteriosclerosis. Report of a prospective randomised controlled trial in a selected group of patients. *J Vasc Surg* **9**; 1–9, 1989
12. Blair JM, Gwertz BL, Moosa H *et al.*: Percutaneous transluminal angioplasty versus surgery for limb-threatening ischaemia. *J Vasc Surg* 698–703, 1989
13. Ray SA, Minty I, Buckenham TM *et al.*: Clinical outcome and restenosis following percutaneous transluminal angioplasty for ischaemic rest pain or ulceration. *Br J Surg* **82**; 1217–21, 1995
14. Currie IC, Wakely CJ, Cole SEA *et al.*: Femoropopliteal angioplasty for severe limb ischaemia. *Br J Surg* **81**; 191–3, 1994
15. Cooper JC, Welsh CL: The role of percutaneous transluminal angioplasty in the treatment of critical limb ischaemia. *Eur J Vasc Surg* **5**; 261–4, 1991
16. London NJM, Varty K, Sayers RD *et al.*: Percutaneous transluminal angioplasty for lower-limb critical ischaemia. *Br J Surg* **82**; 1232–5, 1995
17. Varty K, Nydahl S, Butterworth P *et al.*: Changes in the management of critical limb ischaemia. *Br J Surg* **83**; 953–6, 1996
18. Sivanathan UM, Browne TF, Thorley PJ, Rees MR: Percutaneous transluminal angioplasty of the tibial arteries. *Br J Surg* **81**; 1282–5, 1994
19. Buckenham T, Loh A, Dormandy JA, Taylor RS: Infrapopliteal angioplasty for limb salvage. *Eur J Vasc Surg* **7**; 21–5, 1993
20. Varty K, Bolia A, Naylor AR *et al.*: Infra-popliteal percutaneous transluminal angioplasty: a safe and successful procedure. *Eur J Vasc Endovasc Surg* **9**; 341–5, 1995
21. Bolia A, Sayers RD, Thompson MM, Bell PRF: Subintimal and intraluminal recanalisation of occluded crural arteries by percutaneous balloon angioplasty. *Eur J Vasc Surg* **8**; 214–9, 1994
22. Whitely MS, Ray-Chaudari SB, Galland RB: Changing patterns in aorto-iliac reconstruction: a 7-year audit. *Br J Surg* **83**; 1367–9, 1996
23. Pell JP, Whyman MR, Fowkes FGR *et al.*: Trends in vascular surgery since the introduction of percutaneous transluminal angioplasty. *Br J Surg* **81**; 832–5, 1994

24. Hallett JW, Byrne J, Gayari MM *et al.*: Impact of arterial surgery and balloon angioplasty on amputation: A population-based study of 1155 procedures between 1973 and 1992. *J Vasc Surg* **25**; 29–38, 1997
25. Vroegindewij D, Idu M, Buth J *et al.*: The cost-effectiveness of treatment of short occlusive lesions in the femoropopliteal artery: balloon angioplasty versus endarterectomy. *Eur J Vasc Endovasc Surg* **10**; 40–50, 1995
26. Stanley B, Teague B, Raptis S *et al.*: Efficacy of balloon angioplasty of the superficial femoral artery and popliteal artery in the relief of leg ischaemia. *J Vasc Surg* **23**; 769–85, 1996
27. Dotter CT, Judkins MP: Transluminal treatment of arteriosclerotic obstruction. Description of a new technique and a preliminary report of its application. *Circulation* **30**; 654–70, 1964
28. Porter JM: Endovascular arterial intervention. Expression of concern. *J Vasc Surg* **21**; 995–7, 1995
29. Bradbury AW, Ruckley CV: Angioplasty for lower-limb ischaemia: time for randomised controlled trials. *Lancet* **347**; 277–8, 1996

Editorial comments by P.R.F. Bell

This is a very nice chapter reviewing the management of intermittent claudication and I think most practising vascular surgeons would agree that for the majority of claudicators conservative treatment, that is cessation of smoking and exercise, is by far the best form of management. The evidence from the Oxford group in 1990 was most seminal in this matter and demonstrated quite clearly that angioplasty although it was helpful in the short-term was not particularly helpful in the long-term.

This chapter highlights the difficulties of comparing percutaneous transluminal angioplasty with surgery because in most centres the patients who are put forward for one or other of these procedures are not identical but are a mixed bunch and that comparing patients' survival from surgery or percutaneous transluminal angioplasty or by limb salvage from surgery or percutaneous transluminal angioplasty, is meaningless unless we are comparing like with like.

I think most vascular surgeons would agree with Mr Bradbury that percutaneous transluminal angioplasty with or without stent placement has a valuable role to play in the management of peripheral vascular disease but at the moment we are uncertain as to precisely what that role should be. We certainly need proper controlled trials comparing percutaneous transluminal angioplasty with surgery in comparable groups of patients strictly stratified. This will almost certainly need a multicentre trial. In the meantime if I had a lesion that was amenable to angioplasty I am sure I would prefer an angioplasty to be done percutaneously rather than the greater traumas of an open surgical procedure.

How Easy is an Endoscopic Femoropopliteal Vein Bypass? Is it Worth the Training?

David M. Nott

INTRODUCTION

The title 'How easy is an endoscopic femoropopliteal vein bypass? Is it worth the training?' supposes that at the present time the standard method of performing infrainguinal vein bypass is without doubt well established and asks why then make it more difficult. As vascular surgeons we have all seen in our own practice the difference in recovery rates between those patients who have undergone femoropopliteal prosthetic graft bypass compared with those who have had the vein harvested for either *in situ* or reversed vein bypass. The difference between the two relates to the length of the incisions.

With the development of laparoscopic surgery in the early 1990s it soon became obvious that reducing the size of incisions had beneficial effects for the patient regarding both wound infection rates and pain such that today I regularly perform laparoscopic cholecystectomy and laparoscopic hernia repair with 98% of patients discharged as day cases.[1]

Minimally invasive arterial surgery, however, lends itself more to endovascular/radiological procedures such as angioplasty and stenting. This, as we all know, is suitable for short length occlusions of the superficial femoral artery but long occlusions of 10 cm or more, although producing a good radiological result tend to fail within a short period of time. There are therefore very few minimally invasive options for leg revascularization left to the vascular surgeon, apart from prosthetic grafting which has very poor results below the knee.[2]

The long incisions required in vein bypass surgery for both femoropopliteal and distal bypass have complication rates of up to 72%.[3] These include poor skin healing, superficial infection, lymphatic discharges from the groin or worse, undermining of skin flaps causing large haematomas which result in ischaemic necrosis of the thigh wound (Fig. 1). Not only do these complications cause the patient much morbidity, but prolonged hospital stay is both costly and disruptive to the running of a unit. The rationale therefore, for the development of a new technique is reduction in these complications by reducing the length of the incision on the thigh and leg and abolishing the incision in the groin. In an attempt to achieve this aim, a method was developed laparoscopically to mobilize the external iliac artery combined with endoscopic harvesting of the long saphenous vein, followed by a totally laparoscopic intra-abdominal arteriovenous anastomosis between the external iliac artery and the reversed long saphenous vein.

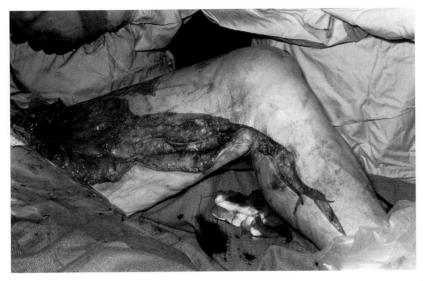

Fig. 1.   Severe undermining of skin flaps in an attempt to follow the course of the
long saphenous vein.

METHODS

A 68-year-old Caucasian male was complaining of severe intermittent claudication
over a distance of 40 yards and of rest pain at night. His ankle brachial pressure index
was 0.7 in the left leg and 0.4 in the right. Intra-arterial digital subtraction
angiography confirmed complete occlusion of the right superficial and popliteal
artery with reconstitution into a single peroneal artery (Fig. 2). The patient was
otherwise very well having no past medical or surgical history.

After obtaining informed consent the patient underwent general anaesthesia with
muscle relaxation. He was prepared with chlorohexidene and placed in the supine
position with the right leg flexed at the knee. A medial calf incision was made and the
long saphenous vein carefully protected as the peroneal artery was exposed and two
slings placed proximally and distally around the area chosen for the arteriotomy.

The long saphenous vein was harvested using an Endopath dissector (Ethicon
Endosurgery Inc.) placed superiorly over the vein in the subcutaneous space between
the vein and the skin. Following removal of that instrument, an Endopath Subcu-
Retractor was inserted which allowed the passage of laparoscopic instruments for
mobilization of the vein (Fig. 3). An endoscopic blunt tip dissector was passed alongside the wide shaft of the subcu-retractor and adhesions overlying the long
saphenous vein were gently mobilized to allow visualization of side branches.
Following this the blunt tip dissector was removed and an endopath vessel dissector
used gently to lift up the vein and assist in the identification of side branches. An
Ethicon allport clip applicator was used to clip the side branch away from the
saphenous vein and the side branch close to the vein divided with laparoscopic

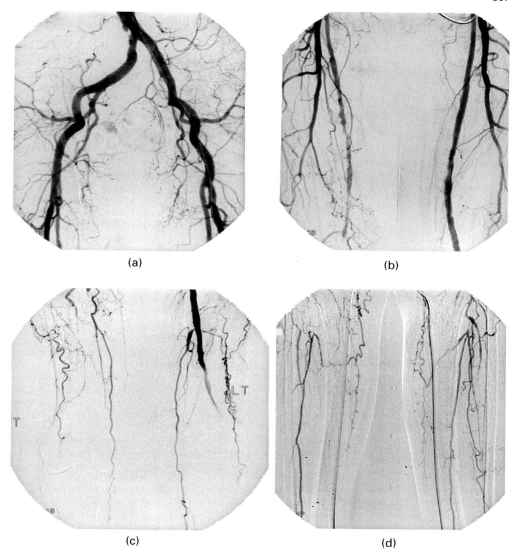

(a)

(b)

(c)

(d)

Fig. 2. Arteriogram of patient under consideration.

scissors (Fig. 4). The Endopath vessel dissector was then used to course up the vein and assist in dissection of the next side branch. The limiting factor in mobilization of the vein was the length of the endopath instruments (31cm).

In order to remove the whole length of the long saphenous vein, three, 2-cm incisions were made. At the groin the long saphenous vein was clipped and divided just beyond the saphenofemoral junction with laparoscopic scissors. By gently pulling the vein from the distal end at the peroneal incision the vein was completely removed in its entirety (Fig. 5).

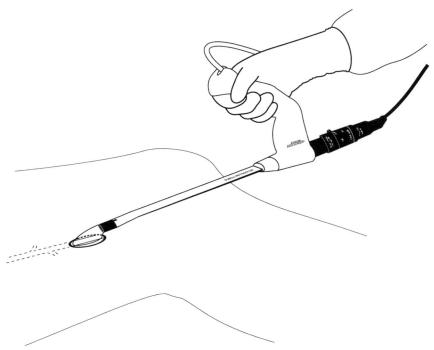

Fig. 3.   Endopath subcu–dissector dissecting to desired tissue plane.

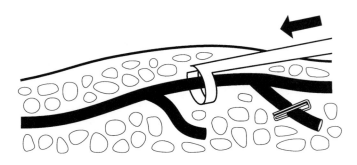

Fig. 4.   Endopath subcu–retractor showing mobilization of the vein
to the next side branch using the vessel dissector with a clip
applied to a side branch.

The vein was reversed and a size 6 umbilical vein catheter was passed down the
vein and heparinized saline flush used to identify all the side branches which were
then ligated with 3/0 silk ties. A fashioning venotomy was made in the long
saphenous vein for the anastomosis with the external iliac artery.

To expose the artery, a subumbilical 1-cm incision was made and a 10-mm port
inserted into the abdomen using the Hassan technique and carbon dioxide instilled

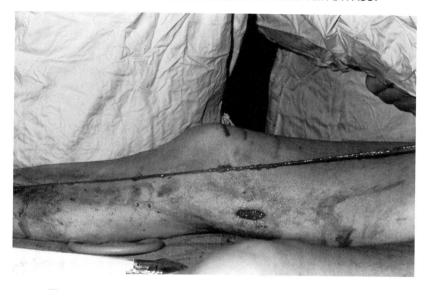

Fig. 5. The long saphenous vein removed in its entirety.

to achieve an intra-abdominal pressure of 15 mm Hg. Two further 10-mm ports were placed in the right and left lumbar area and using laparoscopic dissecting forceps and scissors, the peritoneum was divided over at a distance of 2 cm below the deep inguinal ring to expose the external iliac artery. A pair of blunt tip dissectors were used to free the fascia surrounding the artery until approximately 3 cm of artery was exposed. A tunnel was made with the blunt tip dissector above the external iliac artery such that both the circumflex iliac and superficial epigastric arteries were visualized and the space continued under the inguinal ligament for a distance of 2 cm. A right-angled instrument was passed underneath the artery and two slings were placed proximally and distally around it, two 5-mm ports were inserted into the flanks and the slings brought out for manual control and to aid retraction of the artery (Fig. 6).

Using the tunnel created above the femoral artery, a curved Maryland dissecting forceps was then passed under the inguinal ligament and a 1-cm incision made in the skin, over the tip of dissector on the anterior surface of the thigh. The vein prepared for bypass was grasped with the forceps and carefully withdrawn into the abdomen and laid next to the artery.

The right flank 10-mm port was replaced with a specially designed port with a malleable cannula (Aesculap UK Ltd) which allowed the passage of a laparoscopic satinsky clamp. Through this port a 10-mm instrument was used to position two apply-and-release laparoscopic bull dog vascular clamps both proximally and distally to an area of the artery where the arteriotomy was to be made. Through this same port, the laparoscopic Satinsky clamp was positioned proximally on the artery as a safety clamp. The anaesthetist then gave 5000 units of heparin. A laparoscopic knife within a guarded sheath was passed into the abdomen and following removal of the sheath the knife was released and a 15-mm arteriotomy made in the artery.

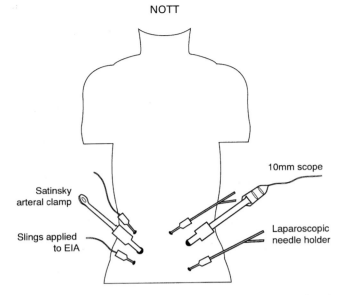

Fig. 6. Positioning of the laparoscopic instruments for intra-corporeal suturing.

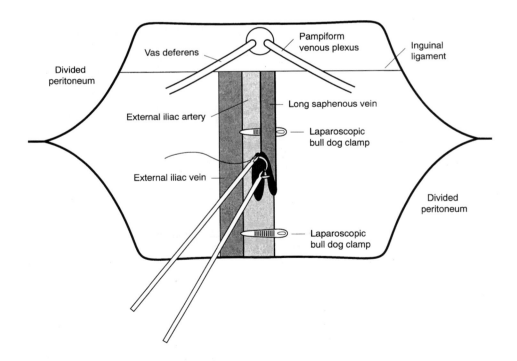

Fig. 7. Intracorporeal anastomosis of the long saphenous vein to the external iliac artery.

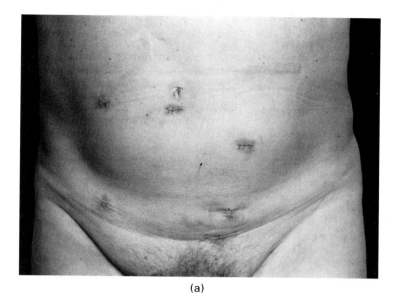

(a)

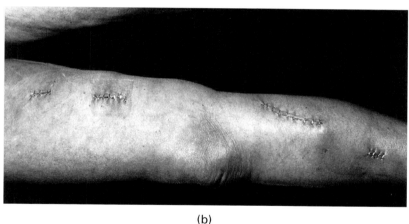

(b)

Fig. 8. Two days after operation showing incisions.

With the use of an Ethicon needle holder and a Storz® flamingo needle holder the vein was sutured onto the artery first at the heel and then around the anastomosis with individually placed 6/0 prolene sutures, each knot tied with a square knot and followed by a securing throw (Fig. 7). Following completion of the anastomosis, another laparoscopic bulldog clamp was placed on the vein graft and the distal arterial clamp taken off first. Any bleeding from the anastomosis was stemmed by pressure from a blunt-tip dissector prior to removal of the proximal clamp. The laparoscopic bulldog clamp on the vein graft was removed and the vein checked externally for good pulsation. A size 4 umbilical vein catheter was passed into one of the side branches and heparinized saline was used to flush the blood out of the vein graft. Following this the laparoscopic bulldog clamp was placed back onto the vein graft just distal to the anastomosis.

A tunnelling device (Impra UK) was passed up the leg from the calf wound overlying the peroneal artery to the small incision in the anterior part of the thigh in the subdermal tunnel created by the Endopath instruments. The vein graft was attached to the tunneller and placed in the subdermal tunnel and laid adjacent to the peroneal artery. An arteriotomy was made in the peroneal artery and a routine hand-sewn arteriovenous anastomosis with 7/0 prolene was made. The laparoscopic clamp was removed and blood allowed to pulsate down the graft. At the end of the operation there was excellent flow down the graft with pulsatile flow palpable within the peroneal artery. The calf wound was closed with running 3/0 PDS sutures and the skin closed with skin clips. One drain was placed in the peroneal wound. The incisions on the leg were closed with skin clips and the 1-cm incisions on the abdomen were closed with a single J shaped Ethibond suture and two skin clips applied to each skin incision and one skin clip applied to the 5-mm incision. The total length of all the incisions was 16 cm and the operating time was 5 hours (Fig. 8).

RESULTS

After surgery the patient was transferred to the high dependency unit for overnight monitoring and was allowed back to the ward the following day. There was no necessity for transfusion. He was mobilized following transfer to the ward and was able to eat and drink later that day. He was discharged on the morning of the 4th day and ankle brachial pressure was 0.95 in the operated leg. The patient was seen 6 weeks and 6 months later in the vascular clinic and ankle brachial pressure index remained at 0.95 and easily palpable pedal pulses as well as a palpable graft medial to the knee joint were noted. He had returned to his part time job as a photographer within 2 weeks of the operation. There was no wound morbidity apart from postperfusion oedema which lasted for 2 months following the operation.

DISCUSSION AND MODIFICATIONS

The operation can be divided into two parts, first the endoscopic vein harvesting, and second the laparoscopic anastomosis vein to artery. Operating time for each procedure was roughly 2 hours. Although I had not performed the procedure on a patient before, I had performed it in a live laboratory setting in Cincinnati some 2 years previously.

Endopath instruments had previously been developed to facilitate vein harvesting for coronary artery bypass grafts where small lengths of vein have been used.[4] This was the first time that the instruments had been used for harvesting of the whole length of the long saphenous vein. The only difficulty encountered with mobilization of the vein was the area around the knee joint where tightness of the skin increased the difficulty of forming a subcutaneous tunnel. Following removal of the vein there was little problem in securing homeostasis, it appeared that the All-port clips provided sufficient compression of the sided branches so that manipulation from the repeated passage of the retractors did not cause dislodgement.

Prior to performing this procedure, laparoscopic mobilization of the external iliac artery had been performed with written consent from six patients. Three underwent extraperitoneal mobilization with the use of an extraperitoneal laparoscopic balloon dissector and three underwent intraperitoneal mobilization. Apart from dissection and mobilization no further laparoscopic procedure was performed and these patients underwent standard bypass surgery. There was little difference in ease of mobilization and dissection of the artery with either method; however the extraperitoneal dissection led to much greater surface bleeding and therefore overall darkening of the picture due to greater absorption of light, hence the intraperitoneal method was chosen in preference.

The most technically demanding part of the procedure was the laparoscopic anastomosis. Laparoscopic suturing is the most demanding of all laparoscopic techniques and to be proficient at this skill requires the operator not only to be experienced in vascular surgery but also in laparoscopic surgery. I am the course convenor in laparoscopic suturing for the Royal College of Surgeons of England and have spent many hours practising anastomosing prosthetic grafts in laparoscopic trainers at the minimal access training unit (Mattu) at the Royal College prior to performing this procedure. After many tribulations I found it better to use individually placed 6/0 prolene sutures rather than a running suture, as better approximation could be made and there were fewer problems should the suture break. Vein harvesting using the Ethicon subcu dissector and retractor also demanded a high degree of hand–eye co-ordination but was certainly technically less demanding.

There is no doubt that the patient made a remarkable recovery following his distal bypass graft which can be directly related to the ethos of minimally invasive surgery, i.e. lack of pain and freedom from problems associated with long wound incisions. The potential for things to go wrong, however, is extremely high and will probably obviate the laparoscopic part of this procedure. Since this first operation which encompassed all the various factors involved with the procedure, subsequent laparoscopic arterial mobilizations have been found to be more technically demanding. Small amounts of calcium in the arterial wall make suturing extremely difficult and short patients with rotund abdomens make the angles required for holding the laparoscopic needle holders very arduous.

With the constraints on time of training, it is unlikely that vascular surgeons will be given time to gain enough experience in specialized laparoscopic techniques to be able to perform the mobilization and arteriovenous anastomosis. However, I feel that endoscopic harvesting of the vein with adequate training is within the scope of all non-trained laparoscopic surgeons although some degree of training with 2D and hand-eye co-ordination is necessary.

At our hospital, for the last 6 months all patients undergoing infrainguinal bypass for femoropopliteal and distal disease have had the long saphenous vein harvested endoscopically. As part of this pilot study 13 patients have been compared with a historical group of sex- and aged-matched patients who over the past year have undergone standard vein harvesting. The femoral artery was exposed routinely in all cases. It was only necessary to abandon the endovein harvesting once because of unsuitability of the vein. Mean operation time from beginning to end of the operation was 193±15 minutes for the endoharvest compared with 152±14 minutes for the conventional procedure. Total wound length was 16±2 cm for the endoharvest group compared with 39±9 cm for the standard group and in-patient stay was 4±2 days compared with 12±5 days for the conventional group. There have been no complications in the endoharvest group compared with two infections in the thigh for the conventional group.

It is important to be sure that all of the side branches of the endoharvested vein have been adequately clipped and divided as on removal of the vein a tear can occur in the vein at the side branch which necessitates repair with 7/0 prolene. If on removal of the vein it appears to be snagged then it is best to reintroduce the endopath instrument and find at clip the side branch.

Because of this problem a further modification of this technique has been introduced. Rather than complete removal and reversing of the endoharvested vein, in the last four patients to undergo infrainguinal bypass the endopath instruments have been used to simply expose the long saphenous vein at the saphenofemoral junction and side branches identified and one occluding clip applied. A 3-cm groin crease incision is then made to divide the new flush with the femoral vein and the common femoral artery dissected to expose a segment for anastomosis. The vein is then anastomosed to the femoral artery with 6/0 prolene. Following this a Hall's valvulotome is introduced from the distal end of the vein bypass and passed proximally. Under direct vision with the endoscope it can be seen that as each valve cusp is disrupted the vein becomes distended with arterial pressure to the next competent valve and again under direct vision this valve is disrupted (Fig. 9). In the event of a missed side branch an endoclip can be applied without recourse to a further skin incision.

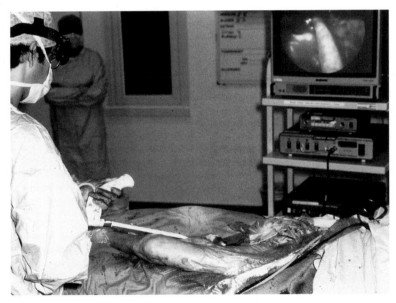

Fig. 9.   Endopath subcu-retractor in position showing arterialized vein graft.

The distal anastomosis is constructed with 6/0 prolene after all the valves have been disrupted and free flow within the graft confirmed. On-table completion angiography is then performed through a side branch at the proximal aspect of the vein to ensure complete valve disruption and to make sure all arteriovenous fistulae due to all unclipped tributaries are dealt with. Mean operating time so far has been 108±6 minutes and the total length of the incisions has been 8±1 cm. There have been no postoperative complications (Fig. 10).

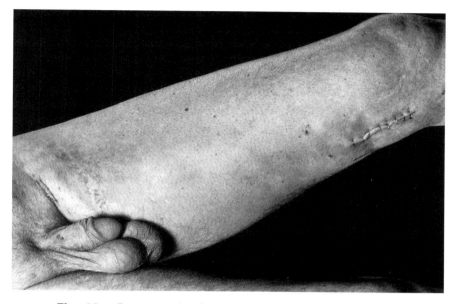

Fig. 10.   Postoperative femeropopliteal vein *in situ* bypass.

CONCLUSIONS

Well, was it all worth the training? There were obviously two parts to the training, one to be a fully trained vascular surgeon which I achieved both at Liverpool and at Charing Cross and the second to be a fully trained laparoscopic surgeon achieved at Charing Cross and Chelsea and Westminster Hospitals. The idea of performing an endoscopic femoropopliteal bypass and achieving the goal and also to appreciate the advantages and disadvantages would not have been possible without proper training in both modalities. With the constraints on early specialization of trainees and constraints on time of training it is unlikely that vascular surgeons will be given the time to gain enough experience in specialized laparoscopic techniques. There is no doubt, however, that a minimally invasive approach to infrainguinal vein grafting is the way forward and I feel that the endoharvest *in situ* vein bypass will become the procedure of choice in the future. So far there have been no complications and patient in-hospital stay has been reduced to a third. I feel that the laparoscopic mobilization of the artery and laparoscopic anastomosis is not the way forward as the training necessary and adverse factors mentioned above mitigate against its routine use. However, endoscopic harvesting of the vein with adequate training is within the scope of all non-trained laparoscopic vascular surgeons who with practice of hand-eye co-ordination at the 2D level will find they will be able to perform the procedure with ease.

REFERENCES

1. Nott DM: Cost implications of laparoscopic surgery. Guest Lecture, Belgian Society of Minimally Invasive Surgeons, Bruge May 1995
2. Harris PL, Bakran A, Enabi L, Nott DM: ePTFE grafts for femoro-crural bypass – improved results with combined adjuvant venous cuff and arterivenous fistula? *Eur J Vasc Surg* **7:** 528–33, 1993
3. Reifsnyder T, Bandyk D, Seabrook G *et al.*: Wound complications of the *in-situ* vein bypass technique. *J Vasc Surg* **15:** 843–50, 1992
4. Lumsden A, Eaves F: Subcutaneous video-assisted saphenous vein harvest. *Perspec Vasc Surg* **7:** 44–55, 1994

Editorial comments by P.R.F. Bell

The author has not really described a femoropopliteal bypass but instead has set out the details required for ileopopliteal bypass using laparoscopic techniques. Mr Nott is clearly a very keen supporter of laparoscopic methods but even he at the end of the day is forced to conclude that he is turning what is a relatively simple procedure into a difficult one by doing a laparoscopic suturing technique above the inquinal ligament. He makes claims about the efficacy and short hospital stay of this method but has only a very limited amount of data to support that view. The main benefit from the procedure is in removing the vein laparoscopically using the Ethicon device. However, equally good results can be obtained using tiny incisions and much simpler methods than he has mentioned here. The operation took 5 hours and I do not think that is a reasonable amount of time for what is a simple procedure. If this method is to be used it should be used with an appropriately randomized study to compare such points as infection, would healing rates and complications in the long term and it should be compared with the best not the worst open techniques. I do not think that Mr Nott has influenced me that this is a good way to go as yet. Smaller incisions in the leg should be better but we do not know if they actually are.

Is the Use of Intravascular Ultrasound Essential for Femoropopliteal Balloon Angioplasty and Stenting?

Marc RHM van Sambeek, Elma J Gussenhoven, Aad van der Lugt, Winnifred van Lankeren and Hero van Urk

INTRODUCTION

Balloon angioplasty is a widely used technique for obstructive disease in the femoropopliteal artery. However, there seems to be a discrepancy between the initial angiographic success and the disappointingly high incidence of re-stenosis (1-year patency rates: 47–73%).[1,2] This promoted the development of alternative endovascular interventions. Parallel with this development there is a need for improved vascular imaging and better diagnostics. Whereas angiography displays a longitudinal silhouette of the vessel lumen, intravascular ultrasound (IVUS) provides histology-like cross-sectional images of the blood vessel, allowing qualitative evaluation of plaque morphology and quantitative measurement of lumen and plaque area by topographic imaging[3-5] (Fig. 1).

Our institution has experience of over 400 endovascular cases in which IVUS was used to guide a variety of vascular interventions.

In this chapter the advantages of IVUS over angiography, the mechanism of balloon angioplasty and stent placement, some aspects of the mechanism of re-stenosis and the IVUS predictors of re-stenosis will be addressed.

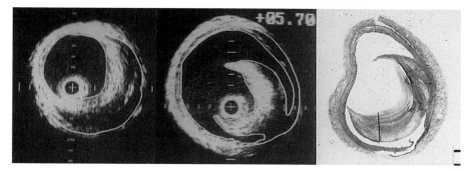

Fig. 1. Intravascular ultrasound images of the femoropopliteal artery obtained *in vitro* before and after balloon angioplasty and corresponding histological section. As a result of the intervention lumen area increase was associated with a dissection. The IVUS cross-sections are contour traced off-line facilitating the recognition of lumen area (inner contour) and media bounded area (outer contour). + = IVUS catheter; calibration = 1mm.

ANGIOGRAPHY VS IVUS

To compare angiographic and IVUS qualitative and quantitative data obtained before
and after percutaneous transluminal angioplasty (PTA) of the femoropopliteal artery,
the records of 135 patients were reviewed.[6] Qualitative and quantitative analysis was
performed on corresponding angiographic and IVUS levels. Presence of a lesion and
amount of plaque was underestimated angiographically (Fig. 2). In angiographic
levels classified as normal, IVUS demonstrated a mean area stenosis of 43%. It was
found that angiography had a poor sensitivity for detection of calcified lesions. On
angiography a calcified lesion was better detected when the arc of calcification
increased in the IVUS cross-sections. A similar relation was found between the
detection of dissection seen by angiography following PTA and the extent of
dissection seen on IVUS. Overall the incidence of vascular damage seen by IVUS
(53%) was higher than seen angiographically (35%).

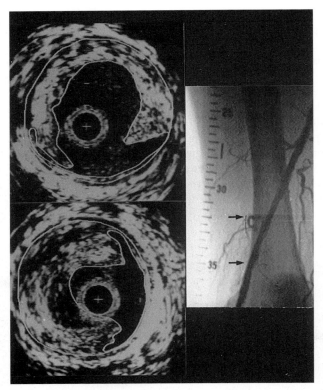

Fig. 2.   Intravascular ultrasound cross-sections and angiogram
obtained from a patient after angiographically defined successful
PTA of the femoropopliteal artery. Note that the presence of a
lesion and amount of plaque seen on IVUS is underestimated on
the angiogram. The IVUS cross-sections are contour traced off-
line facilitating recognition of lumen area (inner contour) and
media-bounded area (outer contour). + = IVUS catheter;
calibration = 1 mm.

Plaque rupture was more frequently seen on IVUS and media rupture was uniquely evidenced by IVUS. Only before PTA there was a good agreement between angiographic diameter stenosis and lumen size seen on IVUS; such a distinct agreement was not seen after PTA. This finding may be related to the vascular damage after PTA, which allows contrast filling of dissection clefts, distorting the luminal silhouette of the angiogram.

MECHANISM OF PTA

The basic mechanism of balloon angioplasty described by Dotter and Judkins in 1964 included plaque compression.[7] Based on histologic sections and angiographic records Castaneda-Zuniga *et al.* proposed that the increase in lumen size is due to media stretch, without significant compression or redistribution of plaque.[8] The introduction of IVUS has enabled the study of the mechanism of balloon angioplasty *in vivo* more precisely. To study the effects of PTA of the femoropopliteal artery with IVUS, corresponding IVUS cross-sections obtained before and after PTA from 115 procedures were analysed. Vascular damage including plaque rupture, media rupture and dissection was assessed. Lumen area, media bounded area (vessel area) and plaque area were measured (Fig. 3). IVUS showed that the increase in vessel area

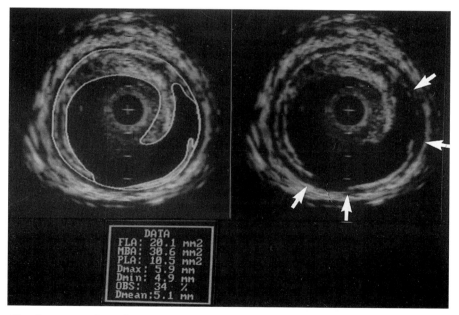

DATA
FLA: 20.1 MM2
MBA: 30.6 MM2
PLA: 10.5 MM2
Dmax: 5.9 MM
Dmin: 4.9 MM
OBS: 34   %
Dmean: 5.1 MM

Fig. 3. Intravascular ultrasound cross-sections obtained after balloon angioplasty showing media rupture and dissection. Left panel: The IVUS cross-section is contour traced off-line facilitating recognition and measurement of lumen area (FLA), vessel area (MBA) and plaque area (PLA). Right panel: White arrows indicate the sections of media rupture. + = IVUS catheter; calibration = 1 mm.

(i.e. media stretch) accounted for 68% of the lumen gain. Overstretching is accompanied almost always by dissection and plaque rupture and occasionally by media rupture[9] (Fig. 4). The relative contribution of plaque reduction was higher at the target sites, suggesting that the plaque at the target site may be crushed more extensively, leading to redistribution of the plaque material.[10]

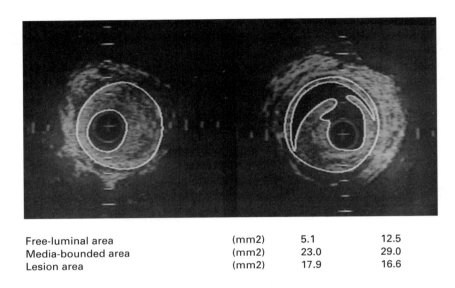

Free-luminal area	(mm2)	5.1	12.5
Media-bounded area	(mm2)	23.0	29.0
Lesion area	(mm2)	17.9	16.6

Fig. 4.   Corresponding intravascular ultrasound cross-sections obtained from a patient before (left panel) and after balloon angioplasty (right panel). The IVUS cross-sections are contour traced off-line facilitating recognition and measurement of lumen area, vessel area and plaque area. Increase in lumen area was associated with significant vessel area increase and minimal plaque area decrease. + = IVUS catheter; calibration = 1 mm.

MECHANISM OF STENTING

Stents were developed in order to prevent recoil after PTA and thus improve the immediate and long-term results of balloon angioplasty in different sites. Intravascular ultrasound in coronary arteries has revealed that stents may be incompletely deployed despite optimal angiographic result.[11] Similar lessons concerning stent placement could perhaps be learned in other parts of the vascular system.

For this purpose we performed an IVUS study to compare the balloon diameter with the immediate outcome following stent placement in 22 patients with peripheral obstructive arterial disease. The results show that well-apposed and symmetrically expanded stents as evidenced angiographically, may vary in lumen dimensions despite the use of adequately sized balloons[12] (Fig. 5). A discrepancy was found between the size of the balloon that was used and resulting smallest stent area

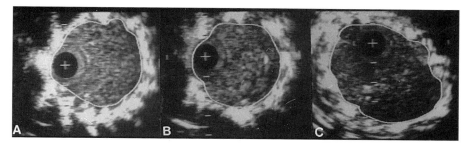

Fig. 5. Intravascular ultrasound cross-sections of the femoropopliteal artery in a patient after stent placement for residual stenosis using a 6-mm balloon. The cross-sections are contour traced off-line showing: the proximal stent edge (A), intra-stent (B) and distal stent edge (C) with mean diameters of 4.5 mm, 4.4 mm and 5.3 mm, respectively. + = IVUS catheter; calibration = 1 mm.

(difference 31%). Moreover, in 52% of the stents a uniform expansion of the stent was found, in 39% a funnel-like shape (one stent edge larger than the dimension in the mid-portion in the stent) was found, while in 9% of the stents both stent edges were larger than the dimension in the mid-portion of the stent. We postulate that inadequate stent expansion may be caused by either a balloon diameter that is too small for the artery, by compression of the stent by the plaque, or by plaque resistance. The observation that dilatation with both compliant balloons and non-compliant balloons frequently resulted in underexpansion of the stents, suggests that the mechanical properties of the balloon that is used for dilatation and delivery of the stent does not influence the outcome.

MECHANISM OF RE-STENOSIS

After PTA

Initially, autopsy studies have shown that intimal hyperplasia is responsible for the decrease in arterial lumen after intervention. Later, serial IVUS studies have suggested that vascular shrinkage may be the predominant factor in the development of re-stenosis.[13] We used IVUS to study the femoropopliteal artery immediately after the initial intervention and at 1-year follow-up. To ensure that IVUS cross-sections obtained after intervention and at follow-up were indeed from corresponding sites, the cross-sections were studied side-by-side and frame-to-frame. The IVUS cross-sections were analysed for change in lumen area, plaque area and vessel area (media-bounded area). Differences were encountered in the extent of intimal hyperplasia and vascular remodeling at the most stenotic site and in the cross-sections just proximal and distal of the most stenotic site. It was found that the lumen area measured from the corresponding cross-sections decreased significantly both at the most stenotic site (–54%) and in the cross-sections just proximal and distal of the most stenotic site (–15%). A significant increase in plaque area was seen both at the most stenotic site (+21%) and in the adjacent cross-sections of the dilated segment (+15%). A significant decrease in vessel area was seen only at the most stenotic site (–9%). The vessel area in the cross-sections adjacent to the dilated segment did not change (1%) (Fig. 6). According to these data, plaque area increase (i.e. intimal hyperplasia) contributed the major part (57%) and vessel area decrease a smaller part (43%) to the lumen area reduction at the most stenotic site.

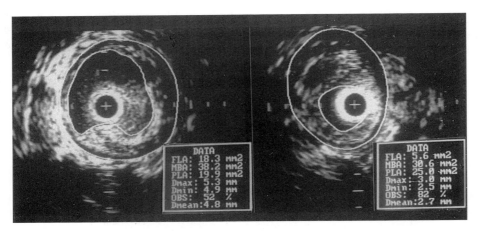

Fig. 6. Intravascular ultrasound cross-sections of the femoropopliteal artery in a patient after PTA (left panel) and at 6-months follow-up (right panel). The cross-sections are contour traced off-line facilitating recognition and measurement of lumen area (FLA, inner contour) and vessel area (MBA, outer contour). The vessel area (MBA) decreased from 38.2 mm^2 to 30.6 mm^2. The lumen area (FLA) decreased from 18.3 mm^2 to 5.6 mm^2. The plaque area increased from 19.9 mm^2 to 25.0 mm^2. + = IVUS catheter; calibration = 1 mm.

Furthermore, it was found that in one-third of the patients an increase of the vessel area at the most stenotic site was found to compensate for the presence of intimal hyperplasia, which resulted in an unchanged lumen area at follow-up. Similarly, an increase in lumen area was seen in one-fifth of the adjacent cross-sections of the dilated segment due to vessel area increase exceeding plaque area increase. From these observations it can be concluded that in the presence of intimal hyperplasia the type of vascular remodelling (enlargement or shrinkage) determined the net lumen change.

After stent placement

As mentioned above, it has been shown that geometrical arterial remodelling may be the dominant factor contributing to re-stenosis after balloon angioplasty. It is postulated that the use of stents may reduce re-stenosis by eliminating this geometrical remodelling. This assumption is supported by serial IVUS analysis after stent placement in coronary arteries, showing that late recoil of Palmaz-Schatz stents rarely occurred (only in 6% of the cases); and when it did occur, late stent recoil was minimal.[14] The dominant mechanism of late lumen loss was intimal hyperplasia.

We performed a serial IVUS analysis in two patients to study the mechanism of re-stenosis after Palmaz stent placement in the femoropopliteal artery.[15] In one patient seven balloon expandable stents were placed with overlap because of a 22-cm long dissection after PTA of a short but high-grade stenosis. After a good initial success the patient returned 5 months later with recurrent disabling claudication. The angiogram showed distinct stenoses at the stent junctions (Fig.7). IVUS images obtained after stent placement and at follow-up were analysed for lumen area, stent area, lesion area, and percentage area stenosis. Both intimal hyperplasia (inside the stent) and stent area

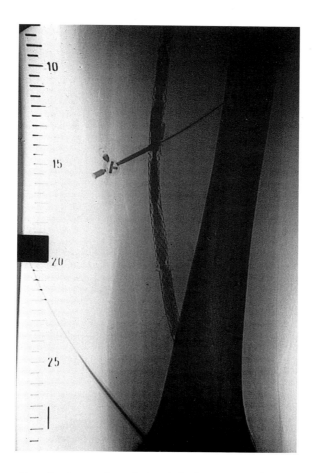

Fig. 7. Angiography of the left femoropopliteal artery obtained at 5-months follow-up showing distinct stenoses at the stent junctions.

reduction were common findings responsible for the late lumen loss. An intriguing finding was that the extent of lumen area reduction, intimal hyperplasia and stent area reduction was more severe at the stent junctions. This raised the question whether the amount of metal struts pressing against the arterial wall, or movement of the stent edges, may be responsible for the increased amount of intimal hyperplasia.

In the second patient, IVUS investigation performed 3 years after stent placement for a stenosis in the femoropopliteal artery revealed that a distinct lumen loss was mainly due to stent area reduction. In this stent only minimal intimal hyperplasia was found (Fig. 8). These two cases illustrate that, in contrast to coronary artery, remodelling of balloon expandable stents contributes to re-stenosis in the femoropopliteal artery.

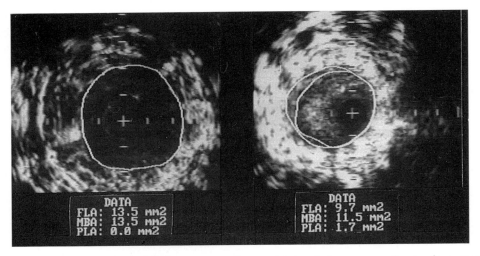

Fig. 8. Corresponding IVUS cross-sections obtained from a patient after stent placement in the femoropopliteal artery (left panel) and at 3-year follow-up (right panel). The cross-sections are contour traced off-line facilitating recognition and measurement. The stent area (MBA) decreased from 13.5 mm^2 to 11.5 mm^2. At follow-up minimal intimal hyperplasia was found (1.7 mm^2).

INTRAVASCULAR ULTRASOUND PREDICTORS OF RE-STENOSIS

In order to determine the additional value of IVUS compared with angiography to predict the outcome following PTA, a multicentre study named EPISODE (Evaluation Peripheral Intravascular Sonography On Dotter Effect) was conducted.[16] The study comprised 39 patients referred for disabling claudication who underwent PTA for femoropopliteal obstructive disease. The intervention was preceded and followed by routine single plane angiography and IVUS investigation. The IVUS parameters selected for analysis included: 1) qualitative and quantitative data obtained at the smallest lumen area before PTA and its matched site after PTA; 2) the mean maximum arc of dissection in the dilated segment; and 3) the presence of dissection and/or media rupture encountered in the dilated segment.

Angiographically, the PTA procedure was classified successful (<50% residual diameter stenosis) in 31 patients and as a failure in eight patients. The 31 patients were followed to show the duration of success and the time of failure up to the census date of 6 months. Success was scored in 14 of the 31 patients (group 1); failure was scored in 17 patients (group 2). The eight patients that were angiographically classified as a failure underwent vascular reconstructive surgery.

As result of PTA, a significant increase in lumen area was noted with IVUS both in group 1 and group 2. In addition, after PTA larger values were encountered in the lumen area in group 1 vs group 2 (6.0 ± 3.6 mm^2 vs 3.6 ± 2.0 mm^2). Differences were encountered in the extent of hard lesion in group 1 vs group 2 ($12° \pm 21°$ vs $57° \pm 93°$). The extent of dissection seen after PTA was significantly less in group 1 vs group 2 ($18° \pm 21°$ vs $78° \pm 69°$).

Recently, the EPISODE study was completed with inclusion of a total of 137 patients.[17] Supplementary conclusions are that media rupture in the dilated segments was less frequently seen in procedures with early re-stenosis than early success, but this difference did not reach a statistically significant level. A larger mean arc of hard lesion was an independent predictor of early re-stenosis.

CLINICAL IMPLICATIONS OF THE USE OF IVUS TO PREDICT RE-STENOSIS INCLUDE

First, in the presence of an extensive hard lesion (i.e. calcification) in the diseased segment other treatment modalities should be considered after initial failure of PTA.

Second, as the presence of a media rupture is beneficial for the outcome, the absence of vascular damage, especially in the presence of a small lumen area or small luminal gain after PTA, is an indication of an inadequate dilatation and may require a repeat PTA. However, the creation of extensive vascular damage, such as a large dissection, creates a dilemma, as a dissection may be a prerequisite for an adequate dilatation while at the same time this may result in an increased probability for late re-stenosis. Large dissections may necessitate the placement of stents to prevent the late re-stenotic process.

Third, maximizing lumen area, and thus minimizing area stenosis, may reduce re-stenosis. In the presence of a large residual stenosis after PTA, a repeat PTA or stent placement may optimize the result.

REFERENCES

1. Matsi PJ, Manninen HI, Vanninen RL et al.: Femoropopliteal angioplasty in patients with claudication: Primary and secondary patency in 140 limbs with 1-3 year follow-up. *Radiology* **191**: 727–33, 1994
2. Vroegindeweij D, Tielbeek AV, Buth J et al.: Directional atherectomy versus balloon angioplasty in segmental femoropopliteal artery disease: Two-year follow-up using color-flow duplex. *J Vasc Surg* **21**: 235–69, 1995
3. Gussenhoven EJ, Essed CE, Frietman P et al.: Intravascular ultrasound imaging: Histologic and echographic correlation. *Eur J Vasc Surg* **3**: 571–6, 1989

4. Gussenhoven WJ, Essed CE, Frietman P *et al.*: Intravascular echographic assessment of vessel wall characteristics: a correlation with histology. *Int J Card Imaging* **4**: 105–116, 1989

5. Gerritsen PG, Gussenhoven EJ, The SHK *et al.*: Intravascular ultrasonography before and after intervention: In vivo comparison with angiography. *J Vasc Surg* **18**: 31–40, 1993

6. van Lankeren W, Gussenhoven EJ, van der Lugt A *et al.*: Comparison of angiography and intravascular ultrasound before and after balloon angioplasty of the femoropopliteal artery. (Submitted for publication.)

7. Dotter CT, Judkins MP: Transluminal treatment of arteriosclerotic obstruction. *Circulation* **30**: 654–70, 1964

8. Castaneda-Zuniga WR, Formanek A, Tadavarthy M *et al.*: The mechanism of balloon angioplasty. *Radiology* **135**: 565–71, 1980

9. The SHK, Gussenhoven EJ, Zhong Y *et al.*: Effect of balloon angioplasty on femoral artery evaluated with intravascular ultrasound imaging. *Circulation* **86**: 483–93, 1992

10. van der Lugt A, Gussenhoven EJ, Mali WPTM *et al.*: Effect of balloon angioplasty in femoropopliteal arteries assessed by intravascular ultrasound. *Eur J Vasc Endovasc Surg* **13**: 549–56, 1997

11. Nakamura S, Colombo A, Gaglione A *et al.*: Intracoronary ultrasound observations during stent implantation. *Circulation* **89**: 2026–34, 1994

12. van Sambeek MRHM, Qureshi A, van Lankeren W *et al.*: Discrepancy between stent deployment and balloon size used assessed by intravascular ultrasound. (in prep.)

13. van Lankeren W, Gussenhoven EJ, van der Lugt A *et al.*: Serial intravascular ultrasound following balloon angioplasty in the femoropopliteal artery: Remodeling or intimal hyperplasia. *Eur Radiol* 7(Suppl 1), S203, 1997

14. Painter JA, Mintz GS, Chiu Wong S *et al.*: Serial intravascular ultrasound studies fail to show evidence of chronic Palmaz-Schatz stent recoil. *Am J Cardiol* **75**: 398–400, 1995

15. van Lankeren W, Gussenhoven EJ, van Kints MJ *et al.*: Stent remodelling contributes to femoropopliteal artery re-stenosis: An intravascular ultrasound study. *J Vasc Surg* **25**: 753–6, 1997

16. Gussenhoven EJ, van de Lugt A, Pasterkamp G *et al.*: Intravascular ultrasound predictors of outcome after peripheral balloon angioplasty. *Eur J Vasc Endovasc Surg* **10**: 279–88, 1995

17. van der Lugt A, Gussenhoven EJ, Pasterkamp G *et al.*: Intravascular ultrasound predictors of restenosis after balloon angioplasty of the femoropopliteal artery. (Submitted for publication.)

Editorial comments by R.M. Greenhalgh

The authors quote the EPISODE Trial really to answer the question posed. This trial was to determine the additional value of intravascular ultrasound over angiography. They clearly conclude that IVUS examination at the time of angioplasty, can identify the patients who will have inadequate outcomes. Therefore by inference IVUS informs these authors whether the angioplasty is well performed and if not what should be done next. In this sense the question is partially answered. It is also appreciated that the more trouble that is taken, e.g. by additional oblique views, by contrast angiography, the better the angioplasty outcome is amended. Some would argue that, with care, a good angiologist can amend PTA outcome and rebound perfectly well without expensive IVUS. Perhaps, at this stage we can say that there is at least some uncertainty on the matter.

Is There a Place for Isolated Profundaplasty in the Treatment of Intermittent Claudication?

Hans O. Myhre, Jarlis Wesche, Tonje Strømholm, Erik S. Haug and Staal Hatlinghus

INTRODUCTION

The profunda femoris artery is the major collateral supply to the lower leg in patients with femoropopliteal occlusive disease (Fig. 1). Its use as a runoff vessel for proximal arterial reconstruction is well established.[1, 2] However, the primary controversy regarding profundaplasty is its use as an isolated procedure for limb revascularization.[3] One reason is the difficulty of predicting which patients could benefit from the procedure. Furthermore, it is difficult to evaluate treatment of intermittent claudication in general, since the symptoms may vary over time.

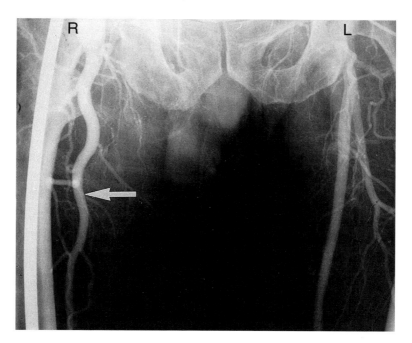

Fig. 1. Arteriogram from a patient who several years previously suffered from a trauma with fracture of the right femur and occlusion of the right superficial femoral artery. The patient is free of symptoms and the right profunda femoris artery (←) has developed, supplying the extremity with sufficient blood to allow heavy excercise. He also has patent pedal pulses.

During recent years, balloon angioplasty of the profunda femoris artery has emerged as an alternative to open profundaplasty.[4, 5] The purpose of this article is to discuss the circumstances in which profundaplasty is indicated as treatment for intermittent claudication.

A so-called isolated profundaplasty can be defined as a reconstruction of the profunda artery itself, primarily by endarterectomy and patch angioplasty. Although the arteriotomy is extended from the profunda femoris artery into the common femoral artery, the proximal arterial tree including the common femoral artery should be relatively free of disease, and no concomitant proximal reconstruction to improve inflow is included in this definition.[6-8] Other investigators include endarterectomy of the common femoral artery in the definition of profundaplasty.[9-11] It can be discussed whether other types of reconstructions performed to relieve stenosis or occlusion of the profunda artery itself could be included in the term profundaplasty, but this was not included in the original definition by Martin *et al.*[9, 10] Bypass grafting from the common femoral artery to the distal part of the profunda is sometimes used in late re-operations, and semi-closed endarterectomy is applied occasionally. Unfortunately, in the reported series of profundaplasty, it is not always specified whether obstruction of the common femoral artery or even the iliac arteries are relieved during the same procedure.

We find that there is a place for isolated profundaplasty in a small, well-defined group of patients with intermittent claudication. Prior to operation for intermittent claudication, conservative measures like abstinence from nicotine and systematic excercise are mandatory. Surgery is only indicated if the patient has a walking distance short enough to interfere significantly with occupation or social life. The indication for surgery is stronger if the patient has progressive symptoms, a walking distance less than 20 meters or an ankle brachial index below 0.5, since there is a tendency for progression to more severe ischaemia in this particular group.[12]

It should be emphasized that in the majority of patients with intermittent claudication due to infrainguinal atherosclerosis, the superficial femoral artery is occluded as well, and femoropopliteal bypass is another alternative which will be discussed. However, isolated profundaplasty seems to be a reasonable alternative to bypass grafting if there is a stenosis of the profunda representing a reduction in vessel diameter of 50% or more. Ideally, only the proximal one-third of the artery should be affected, leaving the distal part relatively free of disease. Although the patency of the popliteal artery is of doubtful significance for the result, a well developed collateral system in continuity with one or more tibial arteries to the foot is of significance for the outcome.[3, 6, 13, 14] Profundaplasty in such patients is an attractive alternative, especially when autologous vein is unavailable due to varicosities or previous vascular surgery (Fig. 2), or if bypass grafting is technically impossible because of popliteal artery occlusion.[15]

Profundaplasty is a relatively minor operative procedure, but in patients with intermittent claudication only, this is perhaps not a strong argument for selecting the procedure. However, the long-term patency rate is usually better than what is obtained by femoropopliteal bypass.[14] It is of note that the long-term results following femoropopliteal bypass in younger patients are less favourable than in elderly individuals.[16] In contrast, it has been reported that profundaplasty has a higher success rate in patients under the age of 60, compared with patients older than 60

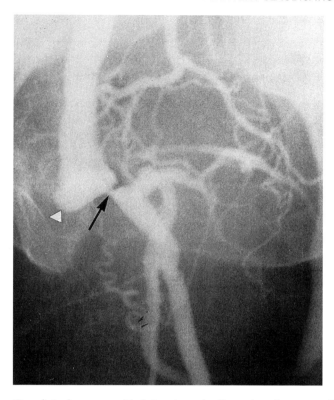

Fig. 2. Arteriogram with lateral projection showing an orifice stenosis of the profunda femoris artery (→). The patient had previously undergone a femoropopliteal bypass grafting, which later occluded (◄). The pressure gradient across the stenosis was 30 mm Hg, increasing to 50 mm Hg after papaverine injection. The patient suffered from severe claudication and became asymptomatic following profundaplasty.

years.[13] There are indications that diabetes may affect profunda artery reconstruction adversely.[17] This is a controversial topic, and we have not taken this factor into consideration in our own experience. Even bearing these criteria in mind, we find that the main problem is to select those patients where the effect of profunda artery reconstruction will give sufficient relief of symptoms.

In patients with intermittent claudication, success can be defined as complete disappearance of claudication or significant increase in the claudication distance. Failure can be defined as a slight increase, no change or a deterioration in claudication distance.[7] In our previous experience, we found that insufficient clinical effect of profundaplasty was experienced by about 20-25% of our patients with critical ischemia, whereas most patients with intermittent claudication improved. [15, 18] The success rate for profundaplasty following intermittent claudication varies significantly, from 50 to 100% in the various clinical series (Table 1). Also the follow-up period varies considerably.[9, 10, 14, 19, 20, 21-27]

Table 1.   Reported results of isolated profundaplasty performed to relieve intermittent claudication

Year	Author (ref.)	Reported results Success/total no.	(%)
1968	Martin et al.[9]	12/14	(86)
1974	Bernhard et al.[41]	9/10	(90)
1974	Morris-Jones and Jones[7]	18/33	(54)
1976	Thompson et al.[22]	16/19	(84)
1977	Harper and Millar[24]	63/93	(68)
1978	Goldstone et al.[21]	20/20	(100)
1979	Heather and Ware[23]	35/45	(78)
1980	Boren et al.[36]	15/15	(100)
1980	Sladen and Burgess[33]	15/16	(94)
1984	Moggi et al.[25]	17/19	(89)
1985	Jennings and Wood[43]	10/12	(83)
1987	Fugger et al.[32]	24/27	(89)
1995	Miani et al.[26]	13/13	(100)
1997	Own series	22/23	(96)
		289/359	(80)

The bottom line shows the summarized results for all these investigations, giving an overall postoperative success rate of profundaplasty in claudicants of 80%. The average follow-up period varies significantly, and is not included.

WHAT ARE THE ALTERNATIVES TO PROFUNDAPLASTY?

One obvious alternative in patients with intermittent claudication is to avoid surgical therapy and rely upon conservative measures only. Abstinence from nicotine and leg excercise have already been mentioned. Pharmacological treatment has so far been of limited value.

Several surgeons claim that they rarely perform operations for intermittent claudication in patients with infrainguinal atherosclerosis. Nevertheless, about 20% of femoropopliteal bypass operations were performed on this indication.[28] The majority of the patients who might be candidates for profundaplasty, in addition to a significant profunda artery stenosis also have occlusion of the femoropopliteal arterial system. Further, in most of these patients, it would be technically possible to do a femoropopliteal bypass, and in general, the long-term patency rate is better in patients with intermittent claudication than in those having more severe ischaemia.[28] With the previously mentioned indications for profundaplasty as the basis, we would, however, regard femoropopliteal bypass grafting as a second choice, because the patency rate following profundaplasty is usually more favourable,[14,29] and it is a minor operation with a lower complication rate. Age under 50 years, the lack of autologous saphenous vein for bypass material and previous ipsilateral infrainguinal reconstruction, make profundaplasty an even more attractive alternative. On the other hand, the advantage of a femoropopliteal bypass is that a more dramatic increase in distal perfusion pressure is obtained. Provided the operation is successful from a technical point of view, the patient will usually be completely free of symptoms.[28] Following profundaplasty, about 80% of the patients can expect to become free of symptoms, or to have a significant increase in their walking distance, and the pedal pulses are restored in 15-20%.[19]

Series of balloon angioplasty for obstructions of the profunda femoris artery have been presented.[4, 5] Most of these series have included angioplasty of arterial obstructions proximal to the profunda artery as well as stenosis of the superficial femoral artery. The number of reopening procedures limited to the profunda femoris artery itself is therefore small. A successful outcome has been described in about 70% of the patients with intermittent claudication.[4, 5] According to our own experience, stenoses of the profunda femoris artery are easily accessible for balloon dilatation. We feel that orifice stenoses are somewhat more difficult to dilate than more distal

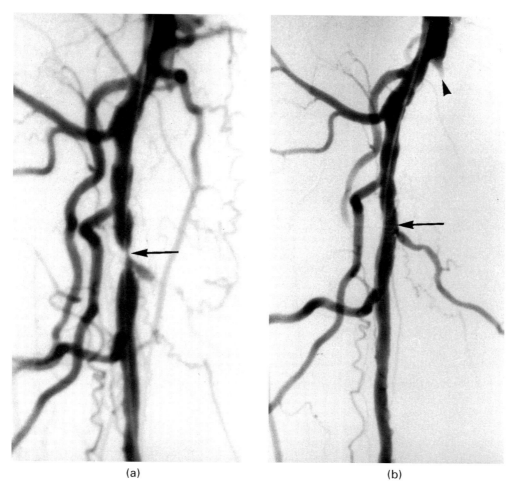

(a)   (b)

Fig. 3. A stenosis distal to the second perforating branch of the profunda femoris artery visualized by arteriography (←). A guide-wire has passed the stenosis (a). The patient who had intermittent claudication and also an occluded superficial femoral artery (◄) became significantly improved after successful balloon angioplasty (←) (b).

stenoses. We have used ipsilateral puncture of the common femoral artery with antegrade catheterization. Access from the contralateral femoral artery across the aortic bifurcation or even the axillary artery are other alternatives.[4] Although we have used balloon angioplasty in elderly high-risk patients with contraindications against direct surgery (Fig. 3), we would at present prefer open profundaplasty in a good-risk patient with intermittent claudication only. In conclusion, most presented series of balloon angioplasty are small, and the follow-up is rather short to define the present role of this technique for the treatment of profunda artery obstructions.

WHICH INVESTIGATIONS CAN BE USED FOR THE SELECTION OF PATIENTS?

When the decision has been made that a re-opening procedure is indicated, arteriography of the lower extremities should include lateral projection of the profunda artery. The orifice of this artery is located on the posterolateral aspect of the common femoral artery, and obstructions of the profunda artery may therefore be hidden on arteriograms taken in the anterolateral plane only. This is an important point, since it has been claimed that the majority of profunda artery obstructions are located in its first part.[9, 10] Beales *et al.* found a narrowing of the origin of the profunda artery in 39% of their patients with lower limb atherosclerosis, and 68% of the narrowed segments were recognized on the oblique or lateral views only.[30] Similar experience has been made by other investigators.[31] The degree of profunda stenosis should be evaluated, since it is generally considered that stenoses with a diameter reduction of 50% or more are haemodynamically significant. This has been a controversial topic, and profundaplasty has been recommended even if no obstruction could be detected by arteriography.[7] Our experience is that profundaplasty for less pronounced obstructions is unlikely to be clinically successful.[15, 18] We find it difficult to quantitate the capacity of the collateral network from the profunda femoris artery to the popliteal artery or leg arteries by arteriographic technique, and we have not included this in our clinical routine. However, both the popliteal artery and the leg arteries should be thoroughly evaluated during the arteriography. Continuity from the collateral circulation to one or more patent leg arteries seems to be a good indicator for a favourable postoperative result.[3, 6, 13, 14, 32, 33]

Ultrasound duplex scanning has been compared with arteriography for the quantification of peripheral arterial lesions.[34, 35] Duplex measurements have shown to be as accurate as arteriography in predicting the presence of stenoses of more than 50% diameter reduction in peripheral arteries. Criteria for such haemodynamically significant stenoses include a 100% increase in peak systolic velocity within the narrowed area, a loss of retrograde flow, and a marked spectral broadening (Fig. 4). However, less stenotic lesions not producing a pressure gradient or flow reduction at rest might become significant at excercise when blood flow demand is increased. Systematic duplex investigations in the diagnosis of stenotic lesions of the profunda femoris artery have been made.[35] The blood velocity pattern of a non-stenotic profunda femoris artery is changed in the presence of a superficial femoral artery occlusion. The overall accuracy and predictive value of time-averaged maximal

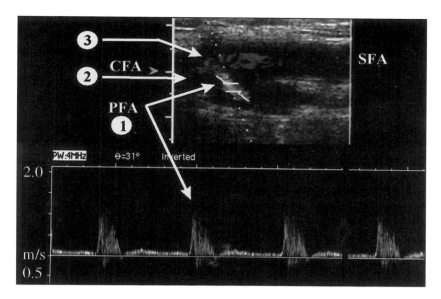

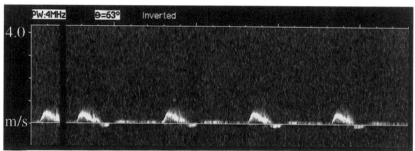

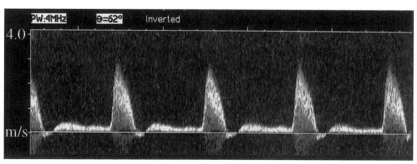

Fig. 4. Duplex scanning from a patient with severe stenosis of the common femoral artery (CFA) and the profunda femoris artery (PFA). In this patient, the superficial femoral artery (SFA) was patent in the proximal part, with occlusion in the mid-portion. The velocity waveform at the profunda orifice was pathological with spectral broadening and irregularities indicating turbulence (1). In the proximal part of the common femoral artery (2), a normal velocity signal was obtained, whereas there was an increased peak systolic velocity as well as spectral broadening in the stenotic part (3). The patient had an intraoperative pressure gradient of 20 mm Hg, and blood flow of the profunda artery of 60 ml per min. Following profundaplasty, basal blood flow was 180 ml per min., increasing to 570 following papaverine injection.

velocity in identifying significant profunda artery stenosis is higher than that of peak systolic velocity. Results of reproducibility and variability of haemodynamic duplex parameters for profunda femoris artery disease compare favourably with similar data obtained in carotid examinations for peak systolic and end diastolic frequencies. Strauss *et al.* also showed that duplex examinations can be applied to document the local haemodynamic improvement of moderate to severe profunda artery orifice stenosis by balloon angioplasty.[35]

The arterial blood pressure in various segments of the lower extremity can be measured using a distal ultrasound sensor and blood pressure cuffs at the thigh, leg and ankle level. By measuring pressure at different levels, one can get an impression of the resistance in the collateral network, from the profunda femoris artery to the more distal arteries in the leg. Various indices have been calculated, but the most reliable seems to be the so-called 'profunda–popliteal collateral index' (PPCI), which is defined as:

$$\frac{\text{The blood pressure at the thigh} - \text{the blood pressure at the leg}}{\text{The blood pressure at the thigh}}$$

This index was originally introduced by Boren *et al.*[36] In patients having a successful outcome following profundaplasty for intermittent claudication, the index averaged 0.18 compared to 0.46 in the clinical failures. In general, higher values were seen in patients with critical limb ischaemia. Other authors have found the thigh–ankle index a reliable indicator for the outcome of profundaplasty, but in this investigation, patients with more severe ischaemia were included.[37]

The value of intraoperative pressure measurements during aortoiliac surgery has been well documented, and intra-arterial pressure measurements have also been used to evaluate the haemodynamic effect of profunda artery stenosis.[38] There are indications that these measurements may be useful for patient selection, and it is likely that in patients with critical ischemia, there should be a pressure gradient during basal conditions before one can expect any benefits from profundaplasty. In patients with intermittent claudication, one can perhaps accept a small pressure gradient at rest, but following the intra-arterial injection of papaverine, an increased pressure gradient could indicate a beneficial clinical effect following profunda artery reconstruction. The papaverine test seems to be an essential part of these measurements.

Measurement of blood flow can be performed after the procedure is completed. The profunda femoris artery has a high blood flow capacity, and the blood flow at rest in patients with occlusion of the superficial femoral artery may be similar to that of the external iliac artery, when the superficial femoral and the profunda femoris arteries are both patent.[18, 39–41] From our own experience, we found a significantly higher blood flow in patients who had a clinical benefit from the procedure, compared with those who were regarded as failures.[18]

Measurement of peripheral vascular resistance has been performed to investigate whether the calculated resistance values could give an indication of the prognosis following femoropopliteal or femorotibial bypass grafting. Recordings of the resistance across obstructions of the profunda femoris artery have been presented. A higher percentage of symptomatic improvement was found in patients where the initial resistance was greater than 0.1 PRU.[42] From a theoretical point of view, intraoperative evaluation of the vascular resistance of the total profunda system seems attractive as a method to evaluate whether isolated profundaplasty would be worthwhile, or whether one should rather proceed with a femoropopliteal reconstruction.

WHAT TRIALS SUPPORT THE USE OF ISOLATED PROFUNDAPLASTY IN PATIENTS WITH INTERMITTENT CLAUDICATION?

In reported series of profundaplasty, there is often a mixture of isolated reconstructions and a combination of aortoiliac re-opening procedures in addition to profundaplasty. Furthermore, the series often contain a majority of patients with critical limb ischaemia, whereas a relatively small number of patients with intermittent claudication has been included. In the following, mainly material of patients with intermittent claudication treated with isolated profundaplasty is discussed.

Jennings and Wood[43] reported 17 patients operated on for intermittent claudication, with a subjective success rate of 83% provided the reconstruction had been closed by a patch angioplasty. This is a prerequisite to obtain a sufficient lumen of the profunda femoris artery. The group operated with patch angioplasty also had a significantly higher increase in ankle brachial index, from 0.52 to 0.8, compared with those operated with endarterectomy and primary closure of the arteriotomy. In another report of claudicants operated with isolated profundaplasty, all patients had either significant improvement or became free of symptoms.[26] All patients in this series had a patent popliteal artery, and at least two patent leg arteries.

In some of the presented series, profundaplasties with and without proximal reconstruction are included. In the series of Martin and Jamieson[29] of 217 revascularizations of the profunda artery, only 44 patients were operated on with profundaplasty only. Out of these a total of 13 (6% of the total series) were operated on for intermittent claudication. This indicates that there are relatively few patients with intermittent claudication who really are candidates for an isolated profundaplasty. Several patients claimed that their intermittent claudication had been improved, although it was impossible to show any improvement by a treadmill test or by measurement of ankle blood pressure index.[29] Fernandez et al.[11] focused on a similar problem; that subjective improvement in intermittent claudication can be obtained without simultaneous improvement in objective tests like measurement of pressure index, fall in ankle pressure after excercise or recovery time. Following successful profundaplasty, however, there was usually a significant increase in ankle brachial index, although the clinical effect in patients with intermittent claudication was moderate.

Correlates of operative results following isolated profundaplasty was investigated by Mitchell et al.,[13] but in their series of 27 patients, only five had intermittent claudication. Two of these became free of symptoms, and the recurrence rate in the total series was 44%. Clinical correlates of success were: age below 60 years, absence of diabetes, the presence of a femoral bruit and an ankle brachial index above 0.25. A common femoral artery reconstruction in addition to the profundaplasty gave better results than profundaplasty alone, indicating that an in-flow obstruction had been relieved during the same procedure in some of these cases. The most reliable criteria were provided by arteriography, and included severe stenosis of the profunda artery of more than 50% diameter stenosis, minimal disease of the distal profunda artery, and disease-free profunda artery collaterals. Furthermore, reconstitution of collaterals into a patent superficial femoral artery or popliteal artery, and good popliteal runoff to the foot by one or more leg arteries were significant indicators of a successful procedure. Only nine patients fulfilled these criteria (33%), and they all became free of symptoms postoperatively. Modgill *et al.* claim that profundaplasty has a place in the surgery of intermittent claudication.[44] In their total series of 45 patients undergoing isolated profundaplasty, only eight had intermittent claudication, and a significant improvement was obtained in all cases. In one of the largest series of 93 patients with intermittent claudication treated with isolated profundaplasty, a 68% clinical improvement was obtained and the average follow-up period was 37 months.[24]

Although most of the presented series are relatively small, satisfactory clinical results are obtained in most patients with intermittent claudication.[21, 22–26] In a series of 106 patients treated with isolated profundaplasty,[45] 43 patients had intermittent claudication, and in this group the average preoperative ankle brachial index was 0.4. A moderate, but significant increase to 0.55 was observed after the operation. Early postoperative improvement of ankle brachial index of more than 0.1 was associated with long-term success in this material. The 3-year follow-up indicated a significantly higher success rate in claudicants compared with those who had more severe ischaemia. There was no significant difference between diabetics and non-diabetics, and patency of the popliteal artery was not a significant predictor of success. However, patients with good out-flow defined as two or three patent tibial arteries had significantly better outcome than those with poor out-flow, as defined by one or no patent tibial arteries. It was concluded that profundaplasty is an alternative for lower limb revascularization, and one advantage is that the possibility for further distal reconstruction is not precluded. The relief of claudication, however, is usually not dramatic. Similar results were obtained by Fugger *et al.* in a series of 133 isolated profundaplasties, where the best results were obtained in patients with intermittent claudication.[32] However, this group only included 27 patients; 89% of them improved, and the best effect was obtained if two or more tibial vessels were patent. It was noted that it often takes weeks for the improvement to become obvious. Half of the patients had a slight increase in ankle pressure index after surgery of 0.12. Others have found limited improvement in most of their cases with intermittent claudication,[11] and it has been claimed that profundaplasty has a limited role in arterial surgery at all.[46] However, in the latter series of 17 reported patients, only three were treated for intermittent claudication, and this series is therefore too small to draw firm conlusions. In the literature, thigh claudication caused by profunda femoris obstruction has been described in spite of patent femoral and popliteal arteries. Such symptoms can be successfully treated by profundaplasty, but this syndrome seems to be extremely rare.[47]

Our own experience is largely in accordance with most published series. During the period 1983-95, altogether 264 reconstructions of the profunda femoris artery were recorded, but only 85 of these were confined to the profunda artery itself. Furthermore, 23 patients were operated on for intermittent claudication with isolated profundaplasty. 22 of the patients had a significant clinical improvement, but only five patients became free of symptoms. The mean follow-up period in this series was 4 years, and the best effect was obtained in the patients who had the most severe stenosis on preoperative arteriograms. Some of the factors of importance for the results following isolated profundaplasty are shown in Fig. 5.

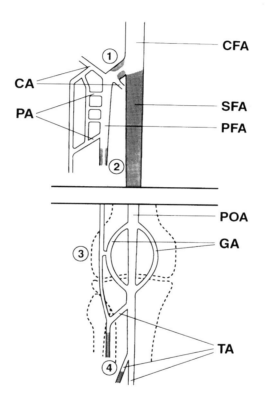

Fig. 5. Schematic illustration of the profunda femoris artery system and its collaterals to the distal arteries of the lower extremity. CFA: common femoral artery; SFA; superficial femoral artery; PFA: profunda femoris artery; POA: popliteal artery; GA: genicular arteries; TA: tibial arteries; CA: circumflex femoral arteries; PA: perforating arteries of the profunda. The following factors are of importance for the outcome of an isolated profundaplasty: 1) the degree of profunda artery stenosis, 2) patency of the peripheral part of the profunda artery, 3) the collateral network communicating with the leg arteries, and 4) patency of the tibial arteries.

WHAT FUTURE TRIALS WOULD BE HELPFUL?

A review of the literature shows that there should be agreement on the definition of isolated profundaplasty, and that these operations should be separated from profundaplasty performed in addition to relief of in-flow obstructions. In the latter category, the extent of the operation should be thoroughly defined. Exact criteria of success and failure from a clinical as well as from a physiological point of view should be defined. It would be advantageous to have a method whereby the resistance of the total profunda artery system, and not only of a localized stenosis, could be evaluated. This might give an indication of the effect of the procedure, and improve the selection of patients.

Results of operations performed for intermittent claudication are often difficult to evaluate. There is often a discrepancy between subjective symptoms and objective recording of the distal circulation. Segmental blood pressure measurements and treadmill testing could improve the evaluation of the effect of isolated profundaplasty. The significance of pre- and postoperative investigation of profunda artery disease by colour-coded duplex scanning should be explored to identify criteria for a haemodynamically significant stenosis.

Rather few patients with intermittent claudication are treated with isolated profundaplasty in each center. Perhaps multicentre trials could be performed to increase the numbers sufficiently to sort out the criteria necessary to expect a beneficial effect of profunda reconstruction only. Today, approximately 20% of the patients have insufficient clinical effect following this operation. In a multicentre study, a thorough arteriographic investigation of relevant arterial segments should be included. Preoperative duplex scanning of the profunda artery and non-invasive segmental blood pressure measurements would be advantageous. Simultaneous intraoperative measurement of pressure gradient and blood flow could provide valuable information. In the postoperative course, objective evaluation of the walking capacity by treadmill testing should be included, and the patient should be followed for a sufficient period of time. Both long-term clinical results as well as the patency rate and the effect of physiological parameters should be recorded.

CONCLUSION

We feel that there is a case for isolated profundaplasty in some patients with intermittent claudication. However, the group of patients where profundaplasty is the first choice is rather small, and probably represents less than 5% of the total population of patients having intermittent claudication caused by infrainguinal atherosclerosis. The best clinical results are obtained if there is a preoperative total occlusion or severe stenosis of the proximal part of the profunda artery, when its distal part is relatively free of disease and if the popliteal runoff is good with two or more patent leg arteries. Success is more likely to be obtained if there is an initial pressure gradient which is increased following the injection of papaverine. With these criteria as basis for selection of patients, most patients can expect to become free of symptoms or feel significant subjective improvement, with a good long-term prognosis.

REFERENCES

1. Leeds FH, Gilfillan RS: Revascularization of the ischemic limb. Importance of profunda femoris artery. *Arch Surg* **82**: 25–31, 1961
2. Morris GC, Edwards W, Cooley DA *et al.*: Surgical importance of profunda femoris artery. *Arch Surg* **82**: 32–7, 1961
3. Tovar-Pardo AE, Bernhard VM: Where the profunda femoris artery fits in the spectrum of lower limb revascularization. *Semin Vasc Surg* **8**: 225–35, 1995
4. Varty K, London NJM, Ratliff DA *et al.*: Percutaneous angioplasty of the profunda femoris artery: A safe and effective endovascular technique. *Eur J Vasc Surg* **7**: 483–7, 1993
5. Dacie JE, Daniell SJN: The value of percutaneous transluminal angioplasty of the profunda femoris artery in threatened limb loss and intermittent claudication. *Clin Radiol* **44**: 311–6, 1991
6. Bernhard VM: The role of profundaplasty in revascularization of the lower extremities. *Surg Clin North Am* **59**: 681–92, 1979
7. Morris-Jones W, Jones CDP: Profundoplasty in the treatment of femoropopliteal occlusion. *Am J Surg* **127**: 680–6, 1974
8. Waibel PP: Autogenous reconstruction of the deep femoral artery. *J Cardiovasc Surg (Torino)* **7**: 179–81, 1966
9. Martin P, Renwick S, Stephenson C: On the surgery of the profunda femoris artery. *Br J Surg* **55**: 539–42, 1968
10. Martin P, Frawley JE, Barabas AP, Rosengarten DS: One the surgery of atherosclerosis of the profunda femoris artery. *Surgery* **71**: 182–9, 1972
11. Fernandez e Fernandez J, Nicolaides AN, Angelides NA, Gordon-Smith IC: An objective assessment of common femoral endarterectomy and profundaplasty in patients with superficial femoral occlusion. *Surgery* **83**: 313–8, 1978
12. Jelnes R, Gaardsting O, Hougaard Jensen K *et al.*: Fate in intermittent claudication: outcome and risk factors. *Br Med J* **293**: 1137–40, 1986
13. Mitchell RA, Bone GE, Bridges R *et al.*: Patient selection for isolated profundaplasty. Arteriographic correlates of operative results. *Am J Surg* **138**: 912–9, 1979
14. Towne JB, Bernhard VM, Rollins DL, Baum PL: Profundaplasty in perspective: Limitations in the long-term management of limb ischemia. *Surgery* **90**: 1037–46, 1981
15. Myhre HO: Has profunda femoris reconstruction a place as alternative to graft thrombectomy and new graft implantation? *Acta Chir Scand* **538** (Suppl): 139–43, 1987
16. Bouhoutsos J, Martin P: The influence of age on prognosis after arterial surgery for atherosclerosis of the lower limb. *Surgery* **74**: 637–40, 1973
17. King TA, DePalma RG: Diabetes mellitus and atherosclerotic involvement of the profunda femoris artery. *Surg Gynecol Obstet* **159**: 553–6, 1984
18. Myhre HO: The place of profundaplasty in surgical treatment of lower limb atherosclerosis. *Acta Chir Scand* **143**: 105–8, 1977
19. Ward AS, Morris-Jones W: The long term results of profundaplasty in femoropopliteal arterial occlusion. *Br J Surg* **64**: 365–7, 1977
20. Jacobs DL, Seabrook GR, Freischlag JA, Towne JB: The current role of profundaplasty in complex peripheral arterial reconstruction. *J Vasc Surg* **18**: 534–5, 1993
21. Goldstone J, Malone JM, Moore WS: Importance of the profunda femoris artery in primary and secondary arterial operations for lower extremity ischemia. *Am J Surg* **136**: 215–20, 1978
22. Thompson BW, Read RC, Campbell GS *et al.*: The role of profundaplasty in revascularization of the lower extremity. *Am J Surg* **132**: 710–5, 1976
23. Heather BP, Ware CC: The non-selective use of profundaplasty in lower limb ischaemia. *Post Grad Med J* **55**: 800–5, 1979
24. Harper DR, Millar DG: Simple conservative profundaplasty in lower limb ischaemia. *J R Coll Surg Edinb* **88**: 197–202, 1977
25. Moggi L, Giustozzi GM, Marianeschi PM *et al.*: Profundaplasty as an alternative to femoropopliteal by-pass in occlusions of the superficial femoral artery. *Panminerva Med* **26**: 9–12, 1984

26. Miani S, Giuffrida GF, Ghilardi G *et al.*: Indications and the role of isolated profundaplasty in patients affected by limb ischemia. *Panminerva Med* **37**: 204–6, 1995

27. Miksic K, Novak B: Profunda femoris revascularization in limb salvage. *J Cardiovasc Surg (Torino)* **27**: 544–52, 1986

28. Myhre HO: Is femoropopliteal bypass surgery indicated for the treatment of intermittent claudication? *Acta Chir Scand* **555** (Suppl): 39–42, 1990

29. Martin P, Jamieson C: The rationale for and measurement after profundaplasty. *Surg Clin North Am* **54**: 95–109, 1974

30. Beales JSM, Adcock FA, Frawley JS *et al.*: The radiological assessment of disease of the profunda femoris artery. *Br J Radiol* **44**: 854–9, 1971

31. McDonald EJ, Malone JM, Gooding GW *et al.*: Stenosis of the deep femoral artery: an evaluation of the accuracy of single-plane, anteroposterior arteriograms. *Br J Radiol* **49**: 932–3, 1976

32. Fugger R, Kretschmer G, Schemper M *et al.*: The place of profundaplasty in the surgical treatment of superficial femoral artery occlusion. *Eur J Vasc Surg* **1**: 187–191, 1987

33. Sladen JG, Burgess JJ: Profundaplasty: Expectations and ominous signs. *Am J Surg* **140**: 242–5: 1980

34. Jager KA, Phillips DJ, Martin RL *et al.*: Noninvasive mapping of lower limb arterial lesions. *Ultrasound Med Biol* **11**: 515–21, 1985

35. Strauss AL, Schäberle W, Rieger H, Roth F-J: Use of duplex scanning in the diagnosis of arteria profunda femoris stenosis. *J Vasc Surg* **13**: 698–704, 1991

36. Boren CH, Towne JB, Bernhard VM, Salles-Cunha S: Profundapopliteal collateral index. A guide to successful profundaplasty. *Arch Surg* **115**: 1366–72, 1980

37. McCoy DM, Sawchuck AP, Schuler JJ *et al.*: The role of isolated profundaplasty for the treatment of rest pain. *Arch Surg* **124**: 441–4, 1989

38. Archie JP Jr, Feldtman RW: Intraoperative assessment of the hemodynamic significance of iliac and profunda femoris artery stenosis. *Surgery* **90**: 876–80, 1981

39. Baron HC, Schwartz M, Batri G: The papaverine test for blood flow potential of the profunda femoris artery. *Surg Gynecol Obstet* **153**: 873–6, 1981

40. Hussain ST, Smith RE, Clark AL, Wood RFM: Blood flow in the lower limb after balloon angioplasty of the superficial femoral artery. *Br J Surg* **83**: 791–5, 1996

41. Bernhard VM, Militello JM, Geringer AM: Repair of the profunda femoris artery. *Am J Surg* **127**: 676–9, 1974

42. Sugden BA, Sheldon CD: Peroperative flow and pressure measurements in profundaplasty. *J Cardiovasc Surg (Torino)* **20**: 185–8, 1979

43. Jennings WC, Wood CD: The role of vein patch angioplasty in isolated operations for profunda femoris stenosis and disabling claudication. *Am J Surg* **150**: 263–5, 1985

44. Modgill VK, Humphrey CS, Shoesmith JH, Kester RC: The value of profundaplasty in the management of severe femoropopliteal occlusion. *Br J Surg* **64**: 362–4, 1977

45. Kalman PG, Johnston KW, Walker PM: The current role of isolated profundaplasty. *J Cardiovasc Surg (Torino)* **31**: 107–11, 1990

46. Harward TRS, Bergan JJ, Yao JST *et al.*: The demise of primary profundaplasty. *Am J Surg* **156**: 126–9, 1988

47. Martin RS: Thigh claudication due to profunda femoris artery occlusion. *J Vasc Surg* **1**: 692–4, 1984

Editorial comments by R.M. Greenhalgh

This chapter is extremely well presented and referenced and the authors comment that their own experiences are largely in accordance with most published series. They report 85 isolated profunda artery reconstructions, of which 23 were operated upon for intermittent claudication, 22 had clinical improvement but only five became free of symptoms. From this one may conclude rather that for a correctly selected patient, intermittent claudication can be improved but not cured. This is because the superficial femoral artery is expected to be occluded in such patients. As far as future trials are concerned the authors stress how difficult it is to assess intermittent claudication and they comment upon the discrepancy between subjective and objective assessments and that a single centre will see rather few of this type of patient. For this reason any trial would need to be multicentre. The authors give the impression that they have a good idea what profundaplasty can do for intermittent claudication and if their views are representative of many of the centres who would be approached, it is possible that there would not be enough enthusiasm to mount a multicentre trial. It seems rather that the selection of the appropriate patient with a haemodynamically significant stenosis in the profunda system should be selected for surgery where the intermittent claudication distance is rather limiting.

Superficial Femoral Artery Stenting: Is It Justified?

Jean Pierre Becquemin, Jerome Cron, Oswaldo Teixeira, Djamel Berrahal and Hicham Kobeiter

INTRODUCTION

Stents have been designed to keep open the lumen of vessels after balloon angioplasty. Interventionalists have enthusiastically accepted the concept of stenting which improves the cosmetic and haemodynamical results of percutaneous transluminal angioplasty (PTA) (Fig. 1). However, stents have some drawbacks: acute occlusion may occur and intimal hyperplasia may develop within the first 6 months (Fig. 2). At present, proof of long-term benefit compared with balloon angioplasty alone remains scarce. In the coronary arteries, two randomized studies have shown that stents improved the results of angioplasty at 6 months.[1,2] In the renal arteries, stenting has also improved the overall patency rate after unsuccessful balloon angioplasty.[3] For lower limb arteries, randomized studies are lacking and decisions are left to the conviction of the individual physician.

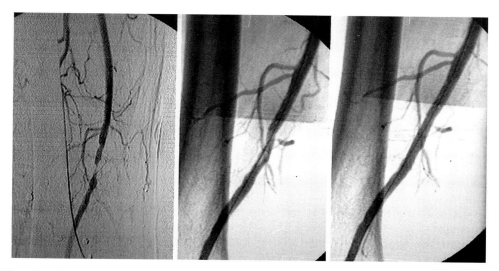

Fig. 1. Pre and peroperative angiograms of a patient treated by Palmaz stent after subobtimal results of PTA for a stenosis of the superficial femoral artery.

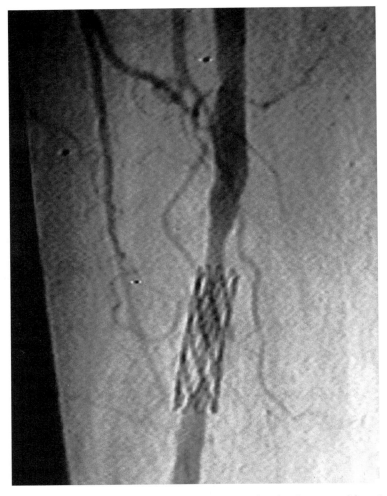

Fig. 2.   Intimal hyperplasia within the stent and at both extremities, 1 year after Palmaz stent placement in a superficial femoral arterial lesion.

Besides efficacy, cost constraint is important for the decision making process. In France, among general measures taken to limit the deficit of the Securite Sociale which is in charge of the Health Care Reimbursement, the price of each stent was fixed to 5500 francs by a government regulation named TIPS. Furthermore, the recommendations of ANDEM,[4] the National Agency for Medical Evaluation, were that the only indication for placing stents in the superficial femoral artery was the occurrence of an occlusion during PTA. Theses recommendations published in 1994 were based on analysis of the literature available at that time. Since then new reports have become available which may alter past conclusions. If efficient, stents may decrease the need for redo-angioplasty and compensate for the extra cost of the material.

AUTHORS' CHOICE OF PROCEDURE

Since 1994 we have chosen to insert a stent selectively in patients who had sub-optimal results after balloon angioplasty mainly in cases of dissection, residual stenosis, or restenosis. This option should be replaced in our general scheme of treating patients with femoropopliteal diseases. Currently, all patients referred to our department for lower limb ischaemia have duplex-scan examination by a certified angiologist. When lesions are limited to the superficial femoral artery, further orientations depend upon the severity of symptoms. Claudicants are advised to stop smoking, to walk regularly, and to take antiplatelet medication for 3 months. Patients with critical ischaemia or failed medical treatment are submitted to an arteriogram, the result of which indicates the therapeutical option.

Patients with short (< 10 cm) and unique stenotic or occlusive superficial femoral artery lesions are treated by PTA, provided that at least one leg artery remains patent. Procedures are done in the operating room under local anaesthesia. The room is equipped with a Diasonic 2000, OCE, comprising a mobile C-arm with digitized imaging, road-mapping and laser film printing. Most lesions are approached from the ipsilateral groin and crossed with a 0.038 Benson or Terumo catheter. Dilatation is performed with Ultra-thin balloon catheters from Boston Scientific, generally 2–4 cm in length and 6–8 mm in diameter. For calcified lesions Blue-max catheters are used. All stages of the procedure are followed on fluoroscopic and road-mapping screens. After balloon deflation a two-plan arteriogram of the dilated artery is obtained as well as images of the popliteal trifurcation (to detect plaque or thrombus dislodgment). If the results are not satisfactory (residual stenosis greater than 30%, plaque dissection), the inflation is repeated. A stent is inserted if defects persist. Usually one Palmaz P394 or P204 stent is used. In a few cases two stents are required to cover the whole lesion. The stents are firmly impacted in the arterial wall inflating the balloon. We have recently started to use the self-expandable nitinol Symphony stent which should not be exposed to stent crushing (an event we have never observed in our series). During procedure, 5000 units of heparin are given intravenously. Low-molecular weight heparin is given for 48 hours and then aspirin 250 mg/day or ticlopidin twice daily, indefinitively. Patients are followed clinically and by duplex scan every 3 months for the first year and yearly thereafter.

Some less favourable lesions are also proposed for PTA such as bifocal short lesions or recent long occlusion (clinical worsening dating less than 15 days). In the latter case thromboaspiration, angioplasty and/or intraoperative thrombolysis are combined to reopen the artery. Again, in these peculiar settings, stents are implanted selectively in the case of residual lesions following PTA. In cases of restenosis after balloon angioplasty a stent is inserted liberally, since PTA alone is associated with poor results.[5]

We do not propose PTA nor PTA and stent for patients with multistenotic lesions, neither for calcified burgeoning plaques, nor in patients with long stenosis or occlusion (> 10 cm). In this group of patients, rehabilitation is indicated when symptoms are mild, and surgery is proposed at first when the complaints are major or when the limb is at risk of amputation. In this scheme, we followed the conclusions drawn by Hunink et al.,[6] who showed that in terms of cost-effectiveness, efficiency and quality of life, surgery was indicated as a first choice in patients with critical ischaemia and superficial femoral arterial occlusion. These conclusions were based on a meta-analysis comparing 4511 bypasses and 4800 PTA for superficial femoral arterial lesions.

ALTERNATIVES AVAILABLE

Rehabilitation

In claudicants, whatever the lesion, rehabilitation is an alternative option. Randomized studies have shown that the walking distance may improve more with rehabilitation than with endovascular treatment.[7,8] Conversely, one randomized study, where walking distance, ankle brachial index and quality of life were the end points, concluded in favour of angioplasty.[9]

Other endovascular options

For short lesions

Since there is no evidence of the role of stent in superficial femoral arteries, angioplasty alone as well as systematic stenting may have defendants.

For long lesions

Recanalization
Despite a poor reputation, recanalization of long lesions has been attempted with favourable results. Using modern guide-wires, Murray *et al.*[10] have treated 44 patients with lesions ranging from 10 to 40cm in length (mean length 24.3 cm) with 93% technical success and 69% cumulative patency rate at 18 months.

Subintimal angioplasty
With the technique of subintimal angioplasty, Bolia[11] treated 200 patients with femoropopliteal occlusion (mean lesion length 11.5 cm) and reported patency rate of 71% at 1 year and 58% at 3 years excluding early failures (20%).

Multiple stenting
Multiple stents or long stents have also been implanted for long lesions. Henry *et al.*[12] reported 75% 2-year primary patency rate with long segments where more than two Palmaz stents were required.

Covered stent graft
Sparse cases have been reported and long-term results are awaited.

Surgery

Best results of bypasses are obtained in patients with claudication and above-the-knee revascularization.[13] A randomized study from Veterans' Hospitals[14] has shown that for short lesions the patency rate of PTA and surgery was the same; however, more redo-procedures were necessary in the PTA group.

EVIDENCE FOR AUTHORS' CHOICE

In 1994 we reported our experience of PTA alone in the superficial femoral artery.[15] The 2-year patency rate was 51%. Probabilities of patency according to significant factors (length, stenosis versus occlusion) were determined by a multifactorial Cox analysis as shown in Fig. 3. One conclusion of this study was that long occlusions should not be treated by PTA. Of note is that the most dramatic fall in patency was due to early failures. Calculations were made according to the intent to treat principle and early failures included impossibility to cross the lesions, failure to crush the plaque, and thrombosis. In patients with early success there was a slow and regular decline in patency afterwards; thus, improving immediate results, as well as improving long-term patency after a successful angioplasty, were for us the main objectives. These were obtained by a better selection of patients, improved technical skills, the use of modern guide-wires and catheters, and by stents for PTA at high risk of failure. For this report we reviewed our recent experience of PTA and selective stenting as described above. Between 1993 and 1997, 188 patients with superficial

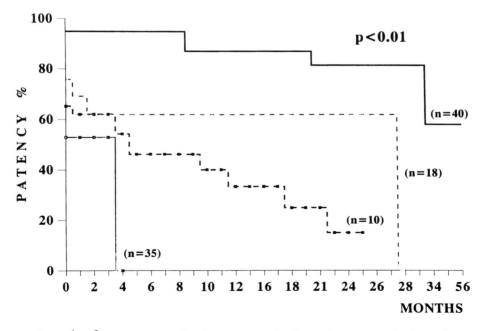

Fig. 3. Probabilities of patency rate according to the combination of length and stenosis vs occlusion in a series of 103 PTA for superficial femoral arterial lesions.

femoral artery lesions were treated by PTA alone (n = 143) or PTA plus stent (n = 45) (23%). There were 120 males and 68 females with a mean age of 69 ± 11 years; 120 were claudicants and 68 had critical ischaemia. There were 111 stenoses and 77 occlusions. The mean length of the lesions was 3.8 cm ± 2.4. Postoperatively two patients died – one of them from myocardial infarction – the remaining one from acute renal failure. The non-fatal general complications were one heart failure, two pulmonary infections, one gastric bleeding, and four urologic infections. These eight complications occurred in five patients who had been treated by angioplasty alone. They were 18 local non-vascular complications (11% for the PTA group, 4% for the stent group). These complications included five infections (only one surgical drainage), 11 haematomas (one surgical suture), and one lymphocoele. There were 14 early reocclusions, 13 in the PTA group (9%) and only one in the stented group (2%). Two residual stenoses were observed in the PTA group. No patient in the stented group and seven patients in the PTA group (4%) were reoperated on (two new PTA, five bypasses) to maintain or restore patency. There was one leg amputation and two foot amputations, all in the PTA group. With a mean follow-up of 12 months, the primary patency rate was 96% in the stented group and 85% in the non-stented group.

WHAT TRIALS SUPPORT AUTHORS' VIEW

No randomized trials comparing PTA vs PTA and stent are currently available so we have to look into series of patients treated by PTA alone and series of patients treated with stent. Among numerous reports on PTA for superficial femoral arterial lesions, the series of Capek *et al.*[16] and those of Johnston[17] are most informative. The Capek series included 217 PTA with a mean follow-up of 7 years. Patency was 73% at 1 year, 55% at 3 years, and 52% at 5 years. Johnston's series included 254 PTA; patency was 62.5% at 1 year, 51% at 3 years, and 38% at 5 years. Table 1 shows the patency obtained at 1 year in recent series using Palmaz, Wallstent, and Strecker stents. In these series, stenting was indicated in cases of suboptimal results of angioplasty. The crude calculations seem in favour of the use of stent. However, conclusions should be made with caution since the series using PTA alone are somewhat older and patient selection as well as techniques have evolved with time. Factors which affect outcome after PTA are currently well identified. Less favourable results are obtained in patients with critical ischaemia as opposed to claudication, occlusive lesions as opposed to stenoses, long lesions as opposed to short lesions and redo-procedures as opposed to first treatments.[15–18] Of note is that these factors are also associated with the poorest results of stent,[19] thus they do not represent a clear indication for stenting. Initial results of PTA are also predictive of outcome. Duplex-scan studies performed the day after PTA, have shown that residual stenosis and dissection were associated with a high rate of failure at 1 year.[20] In that case, insertion of a stent which opens the arterial lumen wide, is appealing. The unanswered question remains the degree of development of intimal hyperplasia in the struts of the stent or at its extremities. If hyperplasia is a significant problem, the utility of stent will be questionable not only as a routine but also in the specific indications listed above.

Table 1. Literature review of recent series of stent for superficial femoral arterial lesions

Authors	Year	No. of limbs	Lesion length	1-year patency (%)
Strecker[21]	93	84	4.8	80
Bergeron[22]	95	42	7.6	81
Bray[23]	95	56	6.8	79
Henry[12]	95	126	3.8	81
Martin[24]	95	96	5.7	61
White[25]	95	32	3.7	75

WHAT FUTURE TRIALS WOULD BE HELPFUL

For short lesion (< 10 cm) comparison of PTA and stent in non-selected patients would be helpful. Such a trial is currently underway in France and Belgium. By October 1997, 213 patients had already been enrolled and treated. All patients will be evaluated clinically and by duplex scan every 3 months for the first year and yearly thereafter for 5 years. An angiogram will be performed at 1 year follow-up in every patient. This trial will answer the question of long-term efficacy of superficial femoral arterial stenting. It may also help to select patients at risk of early failure after PTA and the potential benefit of stent.

For long lesions, comparison of subintimal angioplasty, stenting and surgery would also be of value in choosing the best procedure.

REFERENCES

1. Serruys PW, De Jaegere P, Kiemeneij *et al.*: A comparison of balloon-expandable-stent implantation with balloon angioplasty in patients with coronary artery disease. *New Engl J Med* **331**: 489–95, 1994
2. Fischman DL, Lcon MB, Baim DS *et al.*: A randomized comparison of coronary-stent placement and balloon angioplasty in the treatment of coronary artery disease. *New Engl J Med* **331**: 496–501, 1994
3. Bloom U, Krumme B, Flugel P *et al.*: Treatment of ostial renal artery stenoses with vascular endoprotheses after unsuccessful balloon angioplasty. *New Engl J Med* **336**: 13–20, 1997
4. Bouthillon Y for "L'Agence Nationale pour le Développement de l'Evaluation Médicale": *Evaluation des nouvelles techniques de revascularisation endoluminale des artères des membres inférieurs.* ANDEM, 1993
5. Treiman GS, Ichikawa L, Treiman RL *et al.*: Treatment of recurrent femoral or popliteal artery stenosis after percutaneous transluminal angioplasty. *J Vasc Surg* **20**: 577–87, 1994
6. Hunink MGM, Wong JB, Donaldson MC *et al.*: Revascularization for femoro-popliteal disease: a decision and cost-effectiveness analysis. *J Am Med Ass* **274**: 165–171, 1995
7. Creasy TS, McMillan PJ, Fletcher EWL *et al.*: Is percutaneous transluminal angioplasty better than exercise for claudication? Preliminary results from a prospective randomised trial *Eur J Vasc Surg* **4**: 135–40, 1990
8. Perkins JMT, Collin J, Creasy TS *et al.*: Exercise training versus angioplasty for stable claudication. Long and medium term results of a prospective, randomised trial. *Eur J Vasc Endovasc Surg* **11**: 409–13, 1996

9. Whyman MR, Fowkes FGR, Kerracher EMG *et al.*: Randomized controlled trial of percutaneous transluminal angioplasty for intermittent claudication. *Eur J Vasc Endovasc Surg* **12**: 167–72, 1996

10. Murray JG, Apthorp LA, Wilkins RA. Long-segment (> 10 cm) femoropopliteal angioplasty: improved technical success and long-term patency. *Radiology* **195**: 158–62, 1995

11. Bolia A, Bell PRF. Femoropopliteal and crural artery recanalization using subintimal angioplasty. *Semin Vasc Surg* **8**: 253–64, 1995

12. Henry M, Amor M, Ethevenot G *et al.*: Palmaz stent placement in iliac and femoropopliteal arteries: primary and secondary patency in 310 patients with 2–4 year follow-up. *Radiology* **197**: 167–74, 1995

13. Dalman RL, Taylor LM: Données de base concernant les revascularisations sous-inguinales *Ann Chir Vasc* **4**: 309–12, 1990

14. Wilson SE, Wolf GL, Cross AP: Percutaneous transluminal angioplasty versus operation for peripheral arteriosclerosis: report of a prospective randomized trial in a select group of patients. *J Vasc Surg* **9**: 1–9, 1989

15. Becquemin JP, Cavillon A, Haiduc F: Surgical transluminal femoropopliteal angioplasty: multivariate analysis outcome. *J Vasc Surg* **19**: 495–502, 1994

16. Capek P, McLean GK, Berkowitz HD: Femoropopliteal angioplasty: factors influencing long-term success. *Circulation* **83** (Suppl 1): 70-1-80, 1991

17. Johnston KW: Femoral and popliteal arteries: reanalysis of results of balloon angioplasty. *Radiology* **183**: 767–71, 1992

18. Gray BH, Sullivan TM, Childs MB: High incidence of restenosis/reocclusion of stents in the percutaneous treatment of long-segment superficial femoral artery disease after suboptimal angioplasty. *J Vasc Surg* **25**: 74–83, 1997

19. Gray BH, Olin JW: Limitations of percutaneous transluminal angioplasty with stenting for femoropopliteal arterial occlusive disease. *Semin Vasc Surg* **10**: 8–16, 1997

20. Spijkerboer AM, Nass PC, de Valois JC *et al.*: Evaluation of femoropopliteal arteries with duplex ultrasound after angioplasty. Can we predict results at one year? *Eur J Vasc Endovasc Surg* **12**: 418–23, 1996

21. Strecker EK, Hagan B, Liermann D *et al.*: Iliac and femoropopliteal vascular occlusive disease treated with flexible tantalum stents. *Cardiovasc Intervent Radiol* **16**: 158–64, 1993

22. Bergeron P, Pinot JJ, Poyen V *et al.*: Long-term results with the Palmaz stent in the superficial femoral artery. *J Endovasc Surg* **2**: 161–7, 1995

23. Bray AE, Liu WG, Lewis WA *et al.*: Strecker stents in the femoropopliteal arteries: value of duplex ultrasonography in restenosis assessment. *J Endovasc Surg* **2**: 150–60, 1995

24. Martin EC, Katzen BT, Benenati JF *et al.*: Multicenter trial of the Wallstent in the iliac and femoral arteries. *J Vasc Intervent Radiol* **6**: 843–9, 1995

25. White GH, Liew SCC, Waugh RC *et al.*: Early outcome and intermediate followup of vascular stents in the femoral and popliteal arteries without long-term anticoagulation. *J Vasc Surg* **21**: 270–81, 1995

Editorial comments by R.M. Greenhalgh

The authors have addressed themselves to the question and have indicated that they decide on the basis of angiography if a stent should be used. It seems that they do not use intravascular ultrasound at all. They do stress that they are only interested in superficial femoral artery lesions of less than 10cm and they advise against attempting the longer lesions. As far as the future is concerned they wish to see a trial of superficial femoral artery stenoses managed by angioplasty against angioplasty plus stent in non-selected patients. They mention that such a trial is on the way in France and Belgium and that by October 1997, 213 patients have been allocated.

DISTAL RECONSTRUCTION QUESTIONS AND INDICATIONS

Is Balloon Angioplasty Below the Knee Joint Wise?

David Bergqvist, Sadettin Karacagil and Anee-Marie Löfberg

Balloon angioplasty, most frequently performed percutaneously (percutaneous transluminal angioplasty: PTA) and sometimes intraoperatively, has been available for more than 20 years since the publication on the balloon catheter technique by Grüntzig and Hopff.[1] To start with, however, the balloons were far too large to be used in the crural arteries. More sophisticated and fine calibre catheters and balloon systems and low friction guide-wires were developed, initially to satisfy the use within coronary arteries. In some anatomical areas PTA has become the method of choice with acceptable or even good long-term results, such as iliac, renal or coronary arteries. Today the balloon angioplasty is sometimes combined with stenting, often on the basis of morphological or cosmetic impression of the lesion rather than on the basis of pure scientific knowledge and guidelines. In relation to the large number of publications on angioplasty there are very few randomized trials where the technique has been compared with surgery or with best conservative treatment.[2–5]

To answer the question posed in the title of this chapter – if angioplasty distal to the knee joint is wise or not – is not an easy task, not only because of the philosophical dimension of the question but also because of the relatively low number of studies, which moreover are very unhomogeneous in design. It is also not always clear whether or not below-knee balloon angioplasty has been combined with other reconstructive or reopening procedures – there are actually a number of possible combinations – and whether or not popliteal dilatations are reported together, both above and below the knee joint.

The various possibilities where below-knee angioplasty (popliteal artery, tibioperoneal trunk, anterior tibial, posterior tibial and peroneal arteries) may be used are as follows:

1. Isolated below-knee angioplasty with patent proximal vessels (Fig. 1).
2. Combined angioplasty proximal and distal to the knee joint (Fig. 2).
3. Combined bypass grafting and infrageniculate angioplasty to secure the runoff situation.[6,7]
4. Thrombolysis with angioplasty to treat the cause of thrombotic occlusion or to secure the runoff situation.[7–9]
5. Angioplasty to increase primary assisted or secondary patency in patients with a femorodistal bypass:
   - stenosis in a vein graft below the knee
   - anastomotic stenosis below the knee
   - runoff stenosis because of progressive arteriosclerosis.
   a. As a result of a surveillance programme to prevent failing grafts.[10,11]
   b. As a treatment because of recurrent symptoms.[9,10,12,13]
6. Thrombolytic treatment of an occluded femorodistal bypass with balloon angioplasty to correct the runoff situation (see point 5 above).[14,15]

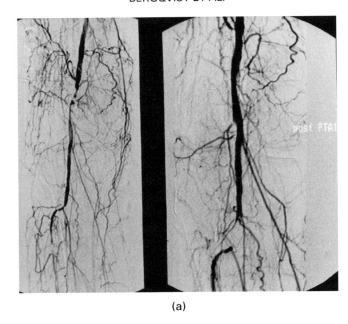

(a)

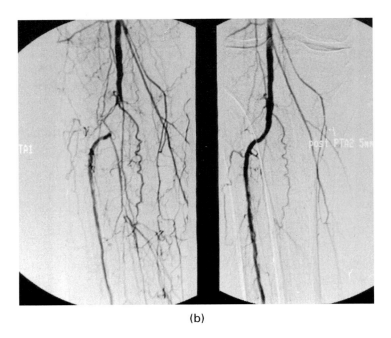

(b)

Fig 1.   A 72-year old man with critical limb ischaemia. (a) Tight stenosis
in the popliteal artery at the knee joint before (left panel) and after (right
panel) PTA. (b) Occlusion of the distal popliteal artery just proximal to the
anterior tibial artery before (left panel) and after (right panel) PTA.

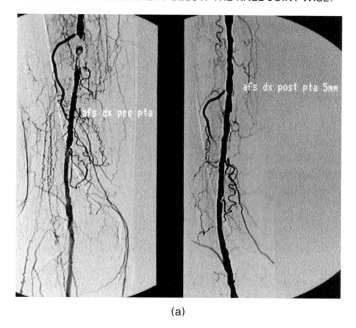

(a)

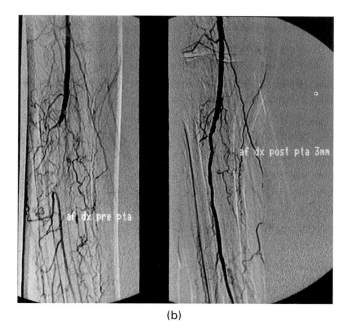

(b)

Fig 2. Female, 90 years old with critical limb ischaemia. (a) Tight stenosis in the superficial femoral artery before (left panel) and after (right panel) PTA. (b) Occlusion of the tibioperoneal trunk and proximal fibular artery before (left panel) and after (right panel) PTA.

Table 1. Studies on below-knee angioplasty with more than 35 patients per study

Author	No of patients	No of legs	No of dilated lesions	Combined proximal procedure		No of diabetic patients	Technical success (%)	No of arteries treated					Follow-up (months)
				A-plasty	Bypass			Popl.	Truncus tib. fib.	Tibial ant.	Tibial post.	Fib.	
Bakal et al.[30]	53	57	76	30	12	45	78	62	22	26	10	18	Short term
Brown et al.[9]	40	?	55		23	35	95						Average 25.8 (1–72)
Bull et al.[22]	168	?	221	87	88	88	89		46	37	11	20	26 (10–70)
Dorros et al.[19]	111	?	168	62		31	90		53	34	45	36	9 ± 6
Flueckiger et al.[32]	91	99	125	86		40	91		62	34	7	22	15 (3–36)
Hold et al.[21]	151	151	151		13	68			36	24	5	11	Median 23
Horvath et al.[35]	71	?	103	59	16	25	96	75	43	30	7	23	Life table to 3 years
Löfberg et al.[34]	82	86	196	55		61	88		21	30	22	51	Life table to 3 years. Mean 16.2 (1–60)
Matsi et al.[16]		?	84				89						Life table to 3 years
Schwarten[13]	96	112	146	7	11	60	97		37	12	36	50	Life table to 3 years (mean 21)
Sivananthan et al.[24]	38	?	73	33		5	96		21	32	16	4	
Varty et al.[23]	38	?	40	19		17	98		8	17	4	7	Life table to 2 years.

aClaudication in 24% of the patients.
bClaudication in 47% of the patients
c4 iliac, 121 femoropopliteal and 84 infrapopliteal dilatations are analysed together.

EPIDEMIOLOGICAL REMARKS

The frequency with which distal balloon angioplasty has been used is not high and only few studies have included more than 35 patients (Table 1). Of PTA in 435 patients undergoing PTA because of chronic lower limb ischaemia, 103 had 117 limbs with critical ischaemia with 209 lesions, 84 being infrapopliteal.[16] During the same period there were 34 bypass operations and 26 amputations.

In another setting 57 of 232 critically ischaemic limbs were dilated (13 infrapopliteally), 149 underwent surgical revascularization, 18 were amputated and 8 treated conservatively.[17] Of 215 patients with critical limb ischaemia, angioplasty was tried in 71, 14 of which were infrapopliteal.[18] Thus, of patients with critical limb ischaemia, some 10% may be suitable for infrageniculate balloon angioplasty.

Looking at nationwide data from Sweden (Swedvasc, Vascular registry in Sweden) until now there have been 4317 procedures involving below-knee outflow, 1549 being endovascular (PTA 1010, peroperative balloon angioplasty 128 and thrombolysis 411). This means that 26% of the procedures are balloon angioplasties.

INDICATION

Most authors agree that below-knee balloon angioplasty should be reserved for critical limb ischaemia, if technically feasible, and probably to increase secondary graft patency although some investigators have also used it in claudicants.[19–23] In a non-randomized but comparative study, however, simple surgical repair came out with better secondary patency than PTA in patients with vein graft stenosis.[11] Although not systematically investigated it may also be used as an adjuvant intraoperative therapy to improve the runoff situation when a distal bypass is performed.

ADJUVANT PHARMACOTHERAPY

There are many protocols, all based on the individual investigator's preferences, and there are no controlled studies helping the clinician in the decision regarding what to use. Heparin as a bolus dose of around 5000 units intra-arterially seems to be the routine procedure, but some use even higher doses such as 10 000 units.[24] Use of heparin injections or infusions later on is not as frequent. Criado *et al.*[25] infused dextran for rheological reasons. Many authors use acetylsalicylic acid from before the balloon procedure with continuation for a variable period of time thereafter[9,16,18,25–29] sometimes with the addition of dipyridamole.[28, 30] Whatever the effect is on the patency of the dilated segment acetylsalicylic acid probably is of benefit to increase survival in this group of patients. In one study oral anticoagulation was used during follow-up.[15]

Some authors use nitroglycerin if there is a spasm during the procedure,[9,16,18,24,26,28,29] others give nifedipin[9,16,28,30] or tolazolin[27,31] to prevent spasm. With the same aim Wack *et al.*[27] mixed the contrast medium with prilocain. A few authors have used prostaglandin injection.[32]

PATIENTS

The patients are typical of those having critical limb ischaemia caused by distal lesions with mean ages around 70 years or more and with a high frequency of diabetes – in some series above 80%.[13,27,30] The usual dominance of males is less obvious, within some series females even outnumbering the males.[11,16]

RESULTS

Technical failure rate varies between 0%[18,29] and 22%,[33] or even higher in the case of occluded vessels (35%).[19,32]
There are three main problems to consider when results are analysed:

1. Diagnostic methodology used for follow-up and whether this is used in a surveillance programme or only when symptoms develop.
2. Definition of success. There are great variations between studies: increase in ankle brachial index together with relief of symptoms,[17,19,34] less than 20% residual narrowing on the post-PTA angiogram,[9] patent vessel,[8] restoration of 75% of vessel lumen diameter,[30] residual stenosis of 30% or less,[13,31,35,36] less than 50% residual stenosis,[11,16,19,24,29,34] no need for surgical revascularization or amputation.[16] In many series the definition of residual stenosis is not clear. The Society of Cardiovascular and Interventional Radiology used technical success as residual narrowing of 20% or less.[37]
3. In patients where several interventions have been combined, from a technical point of view it is important to evaluate each procedure on its own, whereas for the patient the main interest is a preserved leg despite failure of one of the procedures. To analyse below-knee angioplasties separately is difficult. First, because it is not always stated if and to what extent there are combinations with other procedures, and, second, because the series with isolated below-knee angioplasties are few and small.

In Table 2, the results are summarized as far as patency and limb survival are concerned. The figures are based on numerical data from Kaplan-Meier tables or from approximations of Kaplan-Meier curves from the various studies. There is a substantial variation in the time for follow-up (Table 1), and it is obvious that existing data are insufficient both in number and in quality to allow firm conclusions to be drawn. There is a high rate of recurrencies and the secondary patency rate is only around 50% at about 3 years. In one small series the 3-year patency was only 26% and infrageniculate PTA was recommended only to patients with limited life expectancy or contraindications to operation.[28] Results after balloon angioplasty of failing vein grafts seems to be even worse.[9] One year results from the Swedvasc are seen in Table 3. There seems to have been a selection of better cases for PTA.

Table 2. Long-term results after below-knee angioplasty in studies from Table 1 where this information is possible to obtain

| | No of patients | At follow-up (%) | | |
		Primary patency	Secondary patency	Limb salvage
Brown et al.[9]	40	44	?	52
Bull et al.[22]	168	55		80
Flueckiger et al.[32]	91	–	64(?)	71
Hold et al.[21]	151		~35(?)	
Horvath et al.[35]	71		64(?)	75
Löfberg et al.[34]	82	36	44	72
Schwarten[13]	96			83
Sivananthan et al.[24]	38		~54 (?)	
Varty et al.[23]	38	68	79	77

Most of the figures are somewhat uncertain because of lack of information in the original papers. End of follow-up is given in Table 1.

Table 3. Below-knee reconstruction procedures. One-year results from Swedvasc (%)

	Femorodistal bypass (n = 2592)	Popliteodistal bypass (n = 176)	PTA (n = 1010)
Age (years ± SD)	76 ± 9	72 ± 12	75 ± 10
Critical limb ischaemia (%)	98	98	61
Diabetes (%)	42	65	47
Patent graft/improved patient	39	46	55
Unimproved	6	5	16
Amputated	12	8	14
Dead	43	41	15

COMPLICATIONS

When reporting postprocedure mortality it is important to use the same time period as after surgical procedures, usually meaning 30 days. Otherwise comparisons with surgical series are meaningless. Figures vary between 0%[9,12,17,27,36] and 9%.[15,16,18,38] Most deaths have been caused by myocardial infarction.

Other complications are similar to those seen after angiography or other catheter techniques with puncture site haematoma dominating, some needing surgery and/or transfusions. The frequency increases substantially when the procedure is combined with some form of thrombolysis.[9] General complications are mycoardial infarction, reversible or irreversible kidney failure because of the contrast media and rarely allergic reactions.

Local complications have been reported, sometimes leading to amputation:

- Local occlusion where local thrombolysis or aspiration should be tried.[13,24]
- Perforation or rupture of the vessel or graft.[11,24,31,35,38] Sometimes this is seen just as a small amount of contrast extravasation without consequences for the patients.[30] Delayed rupture has been described as a result of a local infection.[9]
- Distal embolization. These emboli can usually be treated with transcatheter embolectomy or local thrombolysis.[24,30,34] When crural PTA was combined with proximal PTA during the same procedure, Löfberg *et al.*[34] reported a lower risk for distal embolization if the crural angioplasty was performed first.
- Deep vein thrombosis.[38]
- Spasm, usually possible to treat with intra-arterial nitroglycerin.
- Dissection.[16,35]

The incidence of local complications is rather high in some series (7%,[29] 8.5%,[34] 9.5%,[27] 14%[30]), but it is not always stated explicitly how complications have been reported or included in the other publications. Nor is it always clear if the complications are reported per patient or per procedure.

THE UPPSALA EXPERIENCE[34]

Methodology

Antegrade puncture of the femoral artery is used for PTA of the crural arteries. Contralateral puncture with crossover technique is used in extremely obese patients and in patients with a femorodistal bypass graft.

Catheterization and PTA is performed through a 6 French (diameter 2 mm) introducer. Stenoses and occlusions are best passed with glide-wires and low-profile balloons used for PTA. The shaft size of the balloons is usually 5 French, and the diameter of the balloons range from 2.5 mm to 4 mm for the crural arteries. The procedure is done with digital subtraction technique and roadmapping of the arteries.

Results

During a 5-year period PTA of the crural arteries was attempted either alone (n = 39) or in combination with proximal PTA (n = 55) in 86 limbs (82 patients, 42 men and 94 procedures) presenting with critical limb ischaemia. In four patients crural artery PTA was performed on both legs. Repeat PTA on the same leg was performed in six patients (twice in four and three times in two patients). The age range was 37–94 years (mean 72). Sixty-one patients (75%) were diabetics, 30 (36%) had hypertension, and 51 (62%) coronary artery disease. The indications for PTA were rest pain in ten (10%), ulcer in 58 (62%) and gangrene in 26 (28%) limbs. Thirty limbs had falsely elevated ankle pressures (>220 mmHg) and in the remaining 56 limbs the mean ankle brachial pressure index (ABPI) was 0.24 (range 0-0.6) before intervention.

A total of 196 PTAs were performed, 71 of which were for occlusions. No attempt was made to recanalize occlusions more than 10 cm long in the superficial femoral and popliteal arteries or more than 5 cm long at the crural level.

A technically successful PTA in at least one crural vessel was achieved in 83 procedures (83/94; 88%). There was technical failure in a total of 27 segments (27/196), 26 of which were at the crural level. Among 11 procedures where no crural artery could be recanalized, one patient underwent acute distal reconstruction, three were amputated, three received elective bypass grafting, two died within 6 months and two were lost to follow-up during the first 3 months after PTA.

Two patients died due to myocardial infarction (post-PTA mortality 2.4%). There was no limb loss as a complication of the PTA procedure. Fourteen patients developed groin haematomas (15%), two undergoing acute surgical intervention.

Cumulative primary clinical success rates at 6, 12, 24 and 36 months were 55%, 51%, 36% and 36%, respectively. Cumulative secondary clinical success and limb salvage rates at 36 months were 44% and 72%, respectively. In ten limbs, secondary crural artery PTA was performed which resulted in a slightly improved patency rate at 36 months (44% compared with 36%). The presence of diabetes, preoperative ABPI less than 0.2, combined femorocrural PTA, type of lesion (occlusion vs stenosis) and the number of patent crural arteries after successful PTA (one vs two or three) did not adversely affect the results. Thirteen patients underwent elective infrainguinal bypass surgery due to reocclusion at a mean of 7.2 months after PTA (range 1 week to 48 months). Twenty patients underwent amputation at a mean of 4.7 months (range 1-37 months) after reocclusion of PTA without any attempt at reconstruction because of severe distal atherosclerotic involvement. Among 49 patients who did not require surgical reconstruction or primary amputation after PTA, 15 died during the follow-up period (mean 10.8 months, range 1-40) and the remaining 34 patients were followed for a mean of 16.2 months (range 1-60 months).

DISCUSSION

There are several problems, some of them indicated in the previous sections, when dealing with analysis of published series on balloon angioplasty below the knee joint. If isolated below-knee angioplasty is considered there are only few series and a few patients reported, and most publications also include patients where crural angioplasty has been combined with some other measures of reopening. This makes analysis very complicated and evidence-based recommendations are hard to make. Some of the difficulties are as follows:

1. Indication for treatment with variations in aggressiveness. Most authors, however, agree that distal angioplasties are not a treatment option for claudication. On the other hand, there may be situations of haemodynamically failing grafts in asymptomatic patients, where distal PTA is done to increase the secondary patency.

2. The frequency and type of adjunctive procedures may not always be clear. There are various combinations with angioplasty, thrombolysis and/or surgery within other segments than the below-knee one. So far stenting of the relevant arteries has only been made exceptionally and with short follow-up.[39] There are also many types of pharmacological treatments which aim at decreasing the risk of

complications and increasing the patency. However, there is a complete lack of controlled trials. On the other hand, such studies would be difficult to perform because of the clinically complicated situation.

3. There are variations in the level and extension of lesions accepted for dilatation. There are also different attitudes towards the angioplasty of occluded segments. As far as the popliteal artery is concerned some reports do not differentiate between above- and below-knee dilatation.[26,36,40,41]

4. There are variations in the technique for angioplasty and this may also vary within one series. So London *et al.*[17] used both conventional and subintimal angioplasty and it is not possible to evaluate the results separately. Recently, Nydahl *et al.*[31] published a series where only subintimal technique was used.

5. Definitions of success and failure vary (see above).

6. There are variations in means of reporting the results although many authors refer to the SVS/ISCVS standards.[37,42,43] It should be possible to distinguish primary and secondary patency as well as limb survival. It is also important to know if there has been a surveillance programme to find haemodynamic recurrencies before symptoms occur and how such lesions have been handled. One problem which is not always clear is if results are given per patient, per limb and/or per lesion treated. There are no systematic studies on surveillance of treated crural lesions with duplex scanning.

7. There are large variations in follow-up times, most studies reporting rather short median times (Table 1).

8. The diagnostic methodology with which results are evaluated differs. With one method there may also be variations in criteria between centres. Some studies are prospective with well defined criteria, others are retrospective where it is not always possible to distinguish the criteria and if there have been variations over time.

The patients in need of below-knee angioplasty belong to a very complicated group concerning both technical possibilities and risk factors. They are often considered not suitable for distal bypass surgery. To perform any form of randomized study vs surgical reconstruction would pose serious problems both in selection of patients and concerning study logistics. The present situation is that patients undergoing bypass surgery and balloon angioplasty belong to different groups of patients and the methods are to be considered complementary. So far the practical conclusion must be that evidence-based recommendations from hard scientific data are impossible to obtain but distal balloon angioplasty is a therapeutic option in some patients, which often has to be combined with other reconstructive modalities. It is technically feasible but also technically demanding with the need for the very best and dedicated interventionists.

SUMMARY AND CONCLUSIONS

In this chapter the following claims have been made:

1. Balloon angioplasty below the knee joint is used by the authors in patients with critical limb ischaemia and in failing grafts where there are short occlusions

(< 5cm) or stenoses, single or multiple, and often in combination (simulanteously or separated) with various proximal reconstructive procedures. Infrageniculate PTA is possible in aorund 10% of patients with critical limb ischaemia. Careful selection of the patients is necessary.

2. Except for balloon angioplasty available alternatives are reconstruction with bypass, conservative treatment (optimizing heart pump function and microcirculatory flow) and primary amputation. Today the choice is often based on clinical impression with a tendency to dilate when the lesions are short.

3. The authors' choice is based on clinical guidelines and experience. There are several uncontrolled trials (Tables 1, 2) showing the feasibility of such an approach.

4. There are no randomized trials comparing the various treatment options in patients with femorocrural occlusive lesions, but again the feasibility is shown in various retrospective analyses (see above).

5. In patients with infrageniculate occlusions or stenoses a randomized study comparing balloon angioplasty and a short bypass would be of interest. The logistics with such a study would, however, be difficult and the necessary sample size would probably be large. Another option, at least when there are no ischaemic ulcerations or tissue loss, would be comparison with best medical treatment but the same difficulties are true for such a study. A third option would be to prospectively follow all patients with critical limb ischaemia within a defined region, whatever treatment is chosen, and analyse the influence on amputation.

ACKNOWLEDGEMENT

Swedish Medical Research Council 00759.

REFERENCES

1. Grüntzig A, Hopff H: Perkutane Rekanalisation chronischer arterieller Verschlusse mit einem neuen Dilatations-Katheter: Modifikation der Dotter-Technik. *Dtsch Med Wchschr* **99**: 2502–5, 1974
2. Wilson SE, Wolf GL, Cross AP: Percutaneous transluminal angioplasty versus operation for peripheral arteriosclerosis. *J Vasc Surg* **9**: 1–9, 1989
3. Holm J, Arfvidsson B, Jivegård L *et al.*: Chronic lower limb ischaemia. A prospective randomised controlled study comparing the 1-year results of vascular surgery and percutaneous transluminal angioplasty (PTA). *Eur J Vasc Surg* **5**: 517–22, 1991
4. Weibull H, Bergqvist D, Bergentz S-E *et al.*: Percutanous transluminal renal angioplasty versus surgical reconstruction of artherosclerotic renal artery stensosis: A prospective randomized study. *J Vasc Surg* **18**: 841–52, 1993
5. Wolf GL, Wilson SE, Cross AP *et al.*: Surgery or balloon angioplasty for peripheral vascular disease: A randomized clinical trial. *JVIR* **4**: 639–48, 1993
6. Lauber A, Marx A, John H *et al.*: Simultane chirurgische und kathetertechnische Revaskularisierung der unteren Extremität. *Helv Chir Acta* **60**: 739–41, 1993/94
7. Schilling JD, Pond GD, Mulcahy MM *et al.*: Catheter-directed urokinase thrombolysis: an

adjunct to PTA/surgery for management of lower extremity thromboembolic disease. *Angiology* **45**: 851–60, 1994

8. Motarjeme A, Gordon GI, Bodenhagen K: Limb salvage: thrombolysangioplasty as an alternative to amputation. *Int Angiol* 12: 281–90, 1993

9. Brown KT, Moore ED, Getrajdman GI, Saddekni S: Infrapopliteal angioplasty: long-term follow-up. *JVR* **4**: 139–44, 1993

10. Lundell A, Lindblad B, Bergqvist D, Hansen F: Femoropopliteal-crural graft patency is improved by an intensive surveillance program: A prospective randomized study. *J Vasc Surg* **21**: 26–34, 1995

11. Sanchez LA, Suggs WD, Marin ML, Panetta TF *et al.*: Is percutaneous balloon angioplasty appropriate in the treatment of graft and anastomotic lesions responsible for failing vein bypasses? *Am J Surg* **168**: 97-101, 1994

12. Wölfle KD, Mayer H, Tietze W *et al.*: Stellenwert interventioneller Verfahren bei der Behandlung von stenosierten und verschlossenen infrainguinaler Gefässbypasses. *Zentralbl Chir* **119**: 115–23, 1994

13. Schwarten DE: Clinical and anatomical consideration for nonoperative therapy in tibial disease and the results of angioplasty. *Circulation* **83** (Suppl I);86–90, 1991

14. Page JE, Buckenham TM: Accelerated thrombolysis facilitated by direct puncture of occluded prosthetic femoral grafts. *Australas Radiol* **36**: 230–33, 1992

15. Bull PG, Guttierez E, Mendel H *et al.*: Thrombolysis combined with angioplasty for failed femorodistal arterial grafts. *Acta Chir Belg* **93**: 276–83, 1993

16. Matsi PJ, Manninen HI, Suhonen MT *et al.*: Chronic critical lower-limb ischemia: prospective trial of angioplasty with 1-36 months follow-up. *Radiology* **188**: 381–87, 1993

17. London NJM, Varty K, Sayers RD *et al.*: Percutaneous transluminal angioplasty for lower-limb critical ischaemia. *Br J Surg* **82**: 1232–35, 1995

18. Buckenham TM, Loh A, Dormandy JA, Taylor RS: Infrapopliteal angioplasty for limb salvage. *Eur J Vasc Surg* **7**: 21–25, 1993

19. Dorros, G, Lewin RF, Jamnadas P, Mathiak LM: Below-the-knee angioplasty: tibioperoneal vessels, the acute outcome. *Cath Cardiovasc Diagn* **19**: 170–8, 1990

20. Favre JP, Malouki I, Sobhy M *et al.*: Angioplasty of distal venous bypasses: is it worth the cost? *J Cardiovasc Surg* **37**: S59–65, 1996

21. Hold M, Mendel H, Raynoschek H *et al.*: Perkutane infragenuale Angioplastien - 5-Jahresergebnis von 151 Fällen. *VASA* **37** (Suppl): 54–56, 1992

22. Bull PG, Mendel H, Hold M *et al.*: Distal popliteal and tibioperoneal transluminal angioplasty: long-term follow-up. *JVIR* **3**: 45–53, 1992

23. Varty K, Bolia A, Naylor AR *et al.*: Infrapopliteal percutanous transluminal angioplasty: A safe and successful procedure. *Eur J Vasc Endovasc Surg* **9**: 341–5, 1995

24. Sivananthan UM, Brown TF, Thorley PJ *et al.*: Percutanous transluminal angioplasty of the tibial arteries. *Br J Surg* **81**: 1281–5, 1994

25. Criado FJ, Queral LA, Patten P, Valentin W: The role of endovascular therapy in lower extremity revascularization. *Int Angiol* **12**: 221–30, 1993

26. Hunink MGM, Donaldson MC, Meyerovitz MF *et al.*: Risks and benefits of femoropopliteal percutanous balloon angioplasty. *J Vasc Surg* **17**: 183–94, 1993

27. Wack C, Wölfle KD, Loeprecht H *et al.*: Perkutane Ballondilatation bei isolierten Läsionen der Unterschenkelarterien mit kritischer Beinischämie. *VASA* **23**: 30–4, 1994

28. Treiman GS, Treiman RL, Ichikawa L, van Allan R: Should percutaneous transluminal angioplasty be recommended for treatment of infrageniculate popliteal artery or tibioperoneal trunk stenosis? *J Vasc Surg* **22**: 457–65, 1995

29. Saab MH, Smith DC, Aka PK *et al.*: Percutanous transluminal angioplasty of tibial arteries for limb salvage. *Cardiovasc Intervent Radiol* **15**: 211–16, 1992

30. Bakal CW, Sprayregen S, Scheinbaum K *et al.*: Percutaneous transluminal angioplasty of infrapopliteal arteries: results in 53 patients. *Am J Roentgenol* **154**: 171–4, 1990

31. Nydahl S, Harthorne T, Bell PRF *et al.*: Subintimal angioplasty of infrapopliteal occlusions in critically ischemic limbs. *Eur J Vasc Endovasc Surg* **14**: 212–16, 1997

32. Flueckiger F, Lammer J, Klein GE *et al.*: Percutaneous transluminal angioplasty of crural arteries. *Acta Radiol* **33**: 152–5, 1992

33. Currie IC, Wakeley CJ, Cole SEA *et al*.: Femoropopliteal angioplasty for severe limb ischaemia. *Br J Surg* **81**: 191–3, 1994
34. Löfberg A-M, Lörelius L-E, Karacagil S *et al*.: The use of below-knee percutanous transluminal angioplasty in arterial occlusive disease causing chronic limb ischemia. *Cardiovasc Intervent Radiol* **19**: 317–22, 1996
35. Horvath W, Oertl M, Haidinger D: Percutanous transluminal angioplasty of crural arteries. *Radiology* **177**: 565–9, 1990
36. Ray SA, Minty I, Buckenham TM *et al*.: Clinical outcome and restenosis following percutaneous transluminal angioplasty for ischaemic rest pain or ulceration. *Br J Surg* **82**: 1217–21, 1995
37. Standards of Practice Committee of the Society of Cardiovascular and Interventional Radiology: Guidelines for percutaneous transluminal angioplasty. *Radiology* **177**: 619–26, 1990
38. Durham JR, Horowitz JD, Wright JD, Smead WL: Percutaneous transluminal angioplasty of tibial arteries for limb salvage in the high-risk diabetic patient. *Ann Vasc Surg* **8**: 48–53, 1994
39. Dorros G, Hall P, Prince C: Successful limb salvage after recanalization of an occluded infrapopliteal artery utilizing a balloon expandable (Palmaz-Schatz) stent. *Cath Cardiovasc Diagn* **28**: 83–8, 1993
40. Brendan S, Teague B, Raptis S *et al*.: Efficacy of balloon angioplasty of the superficialfemoral artery and popliteal artery in the relief of leg ischemia. *J Vasc Surg* **23**: 679–85, 1996
41. Milford MA, Weaver FA, Lundell CJ, Yellin AE: Femoropopliteal percutaneous transluminal angioplasty for limb salvage. *J Vasc Surg* **8**: 292–9, 1988
42. Ahn SS, Rutherford R, Becker GJ: Reporting standards for lower extremity arterial endovascular procedures. *J Vasc Surg* **17**: 1103–7, 1993
43. Rutherford R, Flanigan DP, Gupta SK *et al*.: Suggested standards for reports dealing with lower extremity ischemia. *J Vasc Surg* **4**: 80–90, 1986

Editorial comments by R.M. Greenhalgh

The authors support balloon angioplasty below the knee joint for short occlusions of less than 5 cm or stenoses, single of multiple, or in combination. This is based on the clinical guidelines and experience and the authors are very open to record that there are no randomized trials comparing the various treatment options in patients with femorocrural occlusive lesions. They admit that for infrageniculate occlusions or stenoses, a randomized study between balloon angioplasty and a short bypass would be of interest but admit that this would be difficult logistically.

What Are the Indications for Endovascular Procedures Below The Knee?

Frank J. Criado, Mordechai Twena, Omran Abdul-Khoudoud and Bahaaldin Al-Soufi

INTRODUCTION

It is intriguing that at the dawn of the endovascular era, in the year 1964, two cases of below-knee angioplasty were reported in Dotter's classic paper.[1] Despite this, the crural arteries remain to this day almost forbidden territory for catheter recanalization and are, together with the carotid artery, perhaps the last major arterial segment yet to be conquered by interventional techniques.

Save for a few early attempts,[2-5] transluminal angioplasty in the distal arteries had to await the development of coronary balloon and guide-wire technology in the early 1980s, and further catheter refinements introduced a few years later, which made small-vessel endovascular intervention safer and more attractive.[6,7] Currently available technology has put at our disposal the tools which permit successful recanalization of many stenotic and occluded crural arteries (Figs 1,2): catheters with

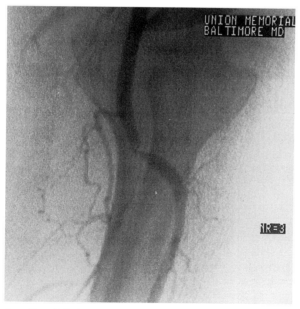

Fig. 1. Focal tight stenosis at origin of anterior tibial artery, associated with total occlusion of the tibioperoneal trunk. Patient presented with non-healing toe amputation site.

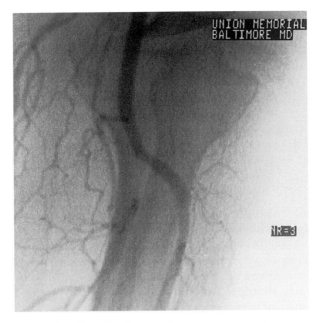

Fig. 2. Angiographic result after PTA.

3-5F shafts, carrying balloons that are wedded to the catheters, resulting in very low smooth profiles, and that can be inflated to 8 atm and more; steerable 0.014–0.018inch guide-wires with fluoroscopically bright platinum tips capable of crossing tight and complex lesions and easily entering angled branch orifices. These guide-wires are stiff enough proximally to safely guide balloon catheters as they track over coaxially. Adjunctive use of effective pharmacologic agents to prevent and overcome vasospasm (vasodilators and calcium-channel blockers) have also contributed significantly to advance the field of distal-limb angioplasty, as have improvements in visualization techniques through fluoroscopic imaging with digital subtraction and roadmapping[8] (Fig. 3a,b).

These technological advances notwithstanding, below-knee angioplasty has been practised only infrequently. More widespread application has been stifled by the perception that:

1. It is technically complex.
2. It carries a high risk of serious complications likely to result in amputation or compromise of a subsequent surgical bypass.
3. Success rates are low or dismal.
4. Occlusive disease in the distal below-knee arteries is often extensive, and not treatable by percutaneous transluminal angioplasty (PTA).
5. Surgical bypass procedures are possible and likely to be successful in the majority of patients.

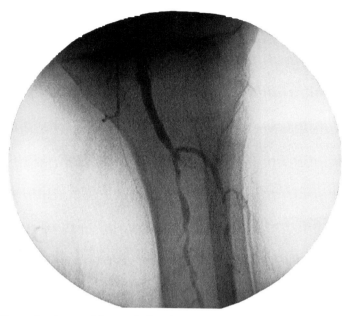

Fig. 3a. Angiographic mask (background) for roadmapping to guide endoluminal manipulations across a diseased segment.

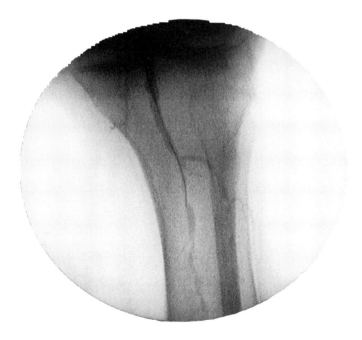

Fig. 3b. 0.018 inch platinum-tip guide-wire traversing lesions as seen utilizing roadmapping technique.

While all of the above points have been traditionally viewed as realistic by both vascular surgeons and radiologists for several years, it is appropriate to revisit them in light of recent reports and current clinical experience.

INTERVENTIONAL TECHNIQUES FOR BELOW-KNEE ANGIOPLASTY

It is undeniable these are complex endovascular procedures, only reasonable for the seasoned interventionist with access to high-quality imaging equipment. As stated, digital subtraction and roadmapping capabilities are highly desirable – if not mandatory.

AUTHORS' TECHNICAL APPROACHES

Endoluminal access

Endoluminal access is by percutaneous antegrade puncture of the common femoral artery (CFA).[9,10] At times, it is easier (or even better) to directly enter the proximal superficial femoral artery (SFA).[10,11] A 5F introducer sheath is advanced over a wire and placed in the lumen of the upper SFA.

Angiography

Angiography is performed by injecting contrast material through the sideport of the sheath. Detailed below-knee visualization is achieved by direct angiographic injection into the distal popliteal artery via a straight catheter placed in that location over a guide-wire (Fig. 4). An arterial map (or mask), with or without digital subtraction, is obtained and, over this background, the real-time manipulations of guide-wire and catheters are displayed (roadmapping).[8]

Nitroglycerin

Nitroglycerin (100 μg) is administered through the sideport of the sheath in order to prevent vasospasm. It may be repeated to a total dose of 300 μg if necessary.

Anticoagulation with heparin

This is induced with a bolus intravenous injection of 3000–5000 units.

Guidewire recanalization

Stenotic lesion

A 0.018 platinum tip guide-wire (Hi-Torque Flex-T, Mallinckrodt) is manoeuvered across the lesion. The straight catheter ('parked' below the knee – see above) may be used to stabilize the wire and facilitate lesion crossing (Fig. 5).

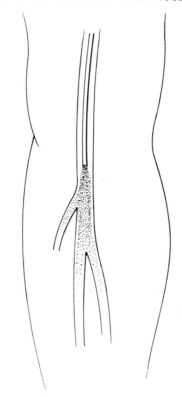

Fig. 4. Selective distal popliteal–crural artery angiography.

Balloon angioplasty

Balloon angioplasty is performed by placing a 2–4 mm diameter balloon (Savvy, Cordis, 105 cm in length, 3.5F shaft) over the platinum tip guide-wire across the lesion. It is inflated applying sufficient pressure to eliminate any waisting on fluoroscopy. Precise monitoring of inflation pressure is felt to be irrelevant.

Total occlusion

A 0.035 inch Terumo Glidewire is preferred for recanalization of occlusive lesions. Once the occlusion is crossed, a 4F straight ('exchange') catheter is passed over the wire in order to exchange it for the 0.018 platinum tip wire referred to above (Fig. 6). The angioplasty then proceeds as described.

Completion angiography

Completion angiography is obtained by injecting contrast through the sideport of the introducer sheath proximally.

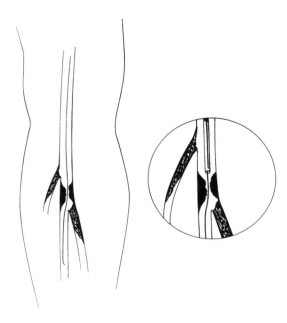

Fig. 5.   0.018 inch guide-wire across tight stenosis. Inset: 4F straight catheter used to stabilize wire.

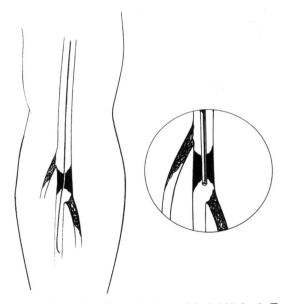

Fig. 6.   Crossing of total occlusion with 0.035 inch Terumo Glidewire. Inset: 4F straight catheter placed over the wire across occlusion, and used to exchange for 0.018 platinum-tip guide-wire.

Intravascular ultrasound

Intravascular ultrasound assessment is often used as it has been found to be of value in small-vessel interventions.

Post-intervention

Patients receive aspirin 325 mg per day, beginning 2 days prior the procedure. On occasion, full anticoagulation with intravenous heparin is maintained for 24-48 hours after recanalization.

AUTHORS' EXPERIENCE (1990-1997)

In the 7-year period, 1990–1997, 26 patients (18 men, eight women) underwent percutaneous balloon angioplasty of one or more native crural arteries. Their mean age was 66 years. Eighteen patients (70%) were diabetic. The expected cardiovascular co-morbidities were present in the majority. Indications for intervention were related to limb-threatening ischaemia, including non-healing ulcers and non-healing minor amputation site (toe or pedal) in 12 (46%), frank digital or partial foot gangrene in nine (35%), and rest pain in five (19%). In every case, limb ischaemia and pattern of occlusive disease were documented by history and physical examination, Doppler segmental pressures, and angiography. With one exception, all patients had continuous arterial perfusion to the below-knee popliteal artery, the major stenotic/occlusive lesions being present only in the tibial/peroneal arteries (including the tibioperoneal trunk). One patient had concomitant distal SFA occlusion which required recanalization ('on the way in') to access the below-knee arteries.

In total, 36 arterial segments (lesions) were treated by endovascular intervention (Table 1). Case selection for angioplasty was based on the presence of normal or near-normal flow to the distal popliteal artery, and focal disease in the crural arteries permitting recanalization of a short segment (3 cm or less) to re-establish direct flow to the ankle level via one continuous vessel, preferably with direct pedal outflow (posterior tibial or anterior tibial arteries). Excluded were patients with extensive arterial calcification as seen on plain radiographs and fluoroscopy. In nine patients, there was absence of a suitable greater saphenous vein for distal bypass grafting, and 12 patients were considered to be extremely high-risk candidates for any kind of vascular reconstructive surgery. Interventions were all performed following the basic technical steps outlined above, and took place in a specially equipped endovascular surgical suite . Local anaesthesia was used for 18 patients, and spinal anaesthesia for eight.

INTERVENTIONAL RESULTS AND CLINICAL OUTCOME (TABLE 1)

Twenty-four of 26 (92%) PTA procedures were technically successful as defined by stenosis improvement to less than 30% residual diameter reduction, or angiographic recanalization of total occlusions with less than 30% residual stenosis and antegrade

Table 1

Patient	Date	Indication	Lesion	Outcome
1	9/90	a	DP/TPT (stenosis)	Healing – BKA at 48 months
2	11/90	a	DP/TPT Peroneal (occlusion)	Healing – Distal bypass at 16 months
3	3/91	b	PTA- 2 lesions (stenosis)	TMA at 12 days – Death
4	7/91	a	PTA (stenosis)	Initial failure/rupture – Distal bypass – Death at 6 months
5	10/91	b	ATA (stenosis)	Success
6	12/91	c	DP/TPT Peroneal (stenosis)	Relieved pain
7	1/92	b	ATA (× 2) (stenoses)	Success
8	4/92	a	PTA (occlusion)	Healing
9	9/92	a	DP/TPT (stenosis)	Healing
10	1/93	c	Peroneal (occlusion)	BKA – Death at 3 months
11	2/93	b	Peroneal (stenosis)	Partial foot amputation – AKA
12	8/93	c	DP/TPT Peroneal (stenoses)	Relieved – BKA at 12 months
13	12/93	b	PTA (occlusion)	Success – Death at 5 months
14	4/94	a	Peroneal (stenosis)	Healing
15	7/94	a	PTA (× 2) (stenoses)	Healing
16	2/95	b	DP/TPT Peroneal (stenosis/ occlusion)	Success – Distal bypass at 18 months
17	3/95	a	ATA (× 2) (stenoses)	Failure – Distal bypass – Death at 24 months
18	5/95	b	Peroneal (stenosis)	Success

Continued

Table 1 – *contd.*

Patient	Date	Indication	Lesion	Outcome
19	10/95	c	Peroneal (stenosis)	Relieved
20	1/96	a	DP/TPT (stenosis)	Healing
21	5/96	c	DP/TPT (occlusion)	Relieved
22	10/96	a	Peroneal (stenosis)	Healing
23	11/96	b	DP/TPT (occlusion)	Success
24	1/97	a	Peroneal (stenosis)	Initial failure – BKA
25	4/97	a	DP/TPT (stenosis)	Healing
26	5/97	b	PTA ($\times$ 2) (stenosis/ occlusion)	Success

Key

Indications	Lesions	Outcome
a: Non-healing lesion	DP: Distal popliteal	BKA: Below-knee amputation
b: Pedal gangrene	TPT: Tibioperoneal trunk	AKA: Above-knee amputation
c: Rest pain	ATA: Anterior tibial artery	TMA: Transmetatarsal amputation
	PTA: Posterior tibial artery	

flow. The two initial failures occurred in one patient with an extremely hard 3 cm occlusion of the peroneal artery which proved resistant to guide-wire recanalization, and on another with a complex stenosis of the origin of the anterior tibial artery (in the presence of total extensive occlusion of the tibioperoneal trunk, peroneal, and posterior tibial arteries); repeated attempts at endovascular therapy resulted in rupture of the proximal anterior tibial. The patient underwent successful vein-graft bypass to the distal anterior tibial artery 2 days later. The former could not be offered limb salvage due to his poor general condition and absence of a suitable saphenous vein; a below-knee amputation was required.

One patient died of acute myocardial infarction 2 weeks after PTA and 12 days after transmetatarsal amputation, for a 30-day mortality of 3.8% (1/26). Procedure-related complications included tibial artery rupture in one (as stated) and puncture-site femoral haematoma in two. Additionally, one diabetic patient with pre-existing mild renal failure (serum creatinine 2.1) experienced significant deterioration of renal function with doubling of the serum creatinine level (to 4.0) which took 3½ weeks to return to baseline.

Success and failure were determined using well-accepted standards.[12,13] Post-intervention assessment included physical examination and segmental Doppler

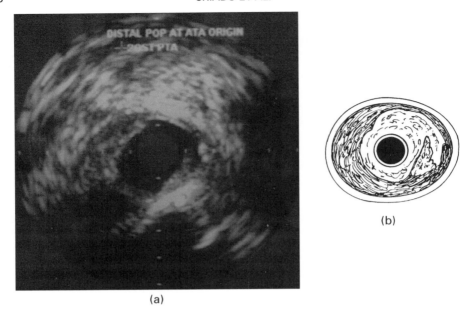

(a)

(b)

Fig. 7. Tight arterial stenosis at distal popliteal/tibioperoneal trunk segment unresponsive to repeated balloon inflations. Note intimal dissection and persistently narrow lumen.

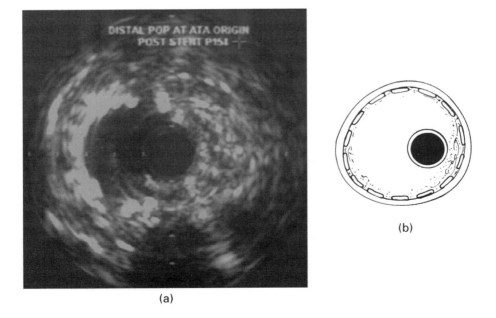

(a)

(b)

Fig. 8. Result obtained with placement of P204 Palmaz stent, balloon expanded to 4 mm.

measurements at 1 day, and then 1, 4, 12 months, and every 6 months thereafter. Color-flow duplex became routine part of this assessment in 1992.

Doppler segmental pressures and indices were evaluable in 20 of the 26 patients. It increased an average of 0.2 (range of 0.1–0.55) in successful PTAs. The other six patients had very calcified arteries with falsely elevated or unmeasurable Doppler pressures; two of these patients experienced immediate failure following angioplasty (described above). In the other four, distal flow enhancement post-PTA was documented by improvements in the amplitude and configuration of the Doppler pulse waveforms.

Overall (intention-to-treat basis), 20/26 patients (77%) had a successful outcome with healing of ischaemic ulcers or minor amputation site (9/12), enabling successful digital or partial foot amputation (7/9), and relieving rest pain (4/5). Three patients had clinical failure following an initially successful endovascular recanalization procedure: a distal bypass was performed in one because of PTA failure to improve flow; two others required amputation, one below-knee (done without attempt at limb salvage), and the other above-knee following failed partial pedal amputation. During a mean follow-up period of 23 months, two additional patients required distal bypass, and two others a below-knee amputation due to severe ischaemia from progressive distal crural arterial occlusive disease. Thus, the long-term limb-salvage rate was 80% (20/25). Late cardiac deaths (from myocardial infarction) occurred in four patients at 3, 5, 6, and 24 months after PTA. No patient received further endovascular treatment. When possible, clinical failures were managed with distal bypass grafting (N4): site of distal anastomosis and type of reconstruction were not adversely affected by the failed or attempted angioplasty in any case.

COMPLICATIONS OF INFRAPOPLITEAL ANGIOPLASTY

Our experience is consistent with that published in the recent literature where the major complication rate has been only 8% in nearly 800 reported procedures, with urgent surgical repair necessary in less than 2% of cases.[4,8,14-24] On balance, it seems that the much anticipated and feared serious potential complications of distal small-vessel PTA have been grossly exaggerated.

FAILED TIBIAL–PERONEAL PTA MAY PRECLUDE OR INCREASE COMPLEXITY OF SUBSEQUENT CRURAL-VESSEL BYPASS GRAFTING

There is little evidence to support such a contention[25] and our experience has certainly been in line with this. It may relate to the fact that most PTA procedures involve the upper and mid-calf arteries leaving the more distal segments nearly intact for bypass anastomosis when necessary. In fact, the presence of nearly intact distal vessels in the lower leg, and with direct pedal outflow (anterior/posterior tibial) in many instances, is obligatory prerequisite for success in well-selected cases for infrapopliteal angioplasty: endoluminal recanalization with sustained patency can only be achieved when stenotic/occlusive lesions are segmental, and continuity with a patent distal artery can be achieved. Almost by definition, then, these distal segments will probably remain patent and be usable as distal anastomotic sites even after failed (more proximal) endovascular intervention.

BELOW-KNEE ANGIOPLASTY PRODUCES SUCH DISMAL RESULTS THAT ITS APPLICATION SHOULD BE RESTRICTED

Available data are very difficult to interpret and final conclusions cannot be drawn due to inadequate reporting standards in many of the radiological publications on the subject. However, there is a growing body of evidence[25] pointing to the fact that patency and limb-salvage rates may well be in the 60–80% range at 3 years on properly selected patients. Our own results tend to corroborate these figures. Other authors[26] have found the clinical efficacy of below-knee PTA to be far less impressive.

MOST PATIENTS WITH CRITICAL LIMB ISCHAEMIA HAVE EXTENSIVE MULTILEVEL OCCLUSIONS NOT AMENABLE TO PTA

This was also our view for many years, until we learned the following:

1. There are patients with critical ischaemia, especially diabetic, who have essentially normal vasculature down to the below-knee popliteal artery. The occlusive process is virtually confined to the distal-most portion of the popliteal artery (at the anterior tibial artery origin) and infrapopliteal crural arteries. Not unusually, there is one (of three) vessel patent with its continuity interrupted by a short (<3 cm) stenotic or occlusive lesion where transluminal recanalization and angioplasty are likely to be successful. We now extend these indications to patients (with such morphology) who may have two focal lesions in tandem in a single crural vessel, or a second lesion in the SFA/popliteal artery which requires treatment to maximize antegrade flow to the leg and to permit unimpeded endoluminal access for infrapopliteal PTA.

2. Patients who have truly extensive crural-artery occlusion have generally been considered beyond the limits of PTA capabilities and, in fact, were not selected for percutaneous therapy in our practice. New information[27,28] now available should make us all re-think such 'conventional wisdom': it seems that 'subintimal angioplasty' indeed may permit successful catheter recanalization in an important number of such cases, with outcomes that promise to match the excellent results obtained with such technique in the iliac and superficial femoral artery territories.[28]

OVERVIEW AND CONCLUSIONS

Current advances with catheter and guide-wire technology, together with pharmacologic adjuncts and improved visualization capabilities, make it logical to re-formulate and further evolve traditional surgical and interventional views on below-knee arterial lesions and their treatment. A new interventional opportunity has emerged with the ability to perform percutaneous recanalization and angioplasty in a significant number of patients. Much of this has occurred as a 'spin-off' of advances in coronary intervention – but, unlike invasive cardiologists, vascular surgeons and peripheral interventionists have been rather shy in their endoluminal approaches to distal limb arteries. In reality, these vessels are very similar to but anatomically simpler than the coronary arteries and, yet, below-knee endovascular therapy has lagged far behind its cardiac counterpart. Crural arteries are relatively straight, 2-4 mm in diameter, not too far from the femoral puncture site, and the calf doesn't beat! The reasons for such paradoxical underutilization of infrapopliteal PTA were discussed briefly in the preceding section. One supporting aspect relates to the insufficiency and softness of the available published information on efficacy of below-knee angioplasty. With this we agree wholeheartedly. However, it is only fair to observe that new facts are gradually coming into light which should help create a different mindset and a new attitude regarding the relative merits of endovascular and surgical revascularization below the knee. In conclusion, when it comes to denying patients the percutaneous endovascular therapeutic alternative, it is almost certain that the following alleged reasons for such posture are untrue and totally unsupported by data:

1. High incidence of serious complications.
2. PTA failures are more difficult to bypass, and bypass success rates will likely be lower.
3. Patency and limb salvage rates are dismal, and therefore below-knee angioplasty cannot be justified.

The authors feel strongly that currently available evidence warrants more aggressive pursuit of percutaneous treatment of critical limb ischaemia, a policy now embraced by increasing numbers of interventionists, and by some surgical groups such as Professor Bell's group in Leicester who claim that PTA is currently used as first-line therapy in 42% of their patients with critical ischaemia.[29]

Having outlined the new philosophy and future interventional strategies for an increasing number of patients, let us now re-emphasize two additional points of the utmost importance:

1. Case selection is paramount. We continue to restrict endovascular treatment to patients with critical limb ischaemia presenting with a disease pattern which (demonstrably) responds quite well to PTA. The occlusive lesions may be extensive but there must be one angiographically visualized below-knee patent artery, preferably with continuous pedal outflow, with focal stenosis or occlusion, and essentially normal proximal flow to the below-knee popliteal artery. We continue to monitor with interest the accumulating data on subintimal recanalization of more extensive occlusions, but do not yet practice it.
2. High-resolution fluoroscopic imaging and endovascular technical expertise are mandatory requirements to achieve success and avoid complications with small-vessel interventions. These procedures are not entry-level, and should not even be attempted without previous vast endovascular experience.

Two related topics of interest were not discussed in this chapter:

1. Use of endoluminal stents in below-knee angioplasty. Available data are purely anecdotal, including our own. We have placed stents in four procedures involving crural-vessel PTA. In all, the indication for stenting was suboptimal angioplasty with extensive flow-limiting dissection and/or marked recoil. Intravascular ultrasound assessment provided valuable information at the time of making a decision to stent (Figs 7,8). In every case, a P154 (N2) or P204 (N2) Palmaz stent was deployed, and balloon-expanded to 4 mm in diameter. Stent technology will probably have a future in these interventions, but its role remains unclear at present. Will data and experience with scaffolding in the coronaries serve as the foundation for future interventional strategies in the calf arteries?

2. Below-knee angioplasty for bypass graft salvage to treat graft or outflow-artery lesions. These were not included in our report as they are felt to belong in a different category. Rationale and strategies for outflow-artery PTA are in every way similar to those outlined in this chapter, with percutaneous endoluminal access obtained through direct puncture of the bypass graft in the groin or thigh.

Finally, this chapter would be incomplete without a statement to the fact that distal bypass grafting remains the gold standard, with which all other lower limb revascularization techniques will have to be compared. When an intact, good-quality saphenous vein is available, surgical bypass is clearly the best possible therapy, offering patients incomparable long-term patency and limb salvage rates. However, there is a price to pay in the form of significant morbidity and even possible mortality which is infrequent but not rare. In addition, there are many patients without adequate saphenous veins for whom other surgical alternatives are far less attractive.

REFERENCES

1. Dotter CT, Judkins MP: Transluminal treatment of arteriosclerotic obstruction; description of a new technique and a preliminary report of its application. *Circulation* **30**: 654–70, 1964
2. Zeitler E: Die perkutane behand lung von arteriellen durchblutungss to rungen der extremitation mit katheter. *Fortschr Geb Roentgenstr Nuklearmed* (Suppl): 225–6, 1973
3. Zeitler E: Complications in and after percutaneous transluminal recanalization. In: Zeitler E, Gruentzig A, Schoop W (Eds), *Percutaneous Vascular Recanalization*. Berlin: Springer, 1978
4. Greenfield AJ: Femoral, popliteal, and tibial arteries: percutaneous transluminal angioplasty. *Am J Roent* **135**: 927–35, 1980
5. Sprayregen S, Sniderman KW, Sos TA *et al.*: Popliteal artery branches: percutaneous transluminal angioplasty. *Am J Roent* **136**: 945–50, 1980
6. Schwarten DE, Cutcliff WB: Arterial occlusive disease below the knee: treatment with percutaneous transluminal angioplasty performed with low-profile catheters and steerable guide wires. *Radiology* **169**: 71–4, 1988
7. Casarella WJ: Percutaneous transluminal angioplasty below the knee: new techniques, excellent results. *Radiology* **169**: 271–2, 1988
8. Gordon RL, Ring EJ: Below-knee angioplasty. *Perspect Vasc Surg* **2**: 67-74, 1989

9. Freiman DB, McLean GK, Oleaga JA *et al.*: Percutaneous transluminal angioplasty. In: Ring EJ, McLean GK (Eds), *Interventional Radiology: Principles and Techniques*. Boston: Little Brown Co, 1981

10. Criado FJ, Queral LA, Patten P: Transluminal recanalization, angioplasty and stenting in endovascular surgery: techniques and applications. In: Greenhalgh RM (Ed), *Vascular and Endovascular Surgical Techniques*. London: WB Saunders Co Ltd, 1994

11. Berman HL, Katz SG, Tihansky DP: Guided direct antegrade puncture of the superficial femoral artery. *Am J Roent* **147**: 632, 1986

12. Ahn SS, Rutherford RB, Becker GJ *et al.*: Reporting standards for lower extremity arterial endovascular procedures. *J Vasc Surg* 17: 1103–07, 1993

13. Rutherford RB: Standards for evaluating results of interventional therapy for peripheral vascular disease. *Circulation* **83** (Suppl 1): I-6–I-11, 1991

14. Schwarten DE: Clinical and anatomical considerations for nonoperative therapy in tibial disease and the results of angioplasty. *Circulation* **83** (Suppl 1): I-I86–I-I90, 1991

15. Brown KT, Moore ED, Getrajdman GI *et al.*: Infrapopliteal angioplasty: long-term follow-up. *JVIR* **4**: 139–44, 1993

16. Brown KT, Schoenberg NY, Moore ED *et al.*: Percutaneous transluminal angioplasty of infrapopliteal vessels: preliminary results and technical considerations. *Radiology* **169**: 75–8, 1988

17. Sanborn TA, Mitty HA, Train JS *et al.*: Infrapopliteal and below-knee popliteal lesions: treatment with sole laser thermal angioplasty. Work in progress. *Radiology* **172**: 89–93, 1989

18. Bakal CW, Sprayregen S, Scheinbaum K *et al.*: Percutaneous transluminal angioplasty of the infrapopliteal arteries: results in 53 patients. *Am J Roent* **154**: 171–4, 1990

19. Dorros G, Lewin RF, Jamnadas P *et al.*: Below-the-knee angioplasty: tibioperoneal vessels, the acute outcome. *Cathet Cardiovasc Diagn* **19**: 170–8, 1990

20. Saab MH, Smith DC, Aka PK *et al.*: Percutaneous transluminal angioplasty of tibial arteries for limb salvage. *Cardiovasc Intervent Radiol* **15**: 211–6, 1992

21. Buckenham TM, Loh A, Dormandy JA *et al.*: Infrapopliteal angioplasty for limb salvage. *Eur J Vasc Surg* **7**: 21–25, 1993

22. Horvath W, Oertl M, Haidinger D: Percutaneous transluminal angioplasty of crural arteries. *Radiology* **177**: 565–9, 1990

23. Bull PG, Mendel H, Hold M *et al.*: Distal popliteal and tibioperoneal transluminal angioplasty: long-term follow-up. *J Vasc Intervent Radiol* **3**: 45–53, 1992

24. Sivananthan UM, Browne TF, Thorley PJ *et al.*: Percutaneous transluminal angioplasty of the tibial arteries. *Br J Surg* **81**: 1282–5, 1994

25. Varty K, Bolia A, Naylor AR *et al.*: Infrapopliteal percutaneous transluminal angioplasty: a safe and successful procedure. *Eur J Vasc Endovasc Surg* **9**: 341–5, 1995

26. Treiman GS, Treiman RL, Ichikawa L *et al.*: Should percutaneous transluminal angioplasty be recommended for treatment of infrageniculate popliteal artery or tibioperoneal trunk stenosis? *J Vasc Surg* **22**: 457–65, 1995

27. Bolia A, Sayers RD, Thompson MM *et al.*: Subintimal and intraluminal recanalisation of occluded crural arteries by percutaneous balloon angioplasty. *Eur J Vasc Surg* **8**: 214–9, 1994

28. Bolia A, Bell PRF: Femoropopliteal and crural artery recanalization using subintimal angioplasty. *Semin Vasc Surg* **8**: 253–64, 1995

29. Varty K, Nydahl S, Butterworth P *et al.*: Changes in the management of critical limb ischemia. *Br J Surg* **82**: 953–6, 1996

Editorial comments by B.R. Hopkinson

In this chapter Dr Criado explores the relatively unconquered areas for angioplasty. There is no doubt that the success of surgical as well as endovascular treatment is far better when applied to the larger vessels than to the smaller ones but there is no reason why endovascular methods should not be attempted in small vessels because the surgical results of bypass to the tribal vessels are by no means the ideal in most ordinary centres. Individual centres give excellent results for surgery as indeed they do for endovascular techniques but in only highly selected cases and with very skilled performers. Dr Criado gives an excellent review of the situation. It is salutary that his own experience of dealing with percutaneous angioplasty in the native crural and tibial vessels only involve 26 patients in a 7-year period. This must be a very small number of the patients presenting with arterial problems during that time. It is of interest that although Dr Criado refers to Dr Bolia's work in Leicester on subintimal angioplasty he does not seem to have actually tried it himself. Reports coming from Leicester are very encouraging for this technique and really should be tried more widely.

This whole field of vascular procedures below the knee is bedevilled very much by the differing features of patients and procedures. We do not have standard patients with standard situations on whom standard procedures can be compared. Until we have better stratification of the risks and problems this area will continue to be an art and as Dr Criado said, will be restricted to treatment of patients with critical limb ischaemia presenting with a disease pattern which (demonstratively) responds well to percutaneous transluminal angioplasty. In other words, the physician will do what he feels best for the individual patient using all the resources available to him at any particular moment in time. We desperately need to have better stratification of the risk of any particular patient with a particular situation in their arteries so that we can best assess the effects of any therapeutic intervention. Until we have this stratification we are at risk of not comparing like with like.

Should We Perform Infrainguinal PTFE Bypass and if so Should a Distal Patch or Cuff be Used?

A.H. Davies

INTRODUCTION

In the case of a patient presenting with a critically ischaemic leg a distal bypass is often required. There is very little discussion that the conduit of choice is autogenous vein, usually the long saphenous vein, for infrapopliteal reconstruction.[1-4] However, many patients present more difficulty for distal reconstruction. They either have unavailable or inadequate vein hence an alternative strategy is required.

AUTHOR'S CHOICE OF PROCEDURE

I have no doubt that patients should be offered infrainguinal–infrapopliteal polytetrafluoroethylene (PTFE) bypass with an adjuvant procedure and I routinely use a Miller cuff and occasionally a Taylor patch, the determinant for this being sufficient vein to make a cuff.

POTENTIAL ALTERNATIVES

1. May be possible to harvest small segments of vein from different sites and perform a composite graft.
2. Synthetic graft without an adjuvant procedure.
3. Synthetic graft with a distal arterovenous fistula.
4. Homograft.
5. Amputation.

EVIDENCE FOR THIS CHOICE

Veith *et al.* reported a primary patency rate of 29% at 3 years for femorocrural PTFE grafts and a 50% primary patency was observed for vein grafts at 3 years.[2] However, in a randomized trial when they looked at limb salvage between randomized vein and PTFE grafts the figures were respectively 61% and 57% at 4 years. The good results shown for the popliteal artery were not found initially when PTFE was used for the femorotibial grafts. This has led to two schools of thoughts to look for possible alternatives or even to offer patients amputation.

However, there have been further studies that have shown that reasonably good results can be obtained for patency to the tibial vessels and there is certainly evidence to suggest that the use of adjuvant procedures and intensive surveillance programmes may well improve the results. Furthermore, many of the studies in which PTFE has been used have been secondary procedures rather than a primary procedures. Schweiger *et al.* reported primary patencies of 42% at 4 years for primary femorotibial PTFE grafts compared with 14% secondary procedures.[5] Christenson *et al.* have also shown that patency can be up to 55% in patients with critical ischaemia dependant on the number of calf vessels which are patent.[6] Further evidence from the Guy's group showed that they have developed a scoring system dividing patients into three groups based on inflow and outflow characteristics and have been able to show that while there was a slight tendency for vein grafts to perform better there was no significant overall difference.[7,8] There is increasing evidence to suggest that the difference in patencies do not occur initially in the first 2 years but become more significant after this. A recent study has shown a significant increase in patency of below-knee femoropopliteal grafts if a vein cuff was used and an improvement in limb salvage found.[9] It should also be noted that many of the people presenting with critical lower limb ischaemia have a life expectancy of less than 2–3 years and so it is probably well justified to offer these people distal reconstruction.

AUTOGENOUS VEIN

This is usually easily obtainable and free. It is the best choice as the bypass conduit distal to the inguinal ligament.[4] This is especially the case for below-knee femoropopliteal grafts. In data accumulated from many series, the 5-year patency for below-knee vein grafts was 68.4% (n=2116) where prosthetic grafts were used an overall 5-year patency of 26.6% (n=1977) was quoted.[4] In the above-knee situation, vein grafts had a 5-year patency of 61.8% (n=881) and prosthetic grafts 43.2% (n=1615). In the above- and below-knee group an overall 1-year occlusion rate of 20.2% and 24.3% was seen respectively. Recent evidence suggests that the newer synthetic grafts may be as effective above the knee as autogenous vein,[10] thus leaving the long saphenous vein to be used either for a subsequent more distal reconstruction or for cardiac surgery. However, the subsequent usage of such saved vein is small.

HOMOGRAFT

Many types of homografts have been used as bypass material: fresh, following treatment with glutaraldehyde, DMSO (dimethyl sulphoxide) and freezing.[11–13] The initial attempts were accompanied by poor graft patency secondary to thrombosis which was thought to be secondary to graft rejection. Immunosuppressive agents have been used with little success. Recent clinical work has shown encouraging results with homograft human vein[14,15] and success may be attributable to the fact that it has been recognized that the endothelial cells are responsible for mediating the immune response and if they are destroyed then the graft loses most of its antigenicity. Further work has shown that the exposed basement membrane is not thrombogenic.[16] Davies and Parums have shown that vein stored in normal saline may meet the criteria for an optimum method of treatment.[17] Glutaraldehyde-treated umbilical vein has been popular if autologous vein is not available. The results, however, are mixed.[4] The original umbilical vein grafts were compromised by late aneurysmal dilatation.[18]

ADJUVANT OPTIONS

Cuff – Miller or Boot – St Marys or Taylor Patch

The use of a vein cuff at the distal end of a prosthetic graft can improve patency in the below-knee and crural position.[19] Furthermore, in the event of an occlusion it preserves the native vessel for secondary intervention.

Tyrrel and Wolfe reported 1-year patency figures of 47% for PTFE/crural grafts on 30 patients using a Miller Cuff.[20] Using the Taylor patch technique in 83 patients gave patency rates of 61% (3 years) and 56% (5-year).[21]

The Joint Vascular Research Group randomized 261 patients undergoing femoropopliteal bypass to cuffed and uncuffed bypass. They were able to show a significantly increased patency in patients with a cuffed anastomosis to the below-knee popliteal and a 20% improvement in limb salvage (Table 1).[9]

Table 1. Results of a randomized control study on the role of a cuff in femoropopliteal bypass[9]

Anastomosis	Primary patency		Limb salvage	
	12	24	12	24
	months		months	
Above-knee popliteal				
Cuffed	80	72	86	82
Uncuffed	84	70	93	91
Below-knee popliteal				
Cuffed	80	52	86	84
Uncuffed	65	29	72	62
	p<0.03		p<0.08	

In a series of 353 PTFE bypasses performed at the Royal Adelaide Hospital, 285 had a cuff. There was no significant difference in primary or secondary patency between the two groups (Table 2).[22]

The authors conclude 'despite no statistically significant differences in patency for cuff versus non-cuff, we feel that the addition of a vein cuff makes a technically difficult tibial anastomosis much easier to perform and preserves run-off should the graft thrombose. This allows easier thrombectomy or chemical thrombolysis.

Table 2. Results of a non-randomized trial on the role of cuffs in femorotibial bypass

Anastomosis	Primary patency		Secondary patency	
	12	60	12	60
	months		months	
Cuffed (n=285)	57	18	64	23
Uncuffed (n=68)	58	27	62	35

Arteriovenous fistula (AVf)

To date there is very little evidence to support the routine use of an arteriovenous fistulae (AVf). The aim of reducing the distal peripheral resistance and hence improving blood is laudible but as yet unproven. Myhre and Saether in a cohort of 80 femorodistal reconstructions within an AVf had an overall patency of 36%.[23] Hinshaw et al. in a small series showed a 75% limb salvage in mainly synthetic grafts over a variable follow-up time of between 4 and 24 months.[24] The use of a distally located AVf[25,26] may be of some added benefit.

Primary amputation

There is increasing evidence to suggest that attempts at distal reconstruction should not be performed at all costs. The evidence for this conclusion is the increased awareness of the importance of quality of life in evaluating patient outcome rather than looking just at patient mortality and limb salvage rates. Those patients with critical lower limb ischaemia who are immobile due to arthritis, neurological compromise and in whom mobility is unimportant may best be served by primary amputation.[27]

CONCLUSION

The above evidence would certainly support the use of a cuff with a PTFE graft when used to the below-knee popliteal artery. To date no randomized data exists to support the use of a cuff when an anastomosis is performed to the tibial vessels, however, the data available would suggest that if PTFE is to be used in the tibial situation then a cuff will improve patency.

Trials

1. Randomized control study of PTFE femorotibial bypass with cuff vs PTFE bypass without cuff.
2. Randomized control study of PTFE femorotibial bypass with cuff/without cuff versus primary amputation.

ACKNOWLEDGEMENTS

My thanks go to Mr PA Stonebridge and Mr R Sayers for allowing me access to data which was in press.

REFERENCES

1. European Working Group on Critical Limb Ischaemia: Second European Concensus Document on critical limb ischaemia. *Eur J Vasc Surg* **6** (Suppl A); 1–31, 1992
2. Veith FJ, Gupta SK, Ascer E *et al.*: Six year prospective multicentre randomised comparison of autologous saphenous vein and expanded PTFE grafts in infrainguinal arterial reconstruction. *J Vasc Surg* **3**; 104–14, 1986
3. Londrey GL, Ramsey DE, Hodgson KJ *et al.*: Infrapopliteal bypass for severe ischaemia: comparison of autogenous vein, composite and prosthetic grafts. *J Vasc Surg* **13**; 631–6, 1991
4. Michaels JM: Choice of materials for above-knee femoro-popliteal bypass graft. *Br J Surg* **76**; 7–14, 1989
5. Schweiger H, Klein P, Lang W: Tibial bypass grafting for limb salvage with ringed PTFE prostheses. Results of primary and secondary procedures. *J Vasc Surg* **18**; 867–74, 1993
6. Christenson JT, Bromme A, Norgren L, Eklof B: Revascularisation of popliteal and below knee arteries with PTFE. *Surgery* **97**; 141–9, 1985
7. Panayiotopoulos YP, Tyrrell MR, Owen SE *et al.*: Outcome and cost analysis after femorocrural and femoro-pedal grafting for lower limb ischaemia. *Br J Surg* **84**; 207–12, 1997
8. Panayiotopoulos YP, Taylor PR: A paper for debate: Vein versus PTFE for critical limb ischaemia – an unfair comparison? *Eur J Vasc Endovasc Surg* **14**; 191–4, 1997
9. Stonebridge PA, Prescott RJ, Ruckley CV: Randomized trial comparing infrainguinal PTFE bypass grafting with and without vein interposition cuff at the distal anastomosis. *J Vasc Surg* (in press) 1998
10. Budd JS, Brennan J, Beard JD *et al.*: Infrainguinal bypass surgery: factors determining late graft patency. *Br J Surg* **77**; 1382–7, 1990
11. Weber TR, Lindenauer SM, Dent TL *et al.*: Longterm patency of vein grafts preserved in liquid nitrogen in dimethyl sulfoxide. *Ann Surg* **184**; 709–12, 1976
12. Oschner JL, Lawson JD, Eskind SJ *et al.*: Homologous veins as an arterial substitute: longterm results. *J Vasc Surg* **1**; 306–13, 1984
13. Sitzmann JV, Imbembo AL, Ricotta JJ *et al.*: Dimethylsulfoxide-treated, cryopreserved venous allografts in the arterial and venous systems. *Surgery* **95**; 154–9, 1984
14. van Reedt Dortland RWH, Schuurman HJ, Slootweg PJ *et al.*: Three years experience with denaturated venous homografts as an arterial substitute: a clinical, pathological and immunological study. *Eur J Vasc Surg* **2**; 233–9, 1988
15. van Reedt Dortland RWH, van Leeuwen MS, Steijling JJF *et al.*: Longterm results with vein homograft in femoro-distal reconstructions. *Eur J Vasc Surg* **5**; 557–64, 1991
16. Buchanan MR, Richardson M, Haas TA *et al.*: The basement membrane underlying the vascular endothelium is not thrombogenic: *in vivo* and *in vitro* studies with rabbit and human tissue. *Thromb Haem* **58**; 698–704, 1987
17. Davies AH, Parums D: Storage of donor long saphenous vein. *J Cardiovasc Surg* **33**; 92–7, 1992
18. Dardik HD, Ibrahim IM, Sprayregen S *et al.*: Clinical experience with modified human umbilical cord vein for arterial bypass. *Surgery* **79**; 618–24, 1976
19. Miller JH, Foreman RK, Ferguson L, Faris I: Interpositon vein cuff for anastomosis of prosthesis to small arteries. *Aust NZ J Surg* **54**; 283–5, 1984
20. Tyrell M, Wolfe JHN: Vein collars and ePTFE grafts. In: Greenhalgh RM, Hollier LH (Eds), *The Maintenance of Arterial Reconstructions* pp. 45–55. London: WB Saunders Co Ltd, 1991

21. Taylor RJ, McFarland RJ, Cox MI *et al.*: Improved technique for PTFE bypass grafting: longterm results using anastomotic vein patches. *Br J Surg* **79**; 398–54, 1992
22. Sayers RD, Raptis S, Berce M *et al.*: Femorotibial bypass: longterm results for vein and polyterafluroethylene (PTFE). *Br J Surg* 1998 (in press)
23. Myrhe HO, Saether OD: When should arteriovenous fistula be used with femorodistal bypass. In: Greenhalgh RM, Hollier L (Eds), *The Maintenance of Arterial Reconstruction.* pp. 421–427. London: WB Saunders Co Ltd, 1995
24. Hinshaw DB, Schmidt CA, Simpson JB: Arteriovenous fistula in arterial reconstruction of the ischaemic limb. *Arch Surg* **118**; 589–92, 1983
25. Shah DM, Patsy PSK, Chang BB *et al.*: Remote distal arteriovenous fistula to improve infrapopliteal bypass patency. In: Veith FJ (Ed.), *Current Critical Problems in Vascular Surgery.* St Louis, Missouri: Quality Medical Publishing, 1989
26. Patsy PSK, Shah DM, Saifi J *et al.*: Remote distal arteriovenous fistula to improve infrapopliteal bypass patency. *J Vasc Surg* **11**; 171–8, 1990
27. Singh S, Beard JD: Is primary amputation ever first choice? In: Greenhalgh RM, Fowkes FGR (Eds), *Trials and Tribulations of Vascular Surgery* pp. 365–372. London: WB Saunders Co Ltd, 1996

Editorial comments by B.R. Hopkinson

This is a nice simple chapter with a simple question and a simple answer. Mr Davies has shown quite clearly that use of a venous cuff above the knee makes little difference to a femoropopliteal bypass but when the bypass is taken below the knee the use of a cuff becomes increasingly important. The work of the joint vascular research group is the main support for this.

When it comes to revascularizing tibial vessels many of us away from the centres of excellence have become quite disillusioned with the use of PTFE with or without cuffs and would strongly support a randomized controlled trial of PTFE femoral tibial bypass with or without a cuff vs a primary amputation in patients for whom there was no suitable long saphenous vein to use for a full length bypass. Indeed there is some anecdotal evidence that patients who have a primary amputation have less anxiety than those who have a reconstruction as they feel that their amputation was at least a single definitive performance whereas if they have a bypass graft they are constantly worried in case it should fail.

When Should We Lyse an Occluded Femoropopliteal Bypass?

Andries Kroese, Lars E. Staxrud and Gunnar Sandbaek

INTRODUCTION

Since the personal and economic consequences of a femoropopliteal graft occlusion are very serious, we should establish criteria for selecting the right patient for the optimal treatment.

Immediate (<48 hours postoperatively) and early graft failures (<30 days) are primarily due to technical surgical error, inflow or runoff conditions and hypercoagulable states. Sometimes graft thrombosis occurs for no apparent reason and may be caused by transient decrease in cardiac output and hypotension. Intermediate failure (<1 year) is usually the result of intimal hyperplasia, mostly at the distal anastomosis, local fibrosis of the venous graft, or progression of atherosclerotic disease. Late failure (>1 year) is mainly related to more extensive atherosclerosis, especially in the crural arteries. Femoropopliteal prosthetic grafts generally show a higher incidence of early and late failure than saphenous veins.[1]

Immediate/early reocclusion generally mandates a re-operation if not contraindicated by an incorrectible poor runoff, because the primary indication for operation usually is critical ischaemia or very disabling intermittent claudication. Coagulation disturbances, e.g. heparin-induced thrombosis, have to be diagnosed and treated, usually by long-term anticoagulation. Surgical revision of the graft is done by balloon catheter thrombectomy and/or rigorous saline irrigation between the opened proximal and distal anastomoses, which minimizes trauma to the venous graft. Technical errors will be addressed, e.g. by revision of an inadequate anastomosis, a residual venous valve, or an arteriovenous fistula of an *in situ* venous bypass. Unfavourable runoff conditions may necessitate conversion to a distal bypass.

Intermediate or late failures do not always threaten limb viability, even though the original operation was performed for critical ischaemia, and these patients should be treated conservatively.[2,3] However, healing of tissue loss will usually require restoration of pulsatile blood flow to the foot, whereas relief of rest pain may be obtained by revascularization to the profunda femoris or an isolated segment of the popliteal artery. In special cases disabling claudication may also warrant further surgical treatment.

A secondary operation is as a rule technically demanding due to surgical scarring, and alternative approaches through virginal tissue planes should be looked for.[3] Revision surgery is associated with high 5-year amputation[4] and mortality rates[5] and 1-year patency may be as poor as 14%.[6]

Results from thrombectomy of autogenous grafts have been disappointing and treatment with repeat autogenous bypass grafting has been recommended instead.

Thus limb salvage rates up to 90% at 5 years have been obtained.[7] Even replacement with a prosthetic graft has resulted in better long-term patency than after thrombectomy.[8] However, mortality rates of redo-surgery may be as high as 26% at 6 months and 88% at 5 years[7]. Under those circumstances primary amputation may be the wisest choice with regard to the patient's quality of life.[9]

The poor results after balloon thrombectomy may be due to incomplete clearing of thrombus in the graft, main runoff arteries and collaterals, in addition to mechanical damage of the arterial wall. Due to these dismal results graft surveillance has been advised especially during the first 2 years after implantation, since graft revision of a 'failing graft' renders far better results than re-operation for an occluded bypass.[4]

Any effective alternative treatment which lessens the extent of surgery and improves the outcome of graft occlusion is most welcome, and proper indications need to be established for such methods. Thrombolysis is such an alternative.

CATHETER DIRECTED THROMBOLYSIS – CONCEPT AND GOALS

Arterial and graft thrombolysis are best accomplished by delivering the thrombolytic agent via a catheter into the thrombus: catheter directed thrombolysis (CDT)[10,11] (Fig. 1). Intravenous application is ineffective by requiring high doses of the the lytic drug, which increases the danger of haemorrhage.[12]

Three main goals for CDT

1. To be a complementary rather than an alternative procedure, by lysing the thrombosed bypass and identifying the cause of graft failure. The magnitude of the subsequent remedial intervention is thereby reduced and an urgent procedure is conversed into an elective one[13–17] (Fig. 2).

2. To lyse collaterals and runoff vessels that are inaccessible to balloon thrombectomy, supplying the surgeon with a 'road map' if graft extension or replacement is indicated (Fig. 3).

3. To avoid damage which a thrombectomy catheter may cause to the wall of a venous graft.[18]

Complications

Major complications associated with CDT are: cerebral, retroperitoneal or intestinal haemorrhage, local haematoma, distal emboli, and renal insufficiency due to the nephrotoxicity associated with the multiple constrast studies required for this method.

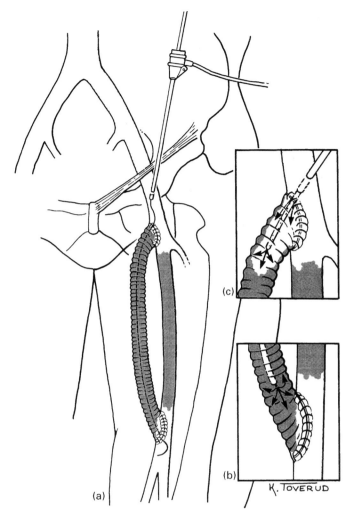

Fig. 1. Antegrade catheter technique for CDT of a thrombosed femoropopliteal graft. The introducer sheath has been placed in the common femoral artery and the guide-wire test is positive (a). The procedure is continued by manoeuvring the catheter tip distally into the thrombus and infusing 5 mg rt-PA while slowly withdrawing the catheter towards the proximal end of the thrombus: 'lacing' (b). With the catheter tip in this position, 5 mg rt-PA is continuously infused during 10 h (c).

General contraindications

The most important contraindications we should consider are: haemostatic defects, severe hypertension, diabetic retinopathy, peptic ulcer and recent cerebral infarction (<6 months), gastrointestinal bleeding (<3 months), or major operation (<1–2 months).

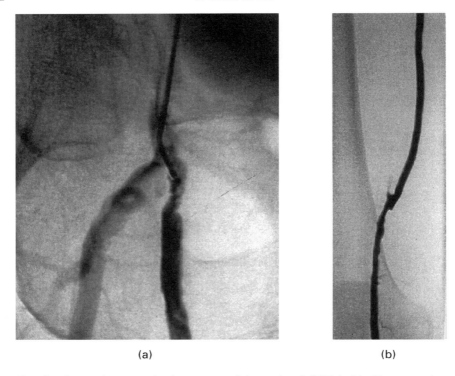

(a)　　　　　　　　　　　　　　　　　　　(b)

Fig. 2. Angiography reveals the successful result of CDT (a,b). No causative distal lesion has been detected after the re-opening of a thrombosed femoropopliteal PTFE graft (b). The residual stenosis at the proximal anastomosis caused by intimal hyperplasia (a), was repaired by local thrombectomy and PTFE patch plasty.

Indications

To evaluate the indications for CDT, we should know the state of the art of endovascular techniques and their efficacy in comparison with alternative treatments. This information can be obtained from non-randomized and randomized studies.

NON-RANDOMIZED STUDIES

Most information on this subject is derived from relatively small, non-randomized, retrospective studies.[19] The variety in patient selection and defined endpoints makes it difficult to compare results and illustrates the need for using proposed reporting

Fig. 3 (*opposite*).　The initial angiogram shows thrombosis of a femoropopliteal PTFE bypass and the crural arteries (a,b,c). After successful CDT of the graft no culprit lesion was visualized, and the patency of the runoff vessels was beautifully restored (d,e,f).

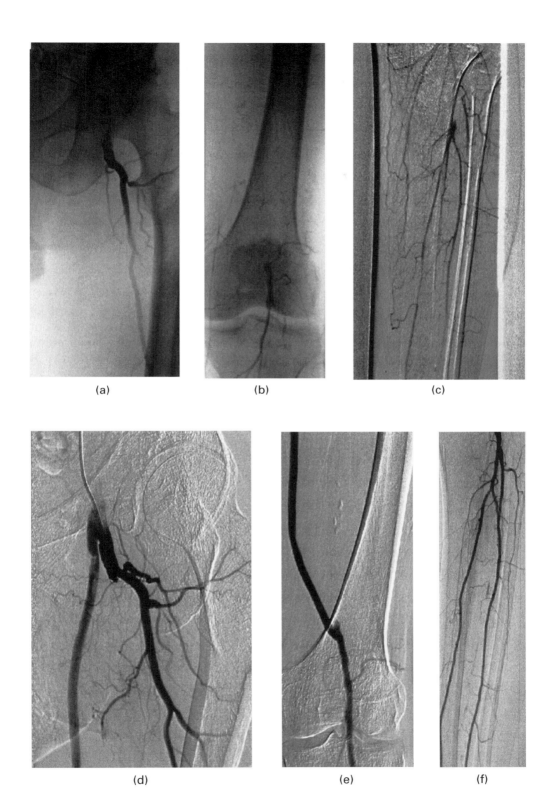

(a) (b) (c)

(d) (e) (f)

standards.[20] Not all studies have been based on the intention-to-treat principle; some have only included patients where successful catheter placement was achieved or in whom the so-called 'guide-wire test' was positive. Neither has 'successful lysis' been uniformly defined. It may refer to percentage of remaining clot, avoidance of operative intervention, improvement of haemodynamic parameters, or limb salvage.

CDT vs surgery

CDT of bypass grafts generally achieves restored patency rates of 60-90%, and may obtain superior 30-day patency and limb retention rates compared with surgical revision alone, whereas the economic impact of these treatments are approximately equal.[21] However, 1-year patency rates of 36–60% have been disappointing.[6,13,16,22–26] Fortunately, limb salvage rates are usually higher than patency rates,[13,17] and most importantly, the survival rates of patients treated with CDT seem to be better than after primary surgery.[27]

Some positive predictors of outcome for CDT have been suggested to improve patient selection. The best results may be obtained in the absence of diabetes and hypercoagulable states, with a 'more mature' (>1 year old) graft, satisfactory crural outflow, and an ankle brachial index >50% after lysis is completed.[17] We found that the ability to penetrate the thrombus with a catheter and patency of the crural arteries were the most important predictive factors.[27] Surprisingly, only few investigators found duration of graft occlusion and pre-existing co-morbidity helpful in predicting the thrombolytic success.[28–30]

Venous vs synthetic grafts

Reports on whether occluded vein, polytetrafluoroethylene (PTFE) or umbilical vein grafts fare better after CDT have been uniquivocal.[22,25,31] Venous grafts most commonly fail as a result of gradual development of a defect in the graft itself, whereas prosthetic grafts fail acutely, presumably because of factors not intrinsic to the graft.[27] Poor 1-year patency rates of 28% or less after CDT of thrombosed venous grafts, have raised serious questions on the cost-benefit of this procedure and on whether secondary vein bypass should be the treatment of choice if autogenous material is available.[4,7,26,32]

More recent information from the literature and our own experience suggest that lysis of synthetic grafts generally is more successful,[13,16,30,33,34] especially if the underlying cause of occlusion is treated effectively.[33]

RANDOMIZED TRIALS

The results of CDT and surgery have been compared in three major prospective, randomized trials, and in one which was too small to draw conclusion upon.[35] It is evident that the results after surgery cannot be compared with those obtained after CDT alone, since additional surgical revision or percutaneous transluminal angioplasty (PTA) are usually required to obtain satisfactory results.[13,14,15,17]

The Rochester study

This trial included 114 patients with embolic or thrombotic, arterial and graft occlusions of less than 7 days duration, half of whom where treated with urokinase (UK) (and surgery/PTA if necessary).[36,37] Clinical success was similar in the CDT and surgery groups, whereas CDT was superior with regard to complications and 1-year mortality. However, occluded grafts were not analysed separately.

The TOPAS study

The TOPAS study (Thrombolysis or Peripheral Artery Surgery) included 213 patients with arterial and graft occlusions of less than 2 weeks duration, with either embolic or non-embolic aetiology. The main object of phase I was to evaluate the safety and efficay of different doses of recombinant urokinase (rUK).[36] It was concluded that CDT is associated with a reduction in the requirement for open surgery, without increasing the risk of death or limb loss. In phase II, patients with occluded grafts are separately analysed, and the results will be reported in the near future.

The STILE study

The STILE (Surgical Revascularization for Ischaemia of the Lower Extremity) multicentre trial comprised 393 patients with non-embolic arterial or graft occlusion, having symptoms of less than 2 weeks duration.[37,38] Either UK or recombinant tissue plasminogen activator (rt-PA) was used. It is the only major randomized study which also focussed on the treatment of graft occlusions. Information from this trial has greatly influenced our indications for CDT.

STILE study – occluded graft subset

In a stratified subset of 124 patients from the STILE trial the fate of bypass graft occlusions of less than 6 months duration was analysed.[37,38] The major findings were:

1. Catheter placement failed in 39% of these 78 patients randomized to CDT, compared with 28% in the total material; a very high technical failure rate. These technical problems were neither related to type or age of graft, nor duration of occlusion. This low technical success rate illustrates one of the disadvantages inherent to large multicentre studies. Experienced endovascular specialists will manage to place the catheter into the thrombus in more than 80% of cases.

2. Restored patency was obtained in 82% of autogenous graft and 85% of prosthetic grafts, following successful catheter placement.

3. An underlying causative lesion was demonstrated in 81% of opened grafts.

4. Significant reduction in anticipated operative procedure was obtained in 42% of the patients treated with CDT.

5. An amputation rate of 19% within 30 days was observed for both venous and PTFE grafts.

6. Outcomes at 1, 6 and 12 months were similar in the CDT and surgical group.

7. Acute ischaemia (<14 days) was treated best with CDT , whereas surgery achieved superior results in patients with chronic (>14 days) graft occlusion.

8. Tibial bypass grafts fared worse than grafts to the popliteal artery, in both the surgery and CDT group. After surgery, amputation rates were 5% and 48%, respectively. When CDT was attempted, ongoing ischaemia rates were 46% and 80%, respectively.

9. Occlusion of native arteries and grafts had a similar prognosis.

10. 'There is a definite indication for CDT' was the main conclusion from STILE. The Clinical Outcome Classification at 30 days for CDT + 'surgery if necessary' was 80% success, compared with 60% after surgical treatment alone.

CDT – LYTIC DRUGS AND TECHNIQUES

Although non-randomized studies have left many questions unanswered , they have provided indispensible information on the value of different CDT techniques. Our present indications and strategy for CDT are based on the evidence from these reports and the randomized trials, in addition to our own experience from approximately 250 patients treated with different lytic drugs and techniques for peripheral arterial and graft occlusions during the last 9 years.

Thrombolytic drugs – indications and complications

All thrombolytic agents act by way of converting plasminogen to plasmin which subsequently hydrolyses fibrin in the thrombus. The three main lytic agents for thrombosed peripheral arteries or grafts are rt-PA, UK and streptokinase (SK). Acylated plasminogen streptokinase activator complex (APSAC) has mainly been applied in the treatment of acute myocardial infarction.

Rt-PA

During the last 2 years we have been using rt-PA, since most studies confirm the superiority of this drug;[39,40] It is more 'fibrin specific' than other thrombolytic agents, having a high affinity for fibrin-bound plasminogen, thus avoiding systemic fibrinogen degradation. Admittedly, this theoretical advantage has not been substantiated in the clinical setting;[41,42] rt-PA may indeed lower plasma fibrinogen concentration.[43] It is easy to administer in dosages independent of the patient's weight. Doses varying from 0.1 to 10 mg/h a 100-fold difference, have been advocated in the literature. We have chosen a very low-dose regimen, which is effective in our experience: 5 mg intra-arterially as a first bolus dose, and subsequently a 0.5 mg/h infusion over a period of 10 h, never exceeding a total dose of 20 mg.[40] Although this is only 1/20 of the dose used for treating myocardial infarction, unfortunately two serious bleeding incidents occurred among the 85 patients we have treated with rt-PA, one of which was a lethal cerebral haemorrhage. An incidence of 1-2% major haemorrhage is quite common for all three major lytic drugs. Although rt-PA is the most expensive clinically used lytic agent, its relatively rapid action[42,43] and the low dosages we have been using, may outweigh this disadvantage.

UK

According to the STILE study the safety (mortality and haemorrhage rates) and efficacy (clot resolution, limb salvage) for UK and rt-PA were equivalent, whereas rt-PA achieved a more rapid lysis than UK: a mean of 8 h vs 18 h.[37] These findings were confirmed in another prospective, randomized comparison of UK with rt-PA.[43] The optimal doses for UK and rt-Pa have not yet been determined in a systematic fashion.[33]

During the last few years UK and rt-PA have been more widely used than SK. UK achieves lysis faster than SK, has higher initial clinical success rates, 90% vs 60%, with a lower incidence of complications,[23,24,33,42-44] and is thus more cost-effective.[42,44,45]

SK

The cheapest and most extensively documented lytic drug is SK. Compared with rt-PA and UK it is less fibrin specific and therefore less efficacious. It initially creates an equimolar SK-plasminogen activator 'complex', on which SK subsequently can act to convert plasminogen to plasmin. This systemic lytic effect may account for the relatively high incidence of bleeding. Furthermore, antibody formation against SK precludes its repetitive use. Additionally, allergic and anaphylactic reactions have been a problem.

Catheterization

The ipsilateral femoral artery may be used to antegradely insert a 6 F co-axial introducer, preferably not puncturing the graft (Fig.1). However, contralateral puncture of the common femoral artery, using the cross-over approach, is generally safer (Fig.4). The benefits and disadvantages of these techniques have to be weighed against each other in each case.

'Guide-wire test'

We initially apply the guide-wire traverse test,[24] where the guide-wire is attempted to be passed through the length of the thrombotic occlusion, prior to embedding the

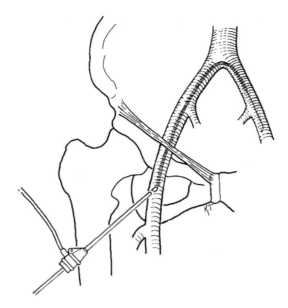

Fig. 4. Retrograde crossover catheter technique where the guide-wire and angiographic catheter have been introduced into the right common femoral artery and fed across the aorta–iliac bifurcation to address an thrombotic occlusion in the left lower limb.

catheter tip in the proximal part of the thrombus (Fig.1a). If the test is positive, successful lysis is five to ten times more likely.[24] We do not deny a trial of lysis if the guide-wire test is negative, but are prepared for failure. Occasionally the catheter is placed against the occlusion and infusion is started, softening the thrombus and allowing later penetration with the guide-wire. However, if the catheter is not able to enter the thrombus, the success rate becomes 0%.[27]

Initial transthrombus bolus: 'lacing'

After the guide-wire is in place, a 5 F catheter with sideholes is advanced almost to the distal end of the thrombus (Fig.1b). While under fluoroscopic monitoring the catheter is slowly withdrawn towards the proximal anastomosis, another 5 mg rt-Pa is infused along the whole length of the thrombus. This so-called 'lacing' reportedly shortens infusion time,[23,46,47] but may cause complications like distal emboli, if not performed carefully.[46]

Drug infusion

Finally, the tip of the catheter is placed into the proximal thrombus and 5 mg of rt-PA diluted in 250 ml of saline is continuously administered by means of an infusion pump in the course of 10 h (Fig.1b). To avoid pericatheter thrombosis and ensuing emboli when the catheter is withdrawn, we infuse heparin co-axially along the catheter. This is probably as effective as systemic administration and causes less bleeding.[48] The absence of branches in a graft obviates the need to adjust the catheter tip with regular intervals to follow the clot interface. This strategy of 'semi-local infusion' simplifies the procedure and regular angiographic follow-up at the angio-laboratory is not necessary, which is cost saving.

If the result of control angiography after 10 h is satisfactory, and a causative lesion is found, further management can be planned. Successful lysis is sometimes defined as restoration of antegrade flow with less than 20% diameter reduction by residual thrombus. Ideally, total lysis should be attempted, since residual thrombosis is potentially thrombogenic.[47] Infusion is stopped if successful lysis is demonstrated, symptoms increase during treatment or major haematomas develop. If no lysis has been achieved, infusion with additional 5 mg rt-PA is continued for a further 10 h. Reperfusion should be established within 12-18 hours; continued lytic therapy is usually unsuccessful.[27] In addition, the probability for major bleeding complications tends to increase with infusion time.[23]

Anticoagulation

Immediate rethrombosis may occur in approximately 3% of patients.[24] Interestingly, thrombolysis itself is associated with *in vivo* activation of the coagulation system.[49] Rethrombosis is less likely if heparin is administered concomitantly.[48] After the catheter has been removed, intravenous heparin is given continuously during 48 h, keeping the Cephotest at approximately 70. All patients receive acetylic acid 160 mg daily indefinetely.

Monitoring

The progression of clot lysis can be observed angiographically with different intervals, depending on the available resources of personnel and equipment.

Close clinical observation, preferably in the intensive care unit is mandatory for early diagnosis of complications. Secondary embolization may occur in 5% of cases,[24] as manifested by sudden onset of pain, skin changes or loss of distal pulse. Especially large prosthetic grafts may be prone to this complication. The majority of small emboli will resolve during continued lytic therapy and anticoagulation. If no clinical improvement is noted within 2 h, repositioning of the catheter into the crural arteries may be necessary, and suction through the catheter may be attempted.

Monitoring of coagulation parameters to avoid major haemorrhage has been advocated, especially since the STILE trial documented an association between fibrinogen plasma levels and bleeding complications.[38] Others deny that laboratory tests diminish the risk of bleeding.[50] The most frequent bleeding occurs at the site of arterial cannulation. Since the duration of thrombolysis is correlated with the occurrence of haemorrhage,[23,51] we use rt-Pa and the 'lacing' technique to shorten lysis time.

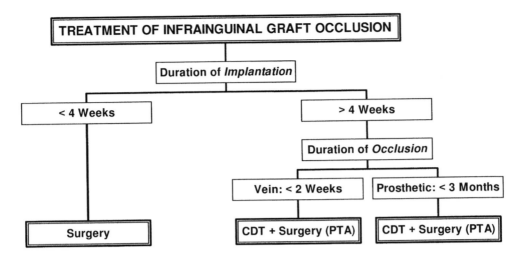

Fig. 5. Algorithm for the treatment of infrainguinal graft occlusion.

Additional surgery or PTA

In some patients the graft is re-opened without finding a culprit lesion (Figs 3, 4). If successful CDT reveals a graft stenosis of more than 50% diameter reduction, PTA or surgery can be performed (Fig. 5). However, growing experience suggests that long-term success after surgical revision of an anastomotic stenosis is greater than after PTA.[11]

Alternative and supplementary catheter techniques

Several techniques have been proposed to shorten the time to achieve initial technical success, e.g. suction thromboembolectomy[52] or mechanical catheter endarterectomy.[53] By using a pulse-spray technique, where the lytic agent is forcefully administered through a multihole catheter along the length of the thrombus, the clot is mechanically disrupted to increase the surface area available for enzymatic action.[54,55] However, it is not certain that lysing time is shortened, whereas the risk of embolization may be increased.[26,55,56] By applying so-called 'burst' therapy the lytic drug is infused intermittently allegedly to avoid bleeding complications. Thrombolysis within a vascular segment enclosed by two balloons is probably more suited for occluded native arteries than grafts.[57] No consistent advantages have been proven with these different catheter techniques.[56]

FUTURE TRIALS

These trials should be on intention-to-treat basis and universally accepted reporting standards should be adhered to.[20] Since institutional expertise varies, participating centres should have well-trained endovascular specialists to avoid a too high percentage of primary technical failure. The following trials are suggested:

1. Compare the efficacy of CDT with surgery and intra-operatively administered lytic agent (rt-PA or UK). If we start with thrombectomy, antegrade flow is rapidly established and the bulk of thrombus is removed, leaving a smaller amount to be lysed.[58] On the other hand, primary lysis reduces the magnitude of surgery. It is relevant to find out which strategy is best.
2. Compare the results of CDT with implantation of a secondary (more distally placed) bypass. Several investigators have pointed out the dismal long-term results of CDT, especially after vein graft thrombosis, and proposed that a secondary bypass operation should be done instead of thrombolysis.
3. New plasminogen activators, techniques to enchance lytic action,[59] methods of drug delivery and mechanical devices to reduce the bulk of thrombus [60,61] will be developed and their efficacy and safety have to be compared appropriately. Alternative surgical treatments like subintimal PTA of the occluded arteries should also be evaluated in this context.

INDICATIONS FOR CDT (Fig. 5)

Occlusion of a femoropopiteal graft which has been implanted for less than 4 weeks requires surgical revision. CDT (+ surgery/PTA, if necessary) is recommended in patients with:

1. Venous graft thrombosis of less than 2 weeks duration.
2. Prosthetic graft thrombosis of less than 3 months duration.

The results after CDT for occluded crural bypasses are discouraging and thrombolysis is therefore only indicated in a very few patients who resist amputation and where other treatment options are lacking.

Optimal patient selection and optimal expertise from vascular and endovascular specialists lead to optimal treatment. Last but not least, the main goal of treatment is not to save a limb, but to help the patient achieve optimal quality of life.

REFERENCES

1. O'Donnell TF, Farber SP, Richmand DM *et al.*: Above-knee polytetrafluoroethylene femoropopliteal bypass graft: Is it a reasonable alternative to the below-knee reverse autogenous vein graft? *Surgery* **94**: 26–31, 1983
2. Green RM, Ouriel K, Ricotta JJ *et al.*: Revision of failed infra-inguinal bypass graft: Principles of management. *Surgery* **100**: 646–53, 1986

3. Veith FJ, Gupta SK, Wengerter KR *et al.*: Management of late failures of femoropopliteal and femorodistal bypasses. In: Kroese AJ, Jorgensen JJ (Eds), *Challenges in Vascular Surgery. 1990 Acta Chir Scand Suppl* **555**: 139–48, 1990

4. Whittemore AD, Clowes AW, Couch NP *et al.*: Secondary femoropopliteal reconstruction. *Ann Surg* **193**: 35–42, 1981

5. Davies AH, Pope I, Collin J *et al.*: Early re-operation after major vascular surgery: a four year prospective analysis. *Br J Surg* **79**: 76–8, 1992

6. Graor RA, Risius B, Young JR *et al.*: Thrombolysis of peripheral arterial bypass grafts: surgical thrombectomy compared with thrombolysis, a preliminary report. *J Vasc Surg* **7**: 347–55, 1988

7. Edwards JE, Taylor LM, Porter JM: Treatment of failed lower extremity bypass grafts with new autogenous vein bypass grafting. *J Vasc Surg* **11**: 136–45, 1990

8. Ascer E, Collier P, Gupta SK *et al.*: Reoperation for polytetrafluoroethylene bypass failure: the importance of distal outflow site and operative technique in determining outcome. *J Vasc Surg* **5**: 298–310, 1987

9. Singh S, Beard JD: Is primary amputation ever the first choice? In: Greenhalgh RM, Fowkes FGR (Eds), *Trials and Tribulations of Vascular Surgery* pp. 365–72. London: WB Saunders, 1996

10. Dotter CT, Rosch J, Seaman AJ: Selective clot lysis with low-dose streptokinase. *Radiology* **111**: 31–7, 1974

11. McNamara TO, Bomberger RA: Factors affecting initial and six month patency rates after intra-arterial thrombolysis with high dose urokinase. *Am J Surg* **152**: 709–12, 1986

12. Amery A, Deloof W, Vermylen J *et al.*: Outcome of recent thrombo-embolic occlusions of limb arteries treated with streptokinase. *Br Med J* **4**: 639–44, 1970

13. Belkin M, Donaldson MC, Whittemore AD *et al.*: Observations on the use of thrombolytic agents for thrombotic occlusion of infra-inguinal vein grafts. *J Vasc Surg* **11**: 289–96, 1990

14. Gardiner GA Jr, Sullivan KL: Catheter-directed thrombolysis for the failed lower extremity bypass graft. *Semin Vasc Surg* **5**: 99–103, 1992

15. McNamara TO: Thrombolysis as an alternative initial therapy for the acutely ischemic lower limb. *Semin Vasc Surg* **5**: 89–98, 1992

16. Faggioli GL, Peer RM, Pedrini L *et al.*: Failure of thrombolytic therapy to improve long-term vascular patency. *J Vasc Surg* **19**: 289–97, 1994

17. Nackman GB, Walsh DB, Fillinger MF *et al.*: Thrombolysis of occluded infra-inguinal vein grafts: predictors of outcome. *J Vasc Surg* **25**: 1023–32, 1997

18. Chidi CC, DePalma DG: Atherogenic potential of embolectomy catheters. *Surgery* **83**: 549–57, 1978

19. Kroese AJ, Staxrud LE: The results of arterial thrombolysis. *Ann Chir Gyn* **84**: 350–3, 1995

20. Ahn SS, Rutherford RB, Becker GJ *et al.*: Reporting standards for lower extremity arterial endovascular procedures. *J Vasc Surg* **9**: 1103–7, 1993

21. Ouriel K, Kolassa M, DeWeese A *et al.*: Economic implications of thrombolysis or operation as the initial treatment modality in acute peripheral arterial occlusion. *Surgery* **118**: 810–4, 1995

22. Gardiner GA Jr, Harrington DP, Koltun W *et al.*: Salvage of occluded arterial bypass grafts by means of thrombolysis. *J Vasc Surg* **9**: 426–31, 1989

23. Sullivan KL, Gardiner GA, Shapiro MJ *et al.*: Acceleration of thrombolysis wih a high-dose transthrombus bolus technique. *Radiology* **173**: 805–8, 1989

24. McNamara TO, Fisher JR: Thrombolysis in peripheral arterial and graft occlusions: improved results using high dose urokinase. *Am J Roent* **144**: 764–55, 1985

25. Durham JD, Geller SC, Abbott WM *et al.*: Regional infusion of urokinase into occluded lower extremity bypass grafts: long-term clinical results. *Radiology* **172**: 83–7, 1989

26. Hye RJ, Turner C, Valji K *et al.*: Is thrombosis of occluded popliteal and tibial bypass grafts worthwhile? *J Vasc Surg* **20**: 588–97, 1994

27. Ouriel K, Shortell CK, DeWeese JA *et al.*: A comparison of thrombolytic therapy with operative revascularization in the initial treatment of acute peripheral arterial ischemia. *J Vasc Surg* **20**: 588–97, 1994

28. Sandbaek G, Staxrud LE, Rosen L *et al.*: Factors predicting the outcome of intra-arterial thrombolysis in peripheral arterial and graft occlusions. *Acta Radiol* **37**: 299–304, 1996

29. Bhatnagar PK, Ierardi RP, Ikeda Y: The impact of thrombolytic therapy on arterial and graft occlusions: a critical analysis. *J Cardiovasc Surg* **37**: 105–12, 1996
30. May J, Thompson J, Rickard K *et al.*: Isolated limb perfusion with urokinase for acute ischemia. *J Vasc Surg* **17**: 408–13, 1993
31. Sussman B, Dardik H, Ibrahim IM *et al.*: Improved patient selection for enzymatic lysis of peripheral arterial and graft occlusions. *Am J Surg* **148**: 244–8, 1984
32. De Frang RD, Edwards JM, Moneta *et al.*: Repeat leg bypass after multiple prior bypass failures. *J Vasc Surg* **19**: 268–77, 1994
33. Sullivan KL, Gardiner GA, Kandarpa K *et al.*: Efficacy of thrombolysis in infra-inguinal bypass grafts. *Circulation* **83** (Suppl 1); I99–I105, 1991
34. Ikeda Y, Rummel MC, Bhatnagar PK *et al.*: Thrombolysis therapy in patients with femoropopliteal synthetic graft occlusions. *Am J Surg* **171**: 251–4, 1996
35. Nilsson L, Albrechtsson U, Jorung T *et al.*: Surgical treatment versus thrombolysis in acute arterial occlusion: a randomized study. *Eur J Vasc Surg* **6**: 189–93, 1992
36. Ouriel K: Surgery versus thrombolytic therapy in the management of peripheral arterial occlusion. *JVIR* **6**: 48S–54S, 1995
37. The STILE Investigators. Results of a prospective randomized trial evaluating surgery versus thrombolysis for ischemia of the lower extremity: the STILE trial. *Ann Surg* **220**: 251–68, 1994
38. Comerota AJ, Weaver FA, Hosking JD *et al.*: Results of a prospective, randomized trial of surgery versus thrombolysis for occluded lower extremity bypass grafts. *Am J Surg* **172**: 105–12, 1996
39. Berridge DC, Gregson RHS, Hopkinson BR *et al.*: Tissue plasminogen activator in peripheral arterial thrombolysis. *Br J Surg* **77**: 179–82, 1990
40. Lonsdale RJ, Berridge DC, Earnshaw JJ: Recombinant tissue-type plasminogen activator is superior to streptokinase for local intra-arterial thrombolysis. *Br J Surg* **79**: 272–9, 1992
41. Goldhaber SZ, Heit J, Sharma GVRK *et al.*: Randomized controlled trial of recombinant tissue plasminogen activator versus urokinase in the treatment of acute pulmonary embolism. *Lancet* **ii**: 293–8, 1988
42. Graor RA, Olin J, Bartholomew JR *et al.*: Efficacy and safety of intraarterial local infusion of streptokinase, urokinase, or tissue-plasminogen activator for peripheral arterial ocllusion: a retrospective review. *J Vasc Med Biol* **2**: 310–5, 1990
43. Meyerowitz MF, Goldhaber SZ, Regan K *et al.*: Recombinant tissue-plasminogen activator versus urokinase in peripheral arterial and graft occlusions: a randomized trial. *Radiology* **175**: 75–8, 1990
44. Breda A, Groar RA, Katzen BT *et al.*: Relative cost-effectiveness of urokinase versus streptokinase in the threatment of peripheral vascular disease. *JVIR* **2**: 77–87, 1991
45. Jasonik JE, Bettmann MA, Kaul ? *et al.*: Therapeutic alternatives for subacute peripheral arterial occlusion: comparison by outcome, length of stay and hospital charges. *Invest Radiol* **26**: 921–5, 1991
46. Ward AS, Andaz SK, Bygrave S: Thrombolysis with tissue-plasminogen activator: results with a high-dose transthrombus technique. *J Vasc Surg* **19**: 503–8, 1994
47. Kandarpa K: Technical determinants of success in catheter-directed thrombolysis for peripheral arterial occlusions. *JVIR* **6**: 55S–61S, 1995
48. Eskridge JM, Becker, Rabe FE *et al.*: Catheter-related thrombosis and fibrinolytic therapy. *Radiology* **149**: 429–32, 1983
49. Baglin TP, Luddington R, Jennings I *et al.*: Thrombin generation and myocardial infarction during infusion of tissue-plasminogen activator. *Lancet* **341**: 504–5, 1993
50. Marder VJ, Sherr S: Thrombolytic therapy: current status (II). *New Engl J Med* **318**: 1585–95, 1988
51. Marder VJ: Bleeding complications of thrombolytic treatment. *Am J Hosp Pharm* **47**: S15–S19, 1990
52. Nachbur B, Mahler Do-Dai-Do F, Schneider E: Initial lysis and catheter clot removal for occlusive disease in critical ischaemia. In: Greenhalgh RM (Ed), *Vascular and Endovascular Surgical Techniques, an Atlas* pp. 292–9. London: WB Saunders, 1994

53. Misra HP: Revascularization of the limbs with urokinase and TEC catheter endarterectomy for occluded bypass grafts. *Am J Surg* **166**: 756–9, 1993
54. Bookstein JJ, Fellmeth B, Roberts A *et al.*: Pulsed-spray pharmacomechanical thrombolysis: Preliminary clinical results. *Am J Roent* **152**: 1097–100, 1989
55. Yusuf SW, Whitaker SC, Gregson RHS *et al.*: Prospective randomised comparative study of pulse spray and conventional local thrombolysis. *Eur J Vasc Endovasc Surg* **10**: 136–41, 1995
56. Kandarpa K, Chopra PS, Aruny JE *et al.*: Prospective, randomized comparison of forced periodic infusion and conventional slow continuous infusion. *Radiology* **188**: 1–7, 1993
57. Jorgensen B, Tonnessen KH, Nielsen JD *et al.*: Segmentally enclosed thrombolysis in percutaneous transluminal angiolasty for femoropopliteal occlusions: a report from a pilot study. *Cardiovasc Intervent Radiol* **14**: 293–8, 1991
58. Comerota AJ, Rao AK, Throm RC *et al.*: A prospective, randomized, blinded and placebo-controlled trial of intra-operative intra-arterial urokinase infusion during lower extremity revascularizations: regional and systemic effects. *Ann Surg* **218**: 534–9, 1993
59. Tachibana K: Enhancement of fibrinolysis with ultrasound energy. *JVIR* **3**: 299–303, 1992
60. Murray JG, Brown AL, Wilkins RA: Percutaneous aspiration thrombo-embolectomy: a preliminary experience. *Clin Radiol* **49**: 553–8, 1994
61. Drasler WJ, Jenson ML, Wilson GJ *et al.*: Rheolytic catheter for percutaneous removal of thrombus. *Radiology* **63**; 263–7, 1992

Editorial comments by C.V. Ruckley

It remains difficult, in routine clinical practice, to define those patients presenting with graft occlusion who are most appropriately treated with thrombolytic therapy. That this reviewer remains unclear is not the fault of the authors. Kroese *et al.* have drawn attention to the lack of randomized clinical trials of thrombolysis vs surgery capable of providing evidence on which guidelines can be based. They are able to quote only one trial, the STILE trial, which has analysed a subset of patients with occluded grafts separate from acute occlusions in general. Neither the early restoration of patency which was achieved in 82% of autogenous grafts and 85% of prosthetic grafts nor even the 30 day 'success' rates (80% for lysis ± surgery vs 60% for surgery alone) truly reflect the generally disappointing longer term outcomes in this type of patient population. Audit of vascular practice in Edinburgh has shown a fall in the number and proportion of cases of acute ischaemia, including graft occlusion, treated with thrombolytic therapy over the last 3 years. The hazards and costs of thrombolysis, with or without surgery, need to be weighed against the benefits and quality of life issues on a longer time scale.

How do we judge when graft lysis is not worthwhile? Many factors influence clinical decision making: poor inflow, impaired cardiac performance, diseased outflow, poor quality vein, general patient frailty etc. Pre-emption of occlusion is clearly preferable. Unfortunately the failure of synthetic grafts seems frequently capricious and unpredictable such that surveillance programmes achieve little. Surveillance in vein grafts is generally advocated as worthwhile, but does not appear to have been objectively evaluated in cost-benefit terms. the failure of a vein graft is often a gradual process, detectable by surveillance and sometimes correctable.

However, when it is due to deterioration of the runoff vasculature, as is commonly the case in the elderly 'critical ischaemia' group, intervention either before or after the occlusion offers little prospect of durable success, especially as the remaining option is frequently only synthetic replacement. thus the most valuable predictor as to whether it is worthwhile intervening for graft occlusion is often the original preoperative angiogram or the operative completion angiogram. In reported series of graft occlusions we hear little of the patients for whom neither surgery nor thrombolysis are contemplated. Thus the selection policies applied in reported series or in clinical trials do not necessarily reflect day-to-day clinical experience and the overall cost-benefits of the re-intervention options for graft occlusions remain difficult to unravel. The authors' argument that further trials should be on an 'intention to treat' basis and incorporating universally accepted reporting standards is well made.

Kroese *et al.* provide a useful discussion of the choice of agents and administration techniques. Radiologists who can achieve high success rates in ensuring catheter access into the thrombus, who can adjust their techniques to achieve lysis with minimal dosage of lytic agent, who have access to the most effective agent, regardless of cost and who can reach, with their surgical colleagues, well founded decisions as to the nature and timing of post-lysis secondary interventions offer the best prospect of eventually defining the role of thrombolysis for the occluded graft.

VENOUS QUESTIONS AND INDICATIONS

Do We Know if Duplex Should be Used for Varicose Vein Surgery?

Jason Smith, Alun H. Davies and Roger M. Greenhalgh

INTRODUCTION

Varicose veins are very common, affecting about 25% of women and 15% of men in England.[1] Around 56 000 operations are performed per annum in the UK alone for this condition.[2] This contributes a significant demand on the National Health Service, and private health care service resources. It is known that up to 20% of patients are dissatisfied with the surgery that they obtain for their varicose veins.[3-8]

Duplex (meaning 'twofold') ultrasonography was introduced into clinical practice in the early 1980s and involves a combination of real-time B mode ultrasonography with a gated Doppler signal. The more recent addition of colour coding various frequency shifts has prompted some to use the term 'triplex'. This technology has revolutionized the approach to the investigation of both arterial and venous disease and has been the subject of numerous trials. Initially the focus was on arterial assessment, venous interest appearing a few years later. However none of these trials have yet answered the question posed by this chapter title.

The ability to directly visualize by non-invasive methods the deep and superficial veins, their interconnections and whether competent or not would seem to be the best functional method to assess varicose veins preoperatively. This would then allow us to determine the most appropriate method of treatment. To date this concept has not yet been fully realized or set out in a randomized controlled trial.

CURRENT METHODS OF ASSESSMENT

There are many methods available for assessing varicose veins, the most important is still taking a full history and performing a detailed clinical examination. The question of whether or not to use duplex is easily answered if the patient is asymptomatic.

The authors would recommend the following approach to the assessment of varicose veins which should be applicable to all patients.

Primary varicose veins
1. history and clinical examination
2. examination with continuous wave Doppler

Recurrent varicose veins, presence of ulceration or clinical evidence of deep venous disease
1. history, clinical examination and review of notes (if available)
2. examination with colour duplex and preoperative marking with colour duplex
3. (contrast phlebography)

Contrast phlebography should be reserved for those few cases such as when colour duplex is deemed equivocal for whatever reason despite having been performed by an experienced technologist.[9]

ALTERNATIVES TO DUPLEX

There are many alternatives to colour duplex for the assessment of varicose veins;[10] however, only the following will be considered as they are the ones most commonly used in clinical practice. The practicality and evidence to back the use of the tests will be considered in order to justify the above recommendations.

- Clinical examination
- Continuous wave Doppler
- Plethysmography
- Phlebography

Due to the widespread adoption of colour duplex for varicose vein assessment many of the studies described in the following text have used colour duplex as the gold standard rather than contrast phlebography – the currently accepted reference gold standard. Therefore interpreting results can be difficult.

CLINICAL EXAMINATION

Apart from general examination of the legs and abdomen there are the time honoured techniques of Perthe and Brodie–Trendelenberg. Several studies, however, have shown that physical examination alone is poor at predicting the sites of incompetence especially in recurrent varicose veins[9,11,12] (Table 1).

Table 1. Different methods of detecting saphenofemoral junction incompetence in recurrent varicose veins

	Method	*Sens*	*Spec*	*PPV*	*NPV*
Bradbury *et al.*[9]	Clinical	65.4	70	85	43.8
n=36	CWD	88.5	40	79.3	57.1
	Duplex	42.3	100	100	40
	Varicography	73.1	100	100	58.8
Bradbury *et al.*[17]	Clinical	72.5	80	90.2	53.3
n=71	CWD	92.2	55	83.9	73.3
De Palma *et al.*[12]	Clinical	47	60	80	25
n=22	CWD	47	80	89	31

n: Number of limbs; Sens: sensitivity; Spec: specificity; PPV: positive predictive value; NPV: negative predictive value; CWD: continuous wave Doppler. All values are given as percentages.

The highly variable anatomy around the popliteal fossa makes it especially difficult to diagnose saphenopopliteal junction or short saphenous vein incompetence.[13,14] In fact only two-thirds of incompetent saphenofemoral junctions were accurately predicted by clinical examination alone when performed by a very experienced vascular surgeon.[9] The advantages of clinical examination are obvious, every medical student is taught the above tests and therefore every practising surgeon should be able to perform them easily. The disadvantages are that there are several ways of performing the tests and hence they cannot be standardized. Lack of experience (e.g. failure to appreciate normal venous filling), and poor predictive value of the tests will cause differences in results.

CONTINUOUS WAVE DOPPLER

This utilizes a 5–10 MHz hand-held probe which is available in almost all hospitals. The probe has two piezo electric crystals, one of which transmits the ultrasound beam and the other receives it. The problem is that any vessel within the range of the probe (related to its frequency) will be insonated and therefore it can be difficult to decide which vessel you are listening to. Furthermore it takes training to use continuous wave Doppler properly and accurately. Doppler assessment improves the accuracy of clinical examination. This appears to be best for long saphenous vein reflux, but is less so for short saphenous vein and deep venous reflux.

When considering how well Doppler performs against colour duplex McMullin and Coleridge Smith[15] presented their figures in such a way a to allow us to perform a kappa analysis in order to determine agreement between these modalities. These values work out to be 0.52 for long saphenous vein incompetence (moderate agreement), 0.29 for short saphenous vein incompetence (fair agreement), and 0.42 for deep venous incompetence (moderate agreement). A further comparison in the assessment of the saphenofemoral and saphenopopliteal junctions in primary varicose veins Doppler is both sensitive (77% and 83% respectively) specific (91% and 93% respectively)[16] when compared with duplex as the gold standard. Sensitivity starts to fall for long saphenous vein incompetence, and it is an insensitive investigation for short saphenous vein, deep venous and perforator vein incompetence.[15,16] McMullin[15] again reported poor sensitivities for Doppler when compared with duplex when examining for short saphenous and deep venous incompetence (37% and 48%). As a comparison McIrvine[11] reports the ability of Doppler to correctly predict reflux at the saphenofemoral junction compared with operative findings as good (sensitivity 90%, specificity 45%) when using operative findings as the gold standard.

In the assessment of recurrent varicose veins with Doppler, Bradbury et al.[9] report a good sensitivity (89%) for the prediction of saphenofemoral junction incompetence using Doppler with compared operative findings. A further study by Bradbury et al.[17] on a different patient population shows similar results, with a sensitivity of 92% (Table 1), although specificity is low in both studies (40% and 55% respectively).

The problem with Doppler when assessing the saphenofemoral junction (and to a lesser extent the saphenopopliteal junction) is its inability accurately to locate a specific vein. Studies have shown that proximal long saphenous vein reflux can occur with a competent saphenofemoral junction[18,19] (Fig. 1). Within the range of the probe, reflux in the common femoral vein (Fig. 1a) can be mistaken for saphenofemoral junction reflux. This is overcome by the application of a tourniquet to the upper thigh. However, in the case of long saphenous vein reflux and a competent saphenofemoral junction (Fig. 1c) an incorrect diagnosis can be made with Doppler unless the rest of the long saphenous vein is examined. A false signal can be generated by Doppler from either a region in which there is a venous junction between superficial veins or from a descending vein which joins the deep venous system.[9,19,20] In the case of recurrent varicose veins and neovascularization it is easy to see why Doppler can mistake saphenofemoral junction reflux for reflux in other branches.

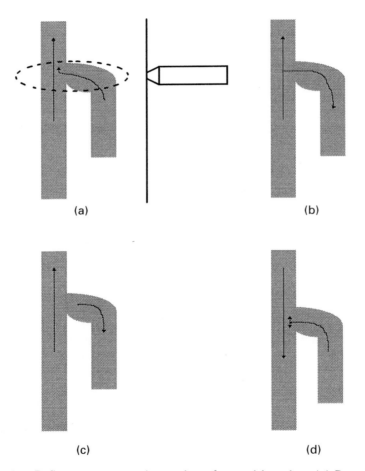

(a)

(b)

(c)

(d)

Fig. 1. Reflux patterns at the saphenofemoral junction. (a) Doppler insonation of the saphenofemoral junction showing range of probe. (b) True saphenofemoral junction reflux. (c) Long saphenous vein reflux with a competent saphenofemoral junction. (d) Deep venous reflux without long saphenous system reflux.

The advantages of Doppler are it is relatively cheap, easy to use, and readily available, and on this basis alone it should be used in the clinic for assessment of all venous patients. Despite this a survey carried out of surgeons in the northern region (UK)[21] showed only 37% used Doppler (increasing to 62% of those with a vascular interest) in the assessment of varicose veins. The disadvantages are that it is very operator dependent and as mentioned above one cannot reliably tell which vessel is being listened to.

PLETHYSMOGRAPHY

Photoplethysmography (PPG) relies on the transmission of light through skin and measures venous refilling time after exercising the limb. Hence it can be used to identify superficial and deep venous incompetence (with the use of tourniquets) but is even less vessel specific than Doppler. Light refraction rheography is a modification using three emitters around one collector and is simpler to use clinically giving results compatible with PPG.[22] Both are more suited to assessing overall venous function of the limb and therefore can be used to assess how well surgery has corrected the venous reflux (shown by increased venous refilling time postoperatively – Fig. 2) Photoplethysmography has been used to assess superficial venous valvular incompetence, but when compared with combined clinical and Doppler examination there was poor agreement, $\kappa=0.30$.[23]

PHLEBOGRAPHY

Phlebography in its various guises has been considered the gold standard in venous assessment for many years. There are inherent problems such as its invasiveness, risk of anaphylaxis, air embolism, thrombosis, pain on injection etc. all of which are rare.

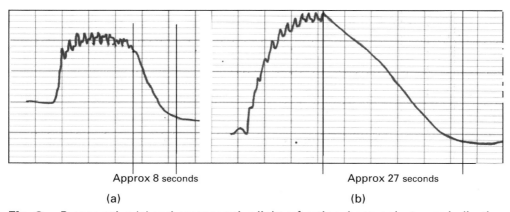

Approx 8 seconds   Approx 27 seconds

(a)   (b)

Fig. 2.   Preoperative (a) and postoperative light refraction rheography traces indicating correction of the venous reflux by increased refilling time.

Ascending venography is used to assess deep venous problems, superficial venous reflux and the calf perforator veins.[24] It is also useful for intraoperative marking of the position of the saphenofemoral and saphenopopliteal junctions.[14] Descending venography is much more invasive and used primarily to assess reflux in deep veins and the long saphenous vein. In the presence of an competent saphenofemoral junction this technique will miss long saphenous vein reflux; it will also miss isolated segmental reflux.

Table 2 shows how well duplex compares with venography[25] with the greater sensitivity in deep venous incompetence for venography. Baldt *et al.*[24] performed a similar study on 137 limbs to compare duplex with descending venography to assess superficial and deep reflux (κ=0.75 and 0.79 respectively) and ascending venography to assess long and short saphenous vein reflux (κ=0.96 and 0.94 respectively). The conclusion was that duplex could replace these more invasive investigations and that contrast studies should be reserved for equivocal duplex results. Another study[26] agrees favourably with the findings of Phillips *et al.*[25] when comparing duplex with venography finding sensitivity and specificity values of 96% and 75% for saphenofemoral junction incompetence, and 90% and 67% for saphenopopliteal junction incompetence.

Table 1 shows how duplex compares with venography in the assessment of saphenofemoral junction incompetence in recurrent varicose veins when assessing the pick-up rate of each test compared with the operative findings.

THE EVIDENCE FOR DUPLEX

One study has been identified where data was provided that allowed a direct comparison between duplex and venography by kappa analysis. Figures taken from Phillips *et al.*[25] show that duplex has a high accuracy in demonstrating saphenofemoral junction incompetence and saphenopopliteal junction incompetence (92% and 95%), but is less useful in demonstrating perforator vein incompetence and

Table 2. Sensitivity and specificity of colour duplex versus venography in diagnosing reflux

	Site	k	Sens (%)	Spec (%)	PPV (%)	NPV (%)
Phillips *et al.*[25]	SFJI	0.74	90.7	83.3	90.7	83.3
(n=84)	SPJI	0.90	95	96.9	90.5	98.4
	DVI	0.42	33.1	98.7	75	92.5
	MTPI	0.63	58.8	97	83.3	90.3
	CPI	−0.21	52.2	17.6	71.4	8.6

n: Total number of limbs; k: kappa value; SFJI: saphenofemoral incompetence; SPJI: saphenopopliteal incompetence; DVI: deep venous incompetence; MTPI: mid-thigh perforator incompetence; CPI: calf perforator incompetence; Sens: sensitivity; Spec: specificity; PPV: positive predictive value; NPV: negative predictive value.

* Values derived from original figures, includes recurrent and primary varicose veins.

deep venous incompetence (61% and 40%) compared with operative findings. In the same study it is seen that duplex is as accurate as venography for demonstrating both saphenofemoral junction incompetence and saphenopopliteal junction incompetence (duplex 92% and 95%, venography 92% and 91%), but is considerably less accurate in diagnosing perforator vein incompetence and deep venous incompetence (duplex 61% and 40%, venography 84% and 90%). Performing a kappa analysis to compare these two test gives the results shown in Table 1. This shows that there is excellent agreement between venography and duplex for saphenofemoral junction incompetence and saphenopopliteal junction incompetence, and moderate agreement for deep venous incompetence.

In a study of recurrent varicose veins the operative findings are compared with duplex prediction for diagnosing saphenofemoral junction incompetence[9] Duplex has a sensitivity of 42% and a specificity of 100% (positive predictive value 100%, negative predictive value 40%) compared with varicography which has values of 73% and 100% respectively (Table 1). The authors of this study were unable to assess 44% of saphenofemoral junctions due to distorted anatomy which could explain the poor sensitivity of duplex. Duplex scanning was able to demonstrate the sites of connection between superficial and deep veins that were responsible for recurrence in over 90% of cases in one series.[27]

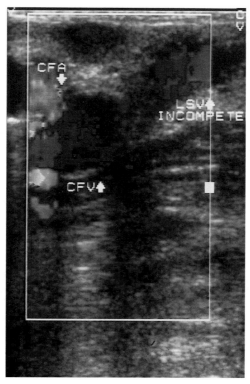

Fig. 3.   Duplex demonstration of reverse flow seen in long saphenous vein.

van der Heijden in their study comparing duplex with clinical findings found that the planned operation was changed in 26% of the legs examined based on the extra information given on duplex scanning.[28]

From these studies it can be inferred that colour duplex can replace the current gold standard in varicose vein assessment; some authors already believe that it has done so.[29] One of the major problems is the definition of reflux is not standardized. Van Bemmelen *et al.*[30] demonstrated that 95% of normal valves in the popliteal fossa close within 0.66s of the cessation of cephalad flow. For this reason some centres use a cut-off of 1s where others use a cut-off of 0.5s. Some centres purely use colour change to define reflux when using a colour duplex scanner (Fig. 3). One of the major advantages of duplex is its ability with an experienced technologist to non-invasively mark the position of the superficial to deep venous connections. This can be done by peroperative venography as mentioned earlier,[14] but duplex has been shown to be as good with an accuracy of 96%.[31] Duplex also has the ability to mark the position of the residual (or neovascularized) long saphenous vein in recurrent varicose vein surgery and to identify its connection to the deep veins and hence can be used to avoid a difficult repeat groin dissection.

A large number of patients are undergoing inadequate first time surgery.[9,17] Is this due to surgical error (poor training or inadequate assessment) or neovascularization? (Fig. 4). Neovascularization does account for some recurrence[32–34] but with reported rates of 5–60% over a 10-year period[3,8,35–42] the results of varicose vein surgery can be improved upon. A thorough and correct preoperative assessment may reduce these figures.

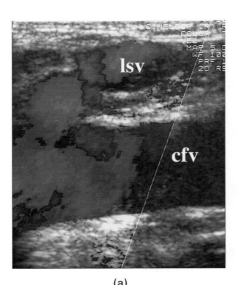
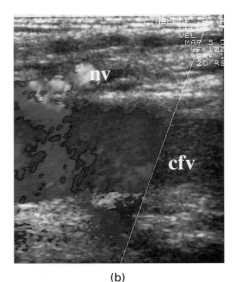

(a)   (b)

Fig. 4.   Duplex demonstration of recurrence at the groin, (a) inadequate first procedure with intact saphenofemoral junction, (b) neovascularization at the saphenofemoral junction. (lsv: long saphenous vein; cfv: common femoral vein; nv: neovascularization.)

SUMMARY

The authors conclude that from the currently available research that all patients presenting with varicose veins should be assessed with continuous wave Doppler and that the assessor should be well trained in its use. The assessment of the long saphenous system and in most cases the location of the saphenopopliteal junction should also be done with Doppler in patients with primary varicose veins. Due to the limitations of Doppler in recurrent varicose veins, colour duplex gives a better idea of the state of the venous system. Colour coded duplex should be used in these patients both to assess and subsequently mark the position of communication of incompetent connections between deep and superficial systems. Due to the variability of the position of the saphenopopliteal junction, unless the operating surgeon is absolutely positive of his/her assessment of its position then even in primary varicose veins its position should be assessed and marked with colour duplex.

Patients rarely get deep venous disease without symptoms or signs and therefore in such patients colour duplex assessment is mandatory and is as good as descending phlebography.[27] Patients have increasing unrealistic expectations from varicose vein surgery and become dissatisfied largely because of the high incidence of minor mobility[43] undoubtedly the high recurrence rate of around 1 in 5 over a 10-year period is also to blame. In a society where litigation is increasing (and this has been attempted for recurrence of varicose veins)[44] it is ever more important to produce a good result first time around. For this reason adequately trained surgeons using the optimum preoperative assessment should be performing the surgery. It has been suggested that vascular surgeons perform varicose vein surgery better than other surgeons without a vascular interest[22] mainly because of the way they assess patients preoperatively. With the drive to improve surgery for our patients and the increasing worry of litigation it may not be too long before varicose vein surgery is a purely 'vascular surgeon' operation.

DO WE KNOW WHETHER DUPLEX MARKING SHOULD BE USED FOR VARICOSE VEIN SURGERY?

This question has still not been answered. Several more studies are needed in order for us to confidently answer this question. The authors would suggest that the following studies are required:

1. How good is preoperative colour duplex marking of saphenofemoral, saphenopopliteal, and perforator vein connections to the deep venous system compared with operative findings?
2. How much better (if at all) is the outcome of varicose vein surgery in patients with duplex assessment/marking and in patients with duplex assessment/ marking and in patients with clinical and Doppler assessment/marking?
3. Should perforator vein surgery be performed by careful colour duplex marking and small incisions or by subfascial endoscopic perforator surgery (SEPS) if at all?

These studies need to be large to be definitive and therefore probably need to be multicentre to finally allow us to answer the question.

REFERENCES

1. Callam MJ: Epidemiology of varicose veins. *Br J Surg* **81:** 167–173, 1994
2. Robbins MA, Frankel SJ, Nanchahal K *et al.*: Varicose vein treatments. *Health care needs assessment: the epidemiologically based needs assessment reviews* (13) Dept of Social Medicine, University of Bristol, 1991
3. Sarin S, Scurr JH, Coleridge-Smith PD: Stripping of the long saphenous vein in the treatment of primary varicose veins. *Br J Surg* **81:** 1455–8, 1994
4. Hammartsen J, Pedersen P, Cederlund CG, Campanello M: Long saphenous vein saving surgery for varicose veins: a long term follow up. *Eur J Vasc Surg* **4:** 361–4, 1990
5. Munn SR, Morton JB, Macbeth WA, Mcleish AR: To strip or not to strip the long saphenous vein? A varicose veins trial. *Br J Surg* **68:** 426–8, 1981
6. Holme JB, Skayaa K, Holme K: Incidence of lesions of the saphenous nerve after partial or complete stripping of the long saphenous vein. *Acta Chir Scand* **156:** 145–8, 1990
7. Koyano K, Sakaguchi S: Selective stripping operation based on Doppler ultrasonic findings for primary varicose veins of the lower extremities. *Surgery* **103:** 615–9, 1988
8. McElwee RS, Maisel B: A study of the results of surgical treatment of varicose veins. *Ann Surg* **126:** 350–7, 1947
9. Bradbury AW, Stonebridge PA, Callam MJ *et al.*: Recurrent varicose veins: assessment of the sapheno-femoral junction. *Br J Surg* **81:** 373–5, 1994
10. Browse NL, Burnand KG, Lea Thomas M. In: *Diseases of the Veins: Pathology, Diagnosis and Treatment* p.181. London: Edward Arnold, 1988
11. McIrvine AJ, Corbett CR, Aston NO *et al.*: The demonstration of sapheno-femoral junction incompetence; Doppler ultrasound compared with clinical tests. *Br J Surg* **71:** 509–10, 1984
12. DePalma RG, Hart MT, Zanin L, Massarin EH: Physical examination, Doppler ultrasound and colour flow duplex scanning: guides to therapy for primary varicose veins. *Phlebology* **8:** 7–11, 1993
13. Burnand KG, Pattison M, Powell S *et al.* Can we diagnose long saphenous vein incompetence correctly? In: Negus D, Jantlet H (Eds), *Phlebology* pp. 101–4. London: John Lindley & Co, 1985
14. Hoare ML, Royle JP: Doppler ultrasound detection of sapheno-femoral and sapheno-popliteal incompetence and operative venography to ensure precise ligation. *Aust NZ J Surg* **54:** 49–52, 1984
15. McMullin GM, Coleridge Smith PD. An evaluation of Doppler ultrasound and photoplethysmography in the investigation of venous insufficiency. *Aust NZ J Surg* **62:** 270–5, 1992
16. Mercer KG, Scott DJ, Berridge DC, Westom M. Outpatient varicose vein assessment: hand held Doppler or duplex scanning. In VSS Abstracts, *Br J Surg* **83:** 563–4, 1996
17. Bradbury AW, Stonebridge PA, Ruckley CV, Beggs I: Recurrent varicose veins: correlation between preoperative clinical and hand held Doppler examination and anatomical findings at surgery. *Br J Surg* **80:** 849–51, 1993
18. Somjen GM, Donlan J, Hurse J *et al.*: Venous reflux at the sapheno-femoral junction. *Phlebology* **10:** 132–5, 1995
19. Abu-Own A, Scurr JH, Coleridge-Smith PD: Saphenous vein reflux without incompetence at the sapheno-femoral junction. *Br J Surg* **81:** 1457–4, 1994
20. Tong Y, Royle J: An anatomic source of false venous reflux with continuous wave Doppler. *J Dermatol Surg Oncol* **20:** 676–8, 1994

21. Lees TA, Holdsworth JD: Assessment and treatment of varicose veins in the northern region. *Phlebology* **10:** 55–61, 1995
22. Williams PM, Barrie WW, Donnelly PK: Light refraction rheography: a simple method of assessing lower limb venous filling. *J R Coll Surg Edinb* **39:** 89–92, 1994
23. Rutgers PH, Kitslarr PJ, Ermers EJ: Photoplethysmography in the diagnosis of superficial venous valvular incompetence. *Br J Surg* **80:** 351–3, 1993
24. Baldt MM, Bohler K, Zontsich *et al.*: Preoperative imaging of lower extremity varicose veins: colour coded duplex sonography or venography. *J Ultrasound Med* **15:** 143–54, 1996
25. Phillips GW, Paige J, Molan MP: A comparison of colour duplex ultrasound with venography and varicography in the assessment of varicose veins. *Clin Radiol* **50:** 20–25, 1995
26. Bork-Wolwer L, Wuppermann T: Improvement in non-invasive diagnosis of the greater and lesser saphenous vein insufficiency with duplex sonography. VASA **20:** 343–7, 1991
27. Myers KA, Zeng GH, Ziegenbien RW, Matthews PG: Duplex ultrasound scanning for chronic venous disease: recurrent varicose veins in the thigh after surgery to the long saphenous vein. *Phlebology* **11:** 125–31, 1996
28. van der Heijden FH, Bruyninckx CM: Pre-operative colour coded duplex scanning in varicose veins of the lower extremity. *Eur J Surg* **159:** 329–33, 1993
29. Campbell WB, Halim AS, Aertson A: The place of duplex scanning for varicose veins and common venous problems. *Ann R Coll Surg Engl* **78:** 490–3, 1996
30. van Bemmelen PS, Bedford G, Beach K, Strandness DE: Quantitative segmental evaluation of venous valvular reflux with duplex ultrasound scanning. *J Vasc Surg* **10:** 425–31, 1989
31. Vasdekis SN, Clarke GH, Nicolaides AN: Evaluation of non-invasive and invasive methods in the assessment of short saphenous vein termination. *Br J Surg* **76:** 929–32, 1989
32. Darke SG: The morphology of recurrent varicose veins. *Eur J Vasc Surg* **7:** 763–4, 1993
33. Jones L, Braithwaite BD, Selwyn D *et al.*: Neovascularisation is the principal cause of varicose vein recurrence: results of a randomised trial of stripping of the long saphenous vein. *Eur J Vasc Endovasc Surg* **12:** 442–5, 1996
34. Glass GM: Neovascularisation in recurrent sapheno-femoral incompetence of varicose veins: anatomy and morphology. *Phlebology* **10:** 136–42, 1995
35. Hammartsen J, Pedersen P, Cederlund CG, Campanello M: Long saphenous vein saving surgery for varicose veins: a long-term follow up. *Eur J Vasc Surg* **4:** 361–4, 1990
36. Munn SR, Morton JB, Macbeth WA, Mcleish AR: To strip or not to strip the long saphenous vein? A varicose veins trial. *Br J Surg* **68:** 426–8, 1981
37. Koyano K, Sakaguchi S: Selective stripping operation based on Doppler ultrasonic findings for primary varicose veins of the lower extremities. *Surgery* **103:** 615–9, 1988
38. Larson RH, Lofgren EP, Myers TT, Lofgren KA: Long term results after vein surgery: A study of 1000 cases after 10 years. *Mayo Clin Proc* **49:** 114–7, 1974
39. Rintoul RF, MacPherson AI: Long-term follow-up of operations for varicose veins. A prospective study. *J R Coll Surg Edinb* **20:** 195–9, 1975
40. Jakobsen BH: The value of different forms of treatment for varicose veins. *Br J Surg* **66:** 182–4, 1979
41. Jarvinen P, Aromaa U, Asp K: Short stay varicose vein surgery. *Ann Chir Gynaecol* **65:** 52–7, 1976
42. Bishop CC, Jarrett PE: Outpatient varicose vein surgery under local anaesthesia. *Br J Surg* **73:** 821–2, 1986
43. Davies AH, Steffen C, Cosgrove C, Wilkins DC: Varicose vein surgery: patient satisfaction. *J R Coll Surg Edinb* **40:** 298–9, 1995
44. Tennant WG, Ruckley CV: Medicolegal action following treatment for varicose veins. *Br J Surg* **83:** 291–2, 1996

Editorial comments by C.V. Ruckley

This question is important, both for patients and for healthcare expenditure. Lothian Surgical Audit shows an average of approximately 1200 varicose vein operations per annum of which 15-20% are for recurrent varices, a figure which could be drastically reduced were the initial preoperative assessment and surgery performed to a higher standard. Primary long saphenous incompetence in a thin patient is not difficult to assess. However, as the authors mention, duplex scanning has shown us that long saphenous reflux can be present below a competent saphenofemoral junction. In a recent cross-sectional survey of the general population of Edinburgh (unpublished data) we have found this to be the case in approximately 25% of individuals with long saphenous system. Such distal reflux feeds from incompetent perforators in thigh or calf. If the surgeon's policy is to strip it may not matter that this subgroup is not defined, but many surgeons choose not to strip, despite the evidence that failure to do so predisposes to recurrence. In future, there may be objections to ablation of the saphenofemoral junction when it is not the site of incompetence.

Short saphenous incompetence is often missed during routine clinical examination and, as the authors point out, continuous wave Doppler is difficult to interpret at popliteal level. The authors argue for routine use of hand held continuous wave Doppler in the clinic. However, they also review the evidence illustrating its limitations The circumstances of many venous clinics and of preoperative vein marking involve reliance on fallible methods followed by inappropriate or incomplete venous surgery. Can we doubt the advantages of a definitive examination carried out in a vascular laboratory by trained sonographers followed by venous surgery targeted with precision at the documented sites of reflux? In this context it is worth remembering that the public are becoming less tolerant of imperfect surgical outcomes and recurrence can be grounds for legal action.

Turning to the management of complex varicose veins, the authors make a clear case for the use of duplex. Recurrent varicose veins and chronic venous insufficiency can be difficult to assess both by clinical examination and by continuous wave Doppler. In patients who present with a groin scar and recurrent varices stemming from the thigh the questions to which the surgeon requires answer are:

1. Does the saphenofemoral junction need to be re-explored?
2. If so what are the anatomical pathways by which the deep and superficial veins remain connected in the groin and thigh.
3. Is there still an incompetent long saphenous vein, in whole or in part, in the thigh?

In studies referenced in this chapter we have found that duplex does not always satisfactorily answer these questions and prefer the additional availability of a road map, i.e. a varicogram, on the viewing box when operating on what can be a difficult category of surgery.

Perhaps the wrong question has been posed? The case for duplex scanning in the management of chronic venous disease cannot seriously be disputed, offering as it does new opportunities for improvements in outcomes. A more pertinent question is: should duplex be recommended for every case of varicose veins? If not, what are the indications? These questions need to be posed and answered in cost benefit terms. Routine duplex assessment of patients with varicose veins for whom surgery is intended might be considered a costly undertaking which few units in the UK could currently undertake. However, the alternative is to condone the continuation of a standard of care which would be unacceptable in other areas of medicine. A case could be made based on potential costs saved by avoidance of re-do surgery plus the benefits in quality of outcome, patient satsfaction and quality of life. It is likely that duplex scanning will come to be regarded as a routine, if not mandatory, preoperative investigation prior to varicose vein surgery which, as the authors suggest, will become the specialist province of the vascular surgeon. The authorsí arguments for multicentre trials to answer basic questions in the management of venous disease are strongly endorsed.

What Are the Indications for Endoscopic Perforator Surgery?

C.V. Ruckley and W.P. Stuart

INTRODUCTION

Subfascial endoscopic perforator surgery (SEPS), practised for more than a decade in some parts of Europe[1,2] has recently gained increasing popularity further afield.[3,4] In common with many modern minimally invasive procedures this trend appears to be technology driven rather than evidence based. At present it is unclear whether there is a role for SEPS and if so in which category of patient.

If SEPS is to be accepted as a valid surgical procedure a number of questions need to be answered:

1. Is perforator surgery, by whatever technique, successful in healing ulcer and preventing recurrence?
2. How does SEPS compare with open operation?
3. Which patients should be selected for SEPS?

This paper examines some of the evidence, presents new data from studies in Edinburgh, and proposes a potential role for perforator surgery.

IS PERFORATOR SURGERY SUCCESSFUL IN HEALING VENOUS ULCER AND PREVENTING RECURRENCE?

The failure of conventional varicose vein surgery (saphenofemoral and saphenopopliteal ligation, stripping etc) to cure lipodermatosclerosis or chronic venous leg ulcer led to a search for other more efficacious techniques.[5,6] The observation that lipodermatosclerosis was commonly associated with enlarged underlying perforating veins was enough to invite surgical attack, despite lack of definition as to the pathophysiological significance of such veins. To locate perforators many surgeons relied on their clinical skills – inspection and palpation, while others endeavoured to improve accuracy by means of phlebography, thermography, fluoescein injection or continuous wave hand-held Doppler.[7-11]

What has changed? Technology has changed. The venous anatomy, normal and abnormal, has become accessible to non-invasive investigation. Not only can a skilled sonographer map the patterns of incompetence in the deep and superficial systems but can detect perforators, measure their size and examine patterns of flow.[12-14] Small perforators of less than 2 mm are not normally detectable by duplex but are unlikely

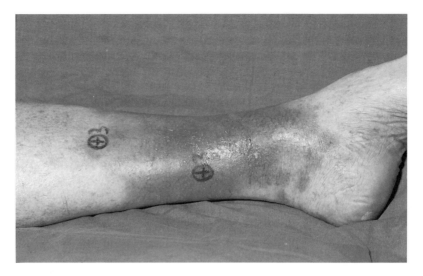

Fig. 1. The position of two incompetent perforators has been marked pre-operatively, by means of duplex scanning, in this patient with active lipodermatosclerosis.

to be of pathological importance. Endoscopic advances mean that the perforator can be viewed and intercepted on camera; SEPS has even entered the realms of ambulatory surgery. Previously, operations devised to deal with perforators had in common large scars and small success. With few exceptions the surgical intervention was by means of direct exposure of the perforators, usually by a subfascial approach via a large incision in the skin and deep fascia.[15–18] This approach generally guaranteed excellent exposure but could not avoid postoperative complications and ulcer recurrence.

The fact that the indications for perforator surgery had never been defined led to a natural reticence on the part of many surgeons to undertake perforator surgery if it meant submitting patients to relatively mutilating operations, a reticence which has now been swept aside by the availability of attractive endoscopic technology. It can be argued, however, that the success of SEPS, in terms of healing ulcer and preventing recurrence, is unlikely to be greater than after operations dealing with perforators by open surgery, and may well be inferior. What then was the success rate of open perforator surgery?

Large numbers of surgical series have been published[19–35] (Table 1). They show extremely variable success rates in terms of ulcer recurrence. These series are difficult to evaluate or to compare, on account of numerous methodogical inconsistencies such as differences in case mix; diagnostic methods; method and duration of follow-up; concurrent surgical operations etc. If we take into account publication bias it is fair to say that this is an area of surgery with a relatively high failure rate.

Table 1.   Series of patients treated by open subfascial ligation

Author/Year	Patients (n)	Limbs (n)	Wound complications (%)	Recurrence (%)	FU/Comment (y: year; m: month)
Silver 1971[19]	28	31	13	10	64% > 5 y
Field 1971[20]	51	57	–	2	1–8y (mean, 6y)
Thurston 1973[21]	89	102	12	13	3–84m (mean 3y)
Bowen 1975[22]	55	71	44	34	6m–15y (48% > 3y)
Blumenberg 1978[23]	16	25	4	4	6m–6y
De Palma 1979[24]	53	68	1	6	6m–12y
Hyde 1981[25]	83	–	13	33	mean 10y
Almgren 1982[26]	57	57	19	9	?
Negus 1983[27]	77	108	19	13	6m–6y, (76% > 3y)
Cheung 1985[28]	32	31	7	11	5m–4y
Johnson 1985[29]	37	47	11	51	1–13y (mean 5y)
Wilkinson 1986[30]	108	134	24	2	6m–9y (80% > 5y)
Szostek 1988[31]	148	148	18	15	105, (6m–10y)
Cikrit 1988[32]	32	–	–	22	6m–10y (mean 4y)
Nash 1991[33]	90	–	–	18	3y
Robison 1992[34]	17	18	56	37	42m (life table)
Bradbury 1993[35]	53	53	–	26	3–144m (mean 5y)

HOW DOES SEPS COMPARE WITH OPEN OPERATION?

There do not appear to have been any comparative studies to determine which type of procedure is the more successful in finding and/or permanently obliterating perforators, assuming that such an objective is desirable. Nor do there appear to have been any randomized trials with the necessary long-term follow-up comparing SEPS with open surgery in terms of therapeutic efficacy. We do, however, have information on early outcome and resource utilization.[36]

We have compared a series of 33 patients suffering from chronic venous insufficiency and/or leg ulcer treated by varicose vein surgery combined with open subfascial surgery ('Linton') with 30 treated by varicose vein surgery combined with the SEPS procedure.[21] This was not a controlled trial, the Linton group antedating the SEPS series.

Table 2 compares the two series. The patients were broadly comparable in terms of age but there were more males in the first series. Numbers of patients with lipodermatosclerosis, open and healed ulcers were similar. Table 3 shows the accompanying procedures carried out on the varicose veins. Stripping refers to thigh stripping of the long saphenous vein only. Many of these patients had previously experienced unsuccessful vein surgery hence the categories of patients who required perforator surgery only and also those who did not have stripping, as the saphenous veins had been previously removed.

The early outcome is summarized in Table 4. Highly significant differences, favouring the SEPS procedure, were observed in the duration of postoperative stay and in calf wound complications: SEPS is a significantly better operation in

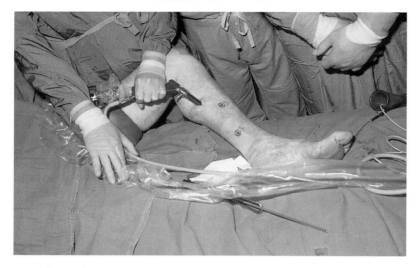

Fig. 2. The endoscope is inserted in the subfascial plane. Note the Lovquist cuff in position.

Table 2. Comparison of patient characteristics.

	Linton	SEPS
Procedures	37	30
Patients	33	30
Median age (range)	57 (37–83)	55(23–82)
Male:Female	27:10	13:17
LDS only	5	5
Open ulcer	12	8
Healed ulcer	20	17

LDS: Lipodermatosclerosis

Table 3. Accompanying procedures

	Linton	SEPS
Perforator ligation only	5	1
SFL + strip	17	26*
SFL, no strip	13	2*
SPL	5	8
Skin graft	4	2

* $p < 0.01$, χ^2 test; SFL: saphenofemoral ligation; SPL: saphenopopliteal ligation.

Table 4. Early outcome

	Linton	SEPS
Postop stay: median (range)	9 (3–36)	2 (1–18)*
Saphenous nerve injury	0	2
DVT/PE	1	1
Calf wound complications	13	1**
Non-healing ulcer	3	1

* p < 0.01 Mann Whitney; ** p < 0.01 Fisher's exact test.
DVT/PE: Deep vein thrombosis/pulmonary embolism.

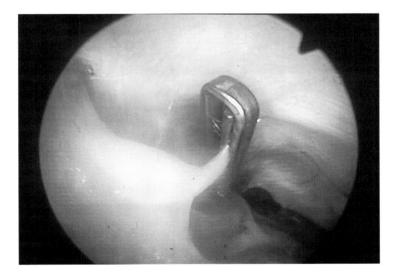

Fig. 3. A clip has been applied to an incompetent perforating vein.

terms of postoperative morbidity and bed occupancy. It remains to be seen whether it is any more successful in healing chronic venous ulcer or in preventing ulcer recurrence.

WHICH PATIENTS SHOULD BE SELECTED FOR SEPS?

We have already noted that the necessary trials have yet to be performed. That being the case one can only take an oblique approach to this question. Clues are provided by the relationship between patterns of venous incompetence, clinical disease and outcome following conservative or surgical therapy.

Patterns of venous incompetence

Several authors have studied the pattern of venous incompetence in patients with chronic venous insuffiency and/or leg ulcer[12,13,37-43] (Table 5). In these series between 27 and 78% limbs have venous incompetence which is limited to the superficial system. To what extent these are real differences reflecting differences in case mix and to what extent they reflect differences in technique and interpretation of duplex sonography is not known. Common to every series, however, is the fact that there are two different populations – i.e. those with and without deep reflux, potentially requiring a different approach to therapy. Is deep incompetence prognostically important? If so approximately 50% of patients with chronic venous insufficiency/venous ulcer may need something more than surgery to their superficial systems alone. Is perforator surgery the answer?

Table 5. The distribution of reflux in patients with venous ulceration by duplex ultrasonography

Author/Year	Limbs (n)	Superficial reflux detected (%)	Deep reflux detected (%)	Superficial reflux only (%)
Van Bemmelen 1990[37]	25	92	92	8
Hanrahan 1991[13]	95	79	50	17
Mastroroberto 1992[38]	51	76	47	4
Shami 1993[39]	79	75	47	53
Lees 1993[40]	25	88	48[a]	52[a]
Van Rij 1994[41]	120			40
Myers 1995[42]	95	86	56	36
Labropoulos 1996[12]	120	90	58	37[a]
Scriven 1997[43]	95	88	43	57[a]
Stuart 1997[b]	69	87	69	31

[a]Including incompetent perforating veins; [b]personal data.

Outcomes

There is considerable evidence that reflux in the deep venous system confers less favourable prognosis for patients with chronic venous insufficiency and ulcer. Substantially more data should be forthcoming in the near future because the availability of duplex ultrasonography has provided the opportunity to correlate outcomes with preoperative non-invasive mapping of venous competence.

Brittenden et al. have analysed the duplex findings in 200 patients with chronic venous leg ulcer managed within a clinical trial of factorial design evaluating drug therapy (oxpentiphylline), multilayer vs single layer bandaging and hydrocolloid vs knitted viscose dressing and were able to demonstrate that impaired ulcer healing was significantly related to reflux in the popliteal vein.[44]

The same is true of surgical outcomes. Before the advent of duplex scanning Burnand et al., in a series of patients with leg ulcer investigated by phlebography and treated with conventional varicose vein surgery, found uniformly poor results in those patients with phlebographically proven deep vein post-phlebitic damage.[45]

Darke and Penfold have categorised chronic leg ulcer patients into those with and without deep venous reflux.[46] They found that venous surgery limited to saphenofemoral ligation and stripping, without perforator surgery, has resulted, on a 3.4 year median follow-up, in a relatively low recurrence rate of 9% in patients with superficial and perforator incompetence alone.

Bradbury *et al.* have analysed the results of a series of 53 patients with an median duration of 60 months follow-up after subfascial perforator surgery by the open ('Linton') technique.[35] The ulcer recurrence rate was 26% and recurrence was significantly associated with reflux in the deep venous system.

WHAT EFFECT DOES SUPERFICIAL VENOUS SURGERY HAVE ON PERFORATOR COMPETENCE?

Campbell has reported a series of 144 patients undergoing conventional superfical varicose vein surgery without perforator interruption.[47] Investigations included pre- and postoperative duplex scanning. It was found that 80% of perforators which had been incompetent preoperatively resumed competence postoperatively.

We have therefore sought to confirm this finding. In a series of 33 patients (50 limbs) with varicose veins and with duplex proven pathological (bidirectional) perforators we have carefully limited the varicose vein surgery to saphenofemoral and or saphenopopliteal ligation, thigh stripping and avulsions avoiding the mapped perforators. We have then reassessed the perforators at a median of 14 weeks (range 6–26) after operation.

The patient characteristics are listed in Table 6. The effects of superficial vein surgery on perforator competence and size are listed in Table 7. It can be seen that superficial venous surgery significantly reduces the median diameter of perforators and restores perforator competence. When postoperative reflux in either deep or superficial veins was correlated with restoration of perforator competence it was found that in nine of ten limbs with persisting perforator incompetence the residual reflux was located in the deep system. We have therefore confirmed that varicose vein surgery limited to the superficial veins restores perforator competence when reflux is limited to the superficial system, but not when there is also deep reflux.

Table 6. Patients undergoing saphenous surgery without perforator interruption

Patients	33 (13m, 20 f)
Limbs	50
Median age (range)	58 (35–77) years
LDS	5
Ulcer history	6
SFL (+ Strip)	45 (+43)
SPL	6
Popliteal reflux	12

LDS: Lipodermatosclerosis; SFL: saphenofemoral ligation; SPL: saphenopopliteal ligation.

Table 7.   Effect of saphenous surgery on number and size of perforators

	Preoperative	Postoperative
Limbs with perforators	48	49
Limbs with IPV	32*	19*
Total number of perforators	108	105
Toal number of IPV	60*	27*
Median perforator diameter	4.00**	3.0**
and range, mm	(1.0–11.0)	(1.0–8.0)

* $p < 0.001$ χ^2; ** $p < 0.01$ Mann Whitney; IPV: incompetent perforating veins.

SUMMARY

1. There is no clinical trial evidence that varicose vein surgery incorporating perforator surgery is more effective in healing chronic venous ulcers or preventing recurrence than either conservative (non-surgical care) or varicose vein surgery without perforator interruption.

2. Published series of open operations on venous perforators are methodologically impossible to compare, but overall show substantial leg ulcer recurrence rates.

3. SEPS carries significant advantages over open operation in terms of wound complications and duration of postoperative stay.

4. When incompetent perforators are present and reflux is otherwise limited to the superficial (saphenous) systems, surgery to those systems will restore perforator competence.

5. Surgery to an incompetent superficial saphenous system will not restore perforator competence in the presence of deep, i.e. popliteal, reflux .

CONCLUSIONS

1. The role of perforator surgery remains ill-defined.

2. The results of open perforator interruptions, in terms of preventing ulcer recurrence, show substantial failure rates.

3. SEPS is safer and incurs less morbidity than open operation. Its long-term efficacy, however, is unproven.

4. Pending clinical trials, the evidence suggests that SEPs is not indicated where incompetence is confined to the superficial system.

5. Trials must therefore categorize patients (and/or limbs) in terms of patterns of reflux and should focus particularly on the group whose perforator incompetence is combined with deep vein reflux.

REFERENCES

1. Hauer G: Die endoscopische subfasciale diszision der perforansvenen: vorlaufige mitteilung (abstract). *Vasa* **14**: 59–61, 1985
2. Jugenheimer M, Junginger T: Endoscopic subfascial sectioning of incompetent veins in treatment of primary varicosis. *World J Surg* **16**: 971–5, 1992
3. Pierik EGJM, Wittens CHA, van Urk H: Subfascial endoscopic ligation in the treatment of incompetent perforating veins. *Eur J Vasc Endovasc Surg* **9**: 38–41, 1995
4. Gloviczki P, Bergan JJ, Menawat S et al.: Safety, feasibility, and early efficacyof subfascial endoscopic perforator surgery: A preliminary report from the North American registry. *J Vasc Surg* **25**: 94–105, 1997
5. Homans J: The operative treatment of varicose veins and ulcers, based upon a classification of these lesions. *Surg Gynec Obst*, **22**: 143–58, 1916
6. Homans J: The eitiology and treatment of varicose ulcer of the leg. *Surg Gynec Obst* **24**: 300–11, 1917
7. Chilvers AS, Thomas MH: Method for the localisation of incompetent perforating veins. *Br Med J* **2**: 577–9, 1970
8. Patil KD,Williams JR: Thermographic localisation of incompetent perforating veins in the leg. *Br Med J* **1**: 195–7, 1970
9. Beesley WH, Fegan WG: An investigation into the localisation of incompetent perforating veins. *Br J Surg* **57**: 30–2, 1970
10. Miller SS, Foote AV: The ultrasonic detection of incompetent perforating veins. *Br J Surg* **61**: 653–6, 1974
11. O'Donnell TF, Burnand KG, Clemenson G, Thomas ML: Doppler examination vs clinical and phlebographic detection of the localisation of incompetent perforating veins: a prospective study. *Arch Surg* **112**: 31–5, 1977
12. Labropoulos N, Delis K, Nicolaides AN et al.: The role of the distribution and anatomic extent of reflux in the development of signs and symptoms in chronic venous disease. *J Vasc Surg* **23**: 504–10, 1996
13. Hanrahan ML, Araki CT, Rodriguez AA, Kechejian GJ et al.: Distribution of valvular incompetence in patients with venous stasis ulceration. *J Vasc Surg* **13**: 805–12, 1991
14. Pierik EGJM, Toonder IM, van Urk H, Wittens CHA: Validation of duplex ultrasonography in detecting competent and incompetent perforating veins in patients with venous ulceration of the lower leg. *J Vasc Surg* **26**: 49–52, 1997
15. Linton RR: The communicating veins of the lower leg and the technique for their ligation. *Ann Surg* **107**: 582–93, 1938
16. Cockett FB: The pathology and treatment of venous ulcers of the leg. *Br J Surg* **43**: 260–278, 1995
17. Dodd H: The diagnosis and ligation of incompetent perforating veins. *Ann R Coll Surg Eng* **34**: 186–96, 1964
18. De Palma RG: Surgical therapy for venous stasis. *Surgery* **76**: 910, 1974
19. Silver D, Gleysteen JJ, Rhodes GR et al.: Surgical treatment of the refractory post-phlebitic ulcer. *Arch Surg* **103**: 554–60, 1971
20. Field P, van Boxel P: The role of the Linton flap procedure in the management of stasis dermatitis and ulceration in the lower limb. *Surgery* **70**: 920–26, 1971
21. Thurston OG, Williams HTG: Chronic venous insufficiency in the lower extremity: pathogenesis and surgical treatment. *Arch Surg* **106**: 537–9, 1973
22. Bowen FH: Subfascial ligation (Linton operation) of the perforating leg veins to treat post-thrombophlebitic syndrome. *Am Surg* **41**: 148–51, 1975
23. Blumenberg RM, Gelfland ML: The posterior stocking seam approach to radical subfascial clipping of perforating veins. *Am J Surg* **136**: 202–5, 1978
24. DePalma RG: Surgical treatment for venous stasis: results of a modified Linton operation. *Am J Surg* **137**: 810–3, 1979
25. Hyde GL, Litton TC, Hull DA: Long-term results of subfascial vein ligation for venous stasis disease. *Surg Gynec Obst* **153**: 683–6, 1981

26. Almgren B, Bowald S, Eriksson I, Forsberg O: The posterior approach for subfascial ligation of perforating veins. *Acta Chir Scand* **148**: 243–5, 1982

27. Negus D, Friedgood A: The effective management of venous ulceration. *Br J Surg* **70**: 623, 1983

28. Cheung P S, Lim S T, Ng A: Evaluation of the posterior approach for subfascial ligation of perforating veins. *Aust N-Z J Surg* **55**: 369–72, 1985

29. Johnson WC, O'Hara ET, Corey C et al.: Venous stasis ulceration: effectiveness of subfascial ligation. *Arch Surg* **120**: 797–800, 1985

30. Wilkinson JE, Maclaren IF: Long term review of procedures for venous perforator insuffiency. *Surg Gynec Obst* **163**: 117–20, 1986

31. Szostek M, Skorski M, Zajac S et al.: Recurrences after surgical treatment of patients with post-thrombotic syndrome of the lower extremities. *Eur J Vasc Surg* **2**: 191–92, 1988

32. Cikrit DF, Nichols WK, Silver D: Surgical management of refractory venous stasis ulceration. *J Vasc Surg* **7**: 473–8, 1988

33. Nash TP: Venous ulceration: factors influencing recurrence after standard surgical procedures. *Med J Aust* **154**: 48–50, 1991

34. Robison J G, Elliot B M, Kaplan A J: Limitations of subfascial ligation for refractory chronic venous stasis ulceration. *Ann Vasc Surg* **6**: 9–14, 1992

35. Bradbury AW, Ruckley CV: Foot volumetry can predict recurrent ulceration after subfascial ligation of perforators and saphenous ligation. *J Vasc Surg* **18**: 789–95, 1993

36. Stuart WP, Adam DJ, Bradbury AW, Ruckley CV: Subfascial Endoscopic perforator surgery is associated with significantly less morbidity and shorter hospital stay than open operation (Linton's procedure). *Br J Surg* **84**: 1364–5, 1997

37. van Bemmelen PS, Bedford G, Beach K, Strandness Jr DE: Status of the valves in the superficial and deep venous system in chronic venous disease. *Surgery* **109**: 730–4, 1990

38. Mastroroberto P, Chello M, Marchese A: (Letter) Distribution of valvular incompetence in patients with venous stasis ulceration. *J Vasc Surg* **16**: 307, 1992

39. Shami SK, Sarir S, Cheatle TR et al.: Venous ulcers and the superficial venous system. *J Vasc Surg* **17**: 487–90, 1993

40. Lees TA, Lambert D: patterns of venous reflux in limbs with skin changes associated with chronic venous insufficiency. *Br J Surg* **80**: 725–8, 1993

41. Van Rij AM, Solomon C, Christie R: Anatomic and physiologic characteristics of venous ulceration. *J Vasc Surg* **81**: 39–41, 1994

42. Myers KA, Ziegenbein RW, Zeng GH, Matthews PG: Duplex ultrasonography scanning for chronic venous disease: Patterns of venous reflux. *J Vasc Surg* **21**: 605–12, 1995

43. Scriven JM, Hartshorne T, Bell PRF et al.: Single-visit venous ulcer clinic: the first year. *Br J Surg* **84**: 334–336, 1997

44. Brittenden J, Bradbury AW, Milne AA et al.: Popliteal reflux demonstrated by duplex ultrasonography is associated with delayed and non-healing of chronic venous ulceration. *Phlebology* (Suppl 1): 796–8: 1995

45. Burnand K, Lea Thomas M, O'Donnell T, Browse NL: Relation between postphlebitic changes in the deep veins and results of surgical treatment of venous ulcers. *Lancet* **i**: 936–8, 1976

46. Darke SG, Penfold C: Venous ulceration and saphenous ligation. *Eur J Vasc Surg* **6**: 4–9, 1992

47. Campbell WA, West A: Duplex ultrasound audit of operative treatment of primary varicose veins. In: Negus D et al. (Eds), *Phlebology '95. Phlebology* (Suppl 1): 407–9, 1995

Editorial comments by R.M. Greenhalgh

The authors underlined from their own data and findings, that incompetence in perforating veins associated with superficial varicose veins only, does not require ligation. They indicate that these perforators become competent when the superficial veins are corrected. The authors claim significant advantages over open operation for the SEPS procedure in terms of complications in duration of postoperative stay. In many ways the chapter offers more questions than solutions but it is extremely valuable to have these lists of conclusions which show really how little is certain at the present time. The first conclusion, *The role of perforator surgery remains ill-defined*, says it all. Clearly the authors favour SEPS as an approach and would confine SEPS to those incompetent perforating veins also associated with incompetence of the deep veins. Clearly there is much to be done, to elucidate further the significance of such incompetent perforating veins in that situation.

When and How Should We Unblock Deep Veins?

K.G. Burnand, F.J. Meyer and A.T. Irvine

INTRODUCTION

The causes of deep venous obstruction can be divided into the following groups: deep venous thrombosis, post-thrombotic obstruction, external compression of the veins, iatrogenic injury and rarely congenital venous aplasia. This chapter will deal with just the first three of these pathologies.

DEEP VENOUS THROMBOSIS

A deep venous thrombus is a solid mass formed within the main stem veins beneath the deep fascia from the constituents of the blood. The true prevalence of this condition is unknown as many cases without symptoms go undetected.[1] Phlebographic studies have suggested that the incidence of spontaneous deep venous thrombosis is about 0.09%.[2] Analyses of hospital computer databases have suggested a prevalence of 70–80 per 100 000 of the population (0.07–0.08%).[3,4] Extrapolating from postoperative studies,[5,6] it is reasonable to assume that at least twice as many patients are having silent thromboses, giving an incidence of no less than 0.27%. In addition to this, one-third of hospital patients with a serious illness or undergoing major surgery develops a deep vein thrombosis,[5] giving an approximate incidence of 0.36% per year. Hopefully the advent of effective prophylaxis will reduce this figure.

Thrombosis in a deep vein occludes its lumen and destroys its valves.[7] Ideally, treatment should restore the veins to complete normality. This requires either removal of the thrombus before it damages the valves or manipulation of the resolution of the thrombus to encourage reopening of the lumen and recovery of the valves. The latter approach is not yet possible. There are two methods for removing thrombus: surgical thrombectomy and pharmacological thrombolysis. Both methods are most effective when thrombus is fresh and non-adherent and when it is often symptomless. Frequently, symptoms do not appear until the thrombus is old and adherent, features which make its removal or dissolution difficult. Alternatively, the thrombus can be left to organize by natural resolution.

The surgical removal of deep vein thrombi was first attempted in the 1920s but was not widely adopted until phlebography improved in the 1940s and 1950s.[8–14] It was improved further in 1963 when Fogarty introduced the balloon catheter.[15–17] There is good experimental evidence which proves that the addition of an arteriovenous fistula below the venotomy anastomosis improves its patency rate[18,19] and may increase the size of collateral formation.[20] Much of the evidence published about venous thrombectomy is anecdotal and has not been scientifically controlled or undertaken as prospective studies.

Pharmacological thrombolysis is achieved by infusion of compounds that actively dissolve thrombi by converting plasminogen to plasmin. Thrombolysis is probably only suitable for use in acute thrombosis, less than 5 days old.[21-23] The thrombolytic agent may be infused directly into the thrombus through an indwelling intravenous catheter.[24,25] Initially, streptokinase, which activates the circulating (intrinsic) fibrinolytic pathway, was used.[26] This also caused allergic reactions in around 30% of patients and significant symptoms, such as rigors and loin pain occurred in about 10% of patients.[20] Recombinant tissue plasminogen activator (rt-PA) is now usually the compound of choice as it is the native activator of the extrinsic fibrinolytic pathway in tissue fluid. Theoretically, tissue plasminogen activator (tPA) only acts on plasminogen bound to thrombus as it is believed to bind solely to fibrin. Therefore, it should not activate circulating plasminogen and so should cause fewer unwanted bleeding complications. Life-endangering haemorrhage still occurs at sites remote from the infusion point of tPA and the risk of haemorrhagic cerebrovascular accident is approximately 2–3%. Heparin should be infused concurrently to reduce the risk of thrombus formation around the catheter,[27] adding to the risk of bleeding.

The main aim of administering thrombolytic therapy is to reduce the incidence of post-thrombotic complications by preserving valvular function as well as restoring vein patency.[22,28] However, this has not been shown in some studies comparing streptokinase infusion with heparin anticoagulation alone.[29] Local catheter-directed thrombolysis is attractive as it delivers the lytic agent directly to the affected area. The risk of valvular damage from this technique is reduced if veins are cannulated in an antegrade manner with respect to their valves.[30] Small, medium-term studies have shown more promising results using tPA thrombolysis with more than 79% of patients having a good result,[25] but follow-up venography is often not performed. Adjuvant venous angioplasty or endovascular stenting[31] (Fig. 1) are now being used to dilate any residual stenosis but there are no adequate long-term studies of these techniques.

The risks of intervention are only acceptable for acute deep venous thrombosis affecting main axial veins such as the iliofemoral or axillary/subclavian segments. Thrombolysis has not yet been compared with thrombectomy and both have their risks and drawbacks. At present, the great majority of patients should be treated with anticoagulants (subcutaneous heparin fragments, such as tinzaparin) until good prospective studies of thrombolysis compared with surgery plus long-term follow-up are available. The risks of thrombolysis cannot be overemphasized and the only justification is a long-term reduction in the incidence of post-thrombotic damage (see below).

POST-THROMBOTIC DEEP VEIN OBSTRUCTION

The post-thrombotic syndrome is a clinical syndrome characterized by an array of changes in the veins, subcutaneous tissues and skin. The exact prevalence of post-thrombotic syndrome is again not known, partly because deep venous thrombosis is often symptomless[1] and many clinicians make the diagnosis in the absence of radiological confirmation of thrombosis. Nevertheless, of patients with phlebographically confirmed thrombosis, 40% at 5 years and 72% at 10 years had

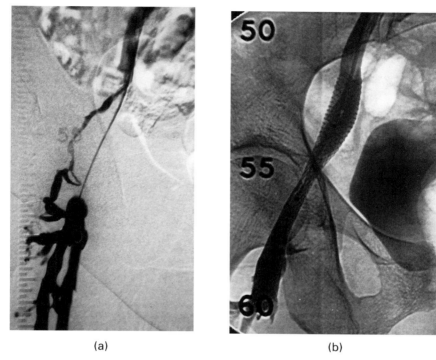

(a)   (b)

Fig. 1. Insertion of a stent into an iliofemoral vein occluded by malignancy. (a) Passage of a guide-wire through the occlusion. (b) Stent deployed and expanded relieving the occlusion.

developed skin and subcutaneous tissue induration.[32] Post-thrombotic obstruction can be treated conservatively or actively.[33] Symptoms may often be palliated by elastic compression using either stockings,[35, 36] bandaging[34] or pneumatic devices.[37] Alternatively, the obstruction can be relieved either radiologically or surgically.

The majority of patients with post-thrombotic venous damage are treated palliatively. Intervention should only be considered when there are severe symptoms, such as venous claudication, and conservative management has failed. Treatment is only possible when there is a localized obstruction. Occlusion of the entire outflow tract is not amenable to cure. The choice of technique largely depends on the site and extent of the occlusion or stenosis.

The principal surgical methods for treating deep venous obstruction comprise some form of bypass. Some short, localized stenoses of the iliac veins have been treated by disobliteration. Bypass surgery is most commonly used to treat isolated iliac or iliofemoral occlusions. Superficial femoral vein obstruction may be bypassed if the popliteal vein is patent. Iliac vein obstruction can be treated by a femorocaval bypass[38] or femorofemoral bypass (Palma operation).[39,40] This is performed by exposing the long saphenous vein of the normal leg, ligating its tributaries and anastomosing its distal end to the healthiest section of the femoral vein of the affected leg (Fig. 2). More recently, polytetrafluoroethylene (PTFE) has been used when the

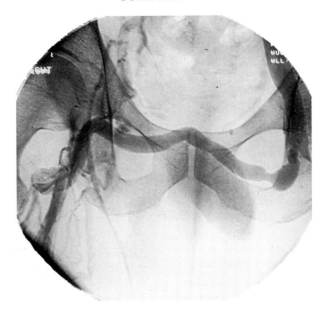

(a)

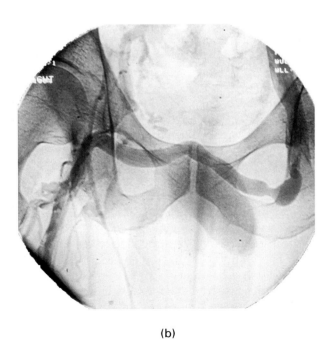

(b)

Fig. 2.   Femorofemoral crossover (Palma) bypass.

long saphenous vein is inadequate.[41,42] Most surgeons also fashion a concomitant arteriovenous fistula just below the anastomosis to increase the venous flow and improve patency.[43-45] This is then ligated after 6 weeks. Patients are usually given anticoagulants for 3–6 months in an attempt to improve patency. The Palma operation should only be considered when there is an abnormal rise in femoral vein pressure during exercise[46,47] and natural collateral pathways (an auto-Palma, Fig. 3) have not developed. Clinical improvement rates exceed graft patency rates. The exact reasons for this are unclear although collateral formation and stocking compliance may be involved. The long-term (5-year) patency rate has been shown to be around 75%[48-50] although about 90% of patients show clinical improvement.[48]

Post-thrombotic obstruction can now be treated by passing a guide-wire through the affected segment under fluoroscopic guidance, dilating the segment and then inserting a balloon expandable, endovascular stent. This has improved the results of angioplasty as venous stenoses are often resistant to dilatation and have a high recurrence rate.[51,52] Initially, stents were used to treat malignant venous strictures[53-55] and then to rescue haemodialysis fistulae.[56,57] More recently, stents with or without angioplasty or thrombolysis have been used to treat benign strictures.[58] Although some have reported cumulative primary stent patency rates of 57% in haemodialysis

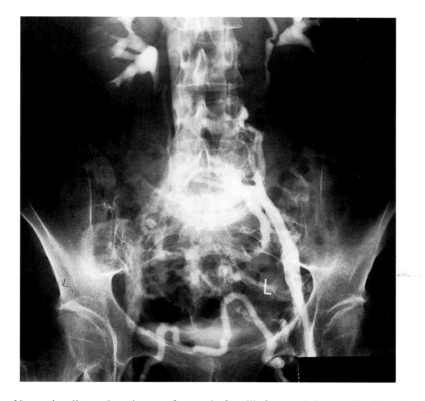

Fig. 3. Natural collateral pathways formed after iliofemoral deep vein thrombosis (an auto-Palma).

patients at 1 year,[59] others have reported patency rates of only 11% at 1 year.[56] There are no long-term results available as yet and the dangers of stenting should not be underestimated (see below). Furthermore there is only anecdotal evidence published about stents for post-thrombotic venous strictures. Stents may, however, prove useful for short segment occlusions or those which are not readily amenable to surgery.

EXTERNAL COMPRESSION OF DEEP VEINS

The deep veins can be obstructed by external compression from surrounding normal or abnormal structures. Examples include: right common iliac artery compression of the left common iliac vein, internal iliac artery compression of the external iliac vein and compression of the femoral vein[60] (Gullmo's phenomenon). These are often incidental findings on phlebography and rarely cause symptoms. Nevertheless, they may predispose to deep venous thrombosis.[61] Extrinsic masses, such as malignant tumours or lymphadenopathy or even adjacent arterial aneurysms, can also compress veins. Other pathologies, such as retroperitoneal fibrosis, may also cause venous obstruction. The axillary/subclavian vein may be kinked as it enters the thoracic inlet by a cervical rib or band and this may lead to thrombosis.[62-64] The superior vena cava can also thrombose (Fig. 4) either as a result of intrathoracic malignancy, for example bronchogenic carcinoma, or occasionally from conditions such as mediastinal fibrosis.[20] Spontaneous superior vena caval thrombosis does occur but it is rare.[20]

Axillary/subclavian vein thrombosis was first described by Sir James Paget in 1875[65] and by von Schroetter in 1884.[66] It often follows physical exertion,[67] although it may solely be the result of external compression.[68-70] Many patients only present some weeks after their initial symptoms. By this time, they have often developed an adequate collateral circulation and conservative treatment with rest and anticoagulants is all that is required.[71] Delayed venous reconstruction can be performed if severe post-thrombotic symptoms develop later.[72] Around 25% of those patients treated conservatively develop persistent symptoms of chronic venous insufficiency[73] although the extent to which these interfere with the patients' lifestyle is debatable.

Various interventional techniques have been used to treat axillary/subclavian thrombosis. These include thrombolysis,[74] thrombectomy[13] and angioplasty[75] with or without subsequent surgical decompression.[70] Thrombolysis is usually performed in the acute phase only, using systemic or catheter-directed thrombolysis. A review of 12 published papers of streptokinase/urokinase fibrinolysis, showed a subjective success rate of between 50 and 100%.[27,76] Few of these patients, however, had follow-up venography. It may be that TPA gives better results, but adequate long-term data are not yet available. Angioplasty or stenting (Fig. 5) may be used[27] after thrombolysis to dilate residual defects although it is unlikely that these techniques will overcome external compression. Venous thrombectomy, with or without subsequent surgical decompression, has yielded disappointing results.[13,70] Long-term studies of angioplasty alone have shown that despite 75% of the patients having successful restoration of patency, 35% are functioning at 1 year and 2-year patency is virtually

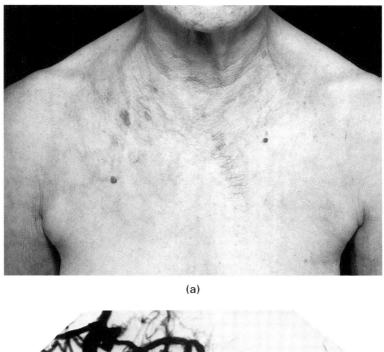

(a)

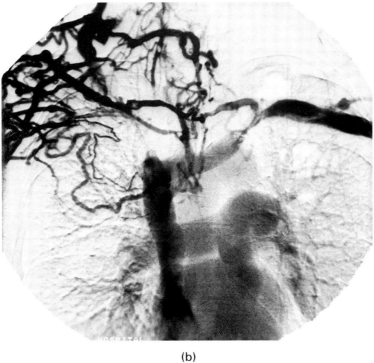

(b)

Fig. 4. Malignant superior vena caval obstruction. (a) Clinical signs of superior vena caval obstruction. (b) Venogram showing superior vena caval obstruction and the formation of collaterals.

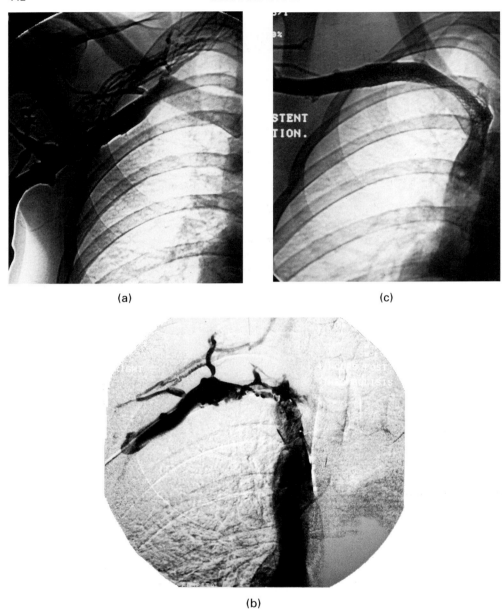

(a)   (c)

(b)

Fig. 5.   Axillary/subclavian vein thrombosis treated with thrombolysis and stenting. (a) Venogram showing initial thrombosis. (b) Suboptimal result following thrombolysis. (c) Placement of stent to dilate residual stenosis.

zero.[75] It may be useful for patients who are likely to suffer repeated occlusions, such as those undergoing renal dialysis. Both thrombectomy and isolated angioplasty have been largely superseded by thrombolysis.

After successful thrombolysis, several studies have demonstrated additional benefit from surgical exploration and decompression.[27,69,71,74,76] However, this is not worthwhile if early management has failed. Various surgical approaches have been used, including first rib resection,[69,77,78] claviculectomy[78] and soft tissue decompression or scalenectomy.[76,78] First rib excision is the treatment of choice. It is the most widely reported technique in the literature and has a good success rate.[69,77,78] Claviculectomy has also produced good results although the number of cases reported is very few because of the mechanical drawbacks (including shoulder joint instability[79]) and unsightliness. Soft tissue decompression has also been reported to have good results[78,80] but unless there is an obvious abnormality, it has to be quite extensive to be successful.[27] At present, the best treatment is probably thrombolysis followed by early first rib excision.

Superior vena caval stenosis is often ameliorated by treating the underlying malignancy, for example irradiation of extensive bronchogenic carcinoma.[20] Surgical bypass has rarely been used so its long-term effectiveness cannot be evaluated.[81] Treatment with endovascular stents has recently been introduced[82,83] but the long-term results of this technique are not yet known. This may not be an important consideration in those patients with malignant disease. There are, however, significant hazards associated with stent employment. Failure of placement or expansion,[83] acute massive venous thrombosis,[84] haemorrhage[84] and native vessel rupture[75] can all occur during stent insertion. Later complications including stent fracture, distal or intracardiac migration, stent embolization, false aneurysm formation, nerve paralysis, intimal hyperplasia, stricture and recurrent thrombosis have all been reported.[83] The role of stents in venous obstruction has yet to be determined.

CONCLUSION

Deep venous obstruction is a relatively common pathology. The presence of good collateral channels makes its effects unpredictable. Surgical thrombectomy and bypass is applicable in few cases. Pharmacological lysis is successful in deep vein thrombosis but its results are far from perfect. Newer techniques of locally delivered lysis, angioplasty and stenting are all experimental and will not restore valve function. Stenting has a definite role in malignant obstruction and surgical bypass may be valuable in a minority of patients with chronic venous obstruction and severe symptoms.

REFERENCES

1. Welch CE, Fexon HH: Thrombophlebitis and pulmonary embolism. *J Am Med Assoc* **117**; 1502, 1941

2. Nylander G, Olivecrona H: The phlebographic pattern of acute leg thrombosis within a defined urban population. *Acta Chir Scand* **142**; 505, 1976
3. Gillum RF: Pulmonary embolism and thrombophlebitis in the United States 1970–1985. *Am Heart J* **114**; 1262–1264,1987
4. Gillum RF: Pulmonary embolism and thrombophlebitis in the United States 1970–1985. *Am Heart J* **120**; 392–395, 1990
5. Bergvist D: *Postoperative Thromboembolism*. Berlin: Springer, 1983
6. Colditz GA, Tuden RA, Oster G: Rates of venous thrombosis after general surgery: combined results of randomised clinical trials. *Lancet* **ii**; 143, 1986
7. Edwards EA, Edwards JE: Effects of thrombophlebitis on venous valves. *Surg Gynec Obstet* **65**; 310, 1937
8. DeWeese JA, Jones TI, Lyon J, Dale W: Evaluation of thrombectomy in the management of iliofemoral venous thrombosis. *Surgery* **47**; 140, 1960
9. Fontaine R: Remarks concerning venous thrombosis and its sequelae. *Surgery* **41**; 6, 1957
10. Haller JA: *Deep Thrombophlebitis*. Philadelphia: WB Saunders, 1967
11. Homans J: Exploration and division of femoral and iliac veins in treatment of thrombo-phlebitis of leg. *New Engl J Med* **224**; 179, 1941
12. Leriche R, Geisendorf W: Resultats d'une thrombectomie precoce avec une resection veineuse dans une phlebite grave des deux membres inferieurs. *Presse Med* **47**; 1239, 1939
13. Mahorner H, Castleberry JW, Coleman WC: Attempts to restore function in major veins which are the site of massive thrombosis. *Ann Surg* **146**; 510, 1957
14. Mahorner H: A new method of management for thrombosis of deep veins of the extremities. *Am Surg* **20**; 487, 1954
15. Fogarty TJ, Cranley JJ, Krause RJ *et al.*: A method for extraction of arterial emboli and thrombi. *Surg Gynec Obstet* **116**; 241, 1963
16. Fogarty TJ, Cranley JJ, Krause RJ *et al.*: Surgical management of phlegmasia cerulea dolens. *Arch Surg* **86**; 256, 1963
17. Fogarty TJ, Krippaehue WW: Catheter technique for venous thrombectomy. *Surg Gynec Obstet* **121**; 362, 1965
18. Ecklof B, Einarsson E, Plate G: Role of thrombectomy and temporary arteriovenous fistula in acute venous thrombosis. In: Bergan JJ, Yao JST (Eds), *Surgery of the Veins*. Orlando: Grune & Stratton, 1985
19. Gruss JD, Lanbach K: Modifikation der operations technik bei TeiferBecken-undoberschenkel venen thrombose. *Thoraxchirurgerie* **19**; 508, 1971
20. Browse NL, Burnand KG, Lea Thomas M: *Disease of the Veins. Pathology, Diagnosis and Treatment*. London: Edward Arnold, 1988
21. Robertson BR, Nilsson IM, Nylander G, Olow B: Effect of streptokinase and heparin on patients with deep venous thrombosis. *Acta Chir Scand* **133**; 205, 1967
22. Browse NL, Lea Thomas M, Pim HP: Streptokinase and deep vein thrombosis. *Br J Med* **3**; 717, 1968
23. Chavatsas D, Martin P: A study of streptokinase in deep vein thrombosis of the lower extremities. *Vasa* **4**; 68, 1975
24. Semba CP, Dake MD: Iliofemoral deep venous thrombosis: Aggressive therapy with catheter directed thrombolysis. *Radiology* **191**; 487–94, 1994
25. Comerota AJ, Aldridge SC, Cohen G *et al.*: A strategy of aggressive regional therapy for acute iliofemoral venous thrombosis with contemporary venous thrombectomy or catheter-directed thrombolysis. *J Vasc Surg* **20**; 244–54, 1994
26. Goldhaber SZ, Buring JE, Lipnick RJ, Hennekens CH: Pooled analyses of randomised trials of streptokinase and heparin in phlebographically documented acute venous thrombosis. *Am J Med* **76**; 393–7, 1984
27. Sanders RJ, Haug C: Subclavian vein obstruction and thoracic outlet syndrome: a review of etiology and management. *Ann Vasc Surg* **4**; 398–403, 1990
28. Robertson BR, Nilsson IM, Nylander G: Value of streptokinase and heparin in treatment of acute deep vein thrombosis. *Acta Chir Scand* **136**; 173, 1968
29. Kakkar VV, Lawrence D: Hemodynamic and clinical assessment after therapy for acute deep vein thrombosis: a prospective study. *Lancet* **150**; 54, 1985

30. Armon MP, Whitaker SC, Tennant WG: Catheter-directed thrombolysis of iliofemoral deep vein thrombosis. A new approach via the posterior tibial vein. *Eur J Vasc Endovasc Surg* **13**; 413–6, 1997

31. Molina JE, Hunter D, Yedlicka JW: Thrombolytic therapy for iliofemoral venous thrombosis. *Vasc Surg* **26**; 630–7, 1992

32. Bauer G: A roentgenological and clinical study of the sequels of thrombosis. *Acta Chir Scand* **86**(Suppl 74); 1, 1942

33. Ackroyd JS, Browse NL: The investigation and surgery of the post-thrombotic syndrome. *J Cardiovasc Surg* **27**; 5, 1986

34. Fentem PH, Goddard M, Gooden BA, Yeung CK: Control of distension of varicose veins achieved by leg bandages as used after sclerotherapy. *Br J Med* **2**; 725, 1976

35. Horner J, Fernandes E, Fernandes J, Nicolaides AN: Value of graded elastic compression stockings in deep venous insufficiency. *Br J Med* **1**; 818, 1980

36. Pierson S, Pierson D, Swallow R, Johnson G Jr: Efficacy of graded elastic compression in the lower leg. *J Am Med Assoc* **249**; 242, 1983

37. Pflug JJ: Intermittent compression of the swollen leg in general practice. *Practitioner* **215**; 69, 1975

38. Hardin C: Bypass saphenous grafts for the relief of venous obstruction of the extremity. *Surg Gynec Obstet* **115**; 709, 1962

39. Palma EC, Esperon R: Tratamiento del sindrome posttromboflebitico mediante transplante de safena interna. *Angiologica* **11**; 87, 1959

40. Palma EC, Esperon R: Vein transplants and grafts in the surgical treatment of the post-phlebitic syndrome. *J Cardiovasc Surg* **1**; 94, 1960

41. Vollmar J: Reconstruction of the iliac vein and inferior vena cava. In: Hobbs JT (Ed.), *The Treatment of Venous Disorders*. Philadelphia: Lippincott, 1977

42. Dale WA: Synthetic grafts in venous reconstruction. In: Bergan JJ, Yao JST (Eds), *Surgery of the Veins*. Orlando: Grune & Stratton, 1985

43. Dumanian AV, Santschi DR, Park K *et al.*: Cross-over saphenous vein graft with a temporary arteriovenous fistula. A case report. *Vasc Surg* **2**; 116, 1968

44. Levin PM, Rich NM, Hutton JE Jr *et al.*: Role of arteriovenous shunts in venous reconstruction *Am J Surg* **122**; 183, 1971

45. Ecklof B, Albrechtson V, Einarsson E, Plate G: The temporary arteriovenous fistula in venous reconstructive surgery. *Int Angiol* **4**; 455, 1985

46. May R, DeWeese JA: Surgery of the pelvic veins. In: May R (Ed.), *Surgery of the Veins of the Leg and Pelvis*. Stuttgart: Georg Thieme, 1974

47. May R: The femoral bypass. *Int Angiol* **4**; 435, 1985

48. Halliday P, Harris J, May J: Femoro-femoral crossover grafts (Palma operation). A long-term follow-up study. In: Bergan JJ, Yao JST (Eds), *Surgery of the Veins*. Orlando: Grune & Stratton, 1985

49. Dale WA: Venous bypass surgery. *Surg Clin N Am* **62**; 391, 1982

50. Husni EA: Reconstruction of the veins, the need for objectivity. *J Cardiovasc Surg* **24**; 525, 1983

51. Wilms G, Baert AL, Nevelsteen A *et al.*: Balloon angioplasty of venous structures. *J Belge Radiol* **72**; 273–7, 1989

52. Hunter DW, Castaneda-Zuniga WR, Coleman CC *et al.*: Failing arteriovenous dialysis fistulas: evaluation and treatment. *Radiology* **152**; 631–5, 1984

53. Watkinson AF, Hansell DM: Expandable wallstent for the treatment of obstruction of the superior vena cava. *Thorax* **48**; 915–20, 1993

54. Dyet JF, Nicholson AA, Cook AM: The use of the wallstent endovascular prosthesis in the treatment of malignant obstruction of the superior vena cava. *Clin Radiol* **48**; 381–5, 1993

55. Entwhistle KG, Watkinson AF, Hibbert J, Adam A: The use of the wallstent endovascular prosthesis in the treatment of malignant inferior vena cava obstruction. *Clin Radiol* **50**; 310–3, 1995

56. Quinn SF, Schuman ES, Demlow TA *et al.*: Percutaneous transluminal angioplasty versus endovascular stent placement in the treatment of venous stenoses in patients undergoing hemodialysis: intermediate results. *J Vasc and Intervent Radiol* **6**; 851–5, 1995

57. Antonucci F, Salomonowitz E, Stuckmann G et al.: Placement of venous stents: clinical experience with a self-expanding prosthesis. Radiology 183; 493–7, 1992
58. Scott-Mackie PL, Irvine AT, Burnand KG: Treatment of benign venous strictures with the wallstent endoprosthesis. Phlebology 11; 106–10, 1996
59. Vorwerk D, Guenther RW, Mann H et al.: Venous stenosis and occlusion in haemodialysis shunts: follow-up results of stent placement in 65 patients. Radiology 195; 140–6, 1995
60. Gullmo A: The strain obstruction syndrome of the femoral vein. Acta Radiol Scand 47; 119, 1957
61. Negus D, Fletcher EWL, Cockett FB, Lea-Thomas M: Compression and band formation at the mouth of the common iliac vein. Br J Surg 55; 369,1968
62. McLeer RS, Kesterson JE, Kirtley JA, Love RB: Subclavian and anterior scalene muscle compression as a cause of intermittent obstruction of the subclavian vein. Ann Surg 133; 588, 1951
63. Adams JT, McEvoy, RK, DeWeese JA: Primary deep venous thrombosis of the upper extremity. Arch Surg 91; 29, 1965
64. DeWeese JA, Adams JT, Gaiser DL: Subclavian venous thrombectomy. Circulation 42; 158, 1970
65. Paget J: Clinical Lectures and Essays. London: Longman's Green, 1875
66. von Schroetter L: Erkrankungen der Gefasse. In: Nothnagel CNH (Ed.), Handbuch der Pathologie und Therapie. Vienna: Holder, 1884
67. Kleinasser LJ: 'Effort' thrombosis of the axillary and subclavian veins. Arch Surg 59; 248, 1949
68. Stevenson IM, Parry EW: Radiological study of the aetiological factor in venous obstruction of the upper limb. J Cardiovasc Surg 16; 580, 1975
69. Dunant JH: Subclavian vein obstruction in thoracic outlet syndrome. Int Angiol 3; 157, 1984
70. Denck H, Fischer M, Kasprzk P: Thrombolysis in acute axillary vein thrombosis. Int Angiol 3; 161, 1984
71. Zimmerman R, Morl H, Harenberg J et al.: Urokinase therapy of axillary-subclavian vein thrombosis. Klin Wochenscher 59; 851, 1981
72. Jacobson JH, Haimov M: Venous revascularisation of the arm. A report of three cases. Surgery 81; 599, 1977
73. Tilney NL, Griffith HJG, Edwards EA: Natural history of major venous thrombosis of the upper extremity. Arch Surg 101; 792, 1970
74. Becker GJ, Holden RW, Rabe FE et al.: Local thrombolytic therapy for subclavian and axillary vein thrombosis. Radiology 149; 419, 1983
75. Glanz S, Gordon DH, Lipkowitz GS et al.: Axillary and subclavian stenosis: percutaneous angioplasty. Radiology 168; 371–3, 1988
76. Malcynski J, O'Donnell TF, Mackey WC, Millan VA: Long-term results of treatment for axillary subclavian vein thrombosis. Can J Surg 36; 365–71, 1993
77. Siegel RS, Steichen FM: Cervicothoracic outlet syndrome: vascular compression caused by congenital abnormality of thoracic ribs. J Bone Joint Surg 49A; 1187–92, 1967
78. Adams JT, DeWeese JA, Mahoney EB, Rob CG: Intermittent subclavian vein obstruction without thrombosis. Surgery 63; 147–65, 1968
79. Pairolero PC, Walls JT, Payne WS et al.: Subclavian-axillary artery aneurysms. Surgery 90; 757–63, 1981
80. Daskalakis E, Bouhoutsos J: Subclavian and axillary compression of musculoskeletal origin. Br J Surg 67; 573–6, 1980
81. Skinner DB, Saltzmann EW, Scannell JG: The challenge of superior vena caval obstruction. J Thoracic Cardiovasc Surg 49; 824, 1965
82. Charsangavej C, Carrasco H, Wallace S et al.: Stenosis of the vena cava: preliminary assessment of treatment with expandable metal stents. Radiology 161; 295–8, 1986
83. Dondelinger RF, Goffette P, Kurdziel JC, Roche A: Expandable metal stents for stenoses of the vena cavae and large veins. Semin Intervent Radiol 8; 252–63, 1991
84. Rîsch J, Hall L, Antonovic R, Uchida BT: Gianturco expandable wire stents (Z stents) in treatment of venous obstructions. Presented at Cardiovascular and Interventional Radiological Society of Europe (CIRSE), Oslo, 1991

Editorial comments by C.V. Ruckley

It was not to be expected that the authors should provide a finite answer to the question posed. What we have, nevertheless, is a succinct and germane review of the issues, in a difficult and largely unresolved area of clinical management. Those of us who run clinics for chronic venous disease are familiar with the patient suffering from disabling post-thrombotic syndrome who might have benefited from a more aggressive approach to their acute deep-vein thrombosis. Such a patient, however, is a rarity and the majority of patients with deep-vein thrombosis, even extensive iliofemoral deep-vein thrombosis, tend to be little affected by post-thrombotic symptoms. Furthermore, those symptoms improve with time in the majority of patients if they are treated with high quality graduated compression. Our first difficulty therefore, as the authors indicate, is to predict which patients actually merit aggressive intervention.

The authors, I believe rightly, feel that there is still an occasional place for venous thrombectomy. One caution. It is commonplace to read in the literature, although not in this chapter, that a definite indication for thrombectomy is the most severe form of acute deep-veined thrombosis, phlegmasia caerulea dolens. In my experience attempts at thrombectomy in such patients usually make matters worse. Phlegmasia caerulea dolens is generally a sign of advanced malignancy or other highly thrombophilic pathology. In such cases there is disseminated thrombus in stem veins, collaterals and microvasculature. Clearance of thrombus sufficient to relieve venous congestion is usually impossible, leaving the patient with a leaking wound in a still swollen leg.

As the authors indicate thrombolysis with tPA shows promise when delivered into thrombus by selective catheter. The difficulty even in the case of local delivery is to get the lytic agent into potentially lysable thrombus throughout the long lengths of vein involved, without damaging valves. There is a need for further studies of limb perfusion, delivering the agent via the arterial side of the circulation, especially if methods can be devised for minimizing complications at the site of vessel puncture and at remote sites, particularly the brain.

Concerning venous thoracic outlet compression, the authors' preference for first rib resection overstenting, assuming that occluding thrombus first can be cleared with lysis, is probably correct on present evidence and considering the underlying anatomical factors.

Index